PHARMACOLOGY MADE INSANELY EASY

Loretta Manning
Sylvia Rayfield

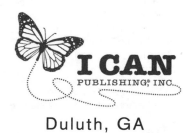

I CAN PUBLISHING®, INC.

Duluth, GA

I CAN Publishing®, Inc.
2650 Chattahoochee Drive • Suite 100
Duluth, GA 30097
866.428.5589

www.icanpublishing.com

Editorial Assistants: Teresa R. Davidson and Jennifer Robinson

Cartoon Illustrations: Teresa R. Davidson, Greensboro, NC; Elizabeth Andrews Lineberry, RN, BSN, Illustrator, Flowery Branch, GA; Children's Medical Group, P.C.; Suwanee, GA; Eileen Burke, Diamond Head, MS

Cover Design: Teresa R. Davidson, Greensboro, NC

Technical Coordinators: Teresa R. Davidson and Jennifer Robinson

Text Layout: Mary Jo Zazueta, To the Point Solutions, Traverse City, MI

Production: Linda Seaman, Bang Printing, Brainerd, MN

Content Reviewers: Pattie Sue Carranza, RPh, CDE and Nicole Blackwelder, PharmD

Printed in the United States of America
ISBN-13: 978-0-9842040-7-6
Library of Congress Control Number: 2012916587

Pharmacology and Medicine are an ever-changing science. The authors and publisher have reviewed current and reliable sources and care has been taken to confirm the accuracy of the information presented and to describe generally accepted practices. The authors, editors, and publisher, however, disclaim all responsibility for errors, omissions, or consequences from application of the information in the book.

Pharmacology Made Insanely Easy has been written to provide general principles of pharmacology and methods to remember this content. This book is not intended as a working guide for client drug administration. Many medications may be prescribed by health care providers for numerous and different indications beyond the scope of this book. Refer to the manufacturer's package insert for recommended drug dosage, route, total list of warnings and undesirable effects, and drug-drug interactions.

The butterfly on the cover signifies transformation. This book has been developed to assist the reader in transforming the study of pharmacology to an exciting and easy process.

I
CAN

Did is a word
of achievement,
Won't is a word
of retreat,
Might is a word
of bereavement
Can't is a word
of defeat,
Ought is a word
of duty,
Try is a word
each hour,
Will is a word
of beauty,
Can is a word
of power.

—Author Unknown

Discovering new ways of learning and teaching pharmacology is a major reason for writing this book. We did not do this by ourselves. Some of these memory tools have been around for generations and we don't know their origins. We want to acknowledge and thank the colleagues, students, and friends who have contributed.

Pattie Akins, RN, MSN
Assistant Professor
Northwestern State University
Shreveport, LA

Julia Aucoin, DNS, RN,-BC, CNE
Chief Knowledge Officer
Practical Success
Durham, NC

Marie Bremner, DSN, RN, CS
Professor of Nursing
Kennesaw State University
Kennesaw, GA

Marianne Call, APRN, APMHNP
Jefferson Parish Human Service Authority
Metairie, LA

Kate K. Chappell, MSN, APRN, CPNP
Clinical Assistant Professor
College of Nursing
University of South Carolina
Columbia, SC

Carol Anne Claxton-Baker, MBA/HA, BSN, BS, RN
Independent Legal Nurse Consultant
Geriatric Nurse Consultant
Duluth, GA

Linda Fisher, RN, BSN, MN
Healthcare Science Instructor
Maxwell High School of Technology
Lawrenceville, GA

Darlene Franklin, RN MSN
Assistant Professor of Nursing Emeritus
Whitson-Hester School of Nursing
Tennessee Technological University
International Nursing Consultant
Sylvia Rayfield & Associates
I CAN Publishing®, Inc.
Cookeville, TN

Joan Galbraith, MSN, RN, CS, GNP, ANP
Carol Woods Retirement Community,
Chapel Hill, NC

Kathy Gallun, MSN, RN
Educational Consultant
Sylvia Rayfield and Associates
I CAN Publishing®, Inc.
Tampa, FL

Melissa J. Geist, EdD, APRN-BC, CNE
Associate Professor of Nursing
Whitson-Hester School of Nursing
Tennessee Technological University
Cookeville, TN

Cecilia Hostetler, BA
Independent Contractor
Suwanee, GA

Melora Mayo, RN, BSN
Yale New Haven Hospital
Children's Clinical Research Center

Jada C. Quinn, DNP, APRN, FNP-BC, ACNP-BC
Clinical Assistant Professor
College of Nursing
University of South Carolina
Columbia, SC

Tina Rayfield, BS, RN, PA-C
President, Sylvia Rayfield & Associates
Pensacola, FL

Vanice Roberts, DSN, RN
Dean School of Nursing
Berry College
Rome, GA

Debra Shelton, EdD, APRN-CNS, CNA,BC, OCN, CNE
Associate Professor, Assistant to the Director for Undergraduate Nursing Programs,
Northwestern State University
Shreveport, LA

Susan Snell, MSN, FNP, BC
Assistant Professor
Northwestern State University,
Shreveport, LA

Mayola L. Villarruel, RN, MSN, ANP-BC, NEA-BC
Director Patient Care Services
Community Hospital
Munster, IN

Lisa T. Williams, DNP, MSN/Ed., MSM, APRN, FNP-BC
Clinical Assistant Professor
College of Nursing
University of South Carolina
Columbia, SC

Larry Zager, MSN
Leadership and Education Consultant
Ridgeway, SC

Lydia R. Zager, MSN, RN, NEA-BC
Education Consultant
Executive Director
Leading Learning LLC
Ridgeway, SC

CONTENTS

Contents

Contents

Contents

Contents

PREFACE

A MESSAGE TO OUR READERS

Pharmacology Made Insanely Easy, 4th Edition has been written as a result of numerous requests from students, graduates, and faculty who have struggled to learn or teach pharmacology. As we work with groups across the country, the common concern is "there is just too much to remember about all the drugs".

While using our teaching strategies during our pharmacology courses, we are told routinely that learners can remember more pharmacology after a few hours with us than they could at the end of a semester of a pharmacology course. Learners report spending hours trying to memorize subtle differences between drugs with similar actions, undesirable effects, etc. We have designed this book, utilizing our strategies, to make life easier for any learner or professional teaching their clients how to safely manage these medications or teaching students pharmacology.

Our experience with thousands of learners each year has helped us develop images and strategies that accelerate the learning process. The format is insanely easy! On the left page is the "bottom line information" about the medications. The image or memory tool is on the right page. Our intent for this book is not for it to be a drug book or pharmacology textbook. This book has been designed to help **simplify** volumes of information as well as to assist you in organizing some of the most pertinent information. In order to assist you in keeping focused on your goal, we have not included exhaustive lists of undesirable effects, doses, routes, or long lists of drug incompatibilities.

We have had a lot of fun working on this project. We look forward to hearing from you. Our web site is www.ican publishing.com. We would love to hear from you regarding recommendations for future editions.

Loretta Manning and Sylvia Rayfield

Belief

is the knowledge that we **CAN** do something.

It's the inner feeling that what we undertake,

we **CAN** accomplish.

For the most part, all of us have the ability

to look at something and know

whether or not we **CAN** do it.

We **CAN** do only what we think we **CAN** do.

We **CAN** be only what we think we **CAN** be.

What we do, what we are, what we accomplish,

all depend on what we think.

So, in belief there is power: our eyes are opened;

our opportunities become plain;

our visions become realities.

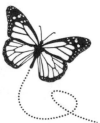

I CAN Publishing®, Inc. has selected the butterfly for our logo since our mission is to help transform your learning from complexity to simplicity! Just as the caterpillar changes into a cocoon, and then emerges as a brilliant butterfly, our mission is to assist you from being overwhelmed to having confidence in your ability to remember and understand pharmacology. Our name, "**I CAN**" is the mnemonic for Creative Approaches to Nursing! We know with "I CAN" you **CAN** learn, have fun, and be successful all at the same time!

ACKNOWLEDGMENTS

We wish to express our appreciation to both of our families and friends for their never ending support and love while we were revising this book.

A special thank you to:

Each of our contributors for the excellent contributions.

Nursing faculty and students who have adapted this book for pharmacology classes.

Our associates who bring the images and words to life during the Pharmacology NCLEX® Review.

HINTS ON HOW TO USE

As we prepared this book, our ultimate goal was to make learning pharmacology fun and easy! As we waded through volumes of research and information on pharmacology, we realized there were some similarities that were applicable to all medications. Rather than repeating these facts with each category and/or medication, we are using the mnemonic "COMPLIANCE". This will assist you in remembering the facts that must be considered for each category of medicines.

When you are reviewing pharmacology, do you ever feel like you are having a "power outage" in your brain? To simplify the content, in several sections of this book we have developed a concept page. This information is pertinent to all of the medications in that category. The left side of the page will review the mnemonic in more detail. This information will not be repeated throughout every category in order to simplify the content. The mnemonic, however, will be referred to in the text of the drug on the left page. The categories that will have these concept pages include: antibiotics, anticoagulants, antidiabetic agents, antidepressants, antimigraine agents, antiparkinson agents antihypertensives, bronchodilators, agents used for chemotherapy, and diuretics.

As we work with graduates across the United States in our review courses, a common request is to have a list outlining the drugs that can cause damage to specific body organs. This has been developed and provided for you in this book. It includes specific drugs that can cause hepatotoxicity, nephrotoxicity, and ototoxicity. Common drug-drug and food-drug interactions are also included. There will be an image of a sun for drugs that may have an undesirable effect of photosensitivity. The Joint Commission on Accreditation of Healthcare Organizations recently released a list of medications with the highest risk of injury when misused. These high-alert medications were divided into six groups: insulins, opiates, antineoplastics, injectable potassium chloride or phosphate, intravenous anticoagulants, and sodium chloride solutions stronger than 0.9%. These categories were established from a study performed by the Institute for Safe Medication Practices. To assist the reader in identifying these drugs, each drug or category will have an image of the yield sign at the top of the page with the words **"HIGH ALERT"**.

We hope you enjoy this book, and it helps you to study and remember facts about pharmacology. Please feel free to notify us if you have additional requests or recommendations for our future publications. We would love to hear from you.

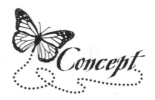
Concept

C hildren—safety

O bserve, report, teach about undesirable effects

M eds—no over-the-counter w/o consultation

P regnancy/lactating are out with meds

L iver must be intact

I nteractions—pharmacological, assess and teach

A llergies—assess; do not administer med if allergic

N utrition must be considered; no crushing sustained release tablets

C ompliance with time and taking full course

E lderly—safety, evaluate outcomes for all meds

"Do Not Use" Abbreviations

Below is a list of frequently used abbreviations that should not be used by institutions as they can be easily misinterpreted:

Abbreviations	Preferred Term
µ (for microgram)	Write **mcg**
T.I.W. for three times weekly	Write **3** (or Three) **Times Weekly**
Trailing zero	Do not use zeros after decimal point (for example, X instead of X.0)
cc for cubic centimeter	Write **ml** for milliliters
IU for International Unit	Write the word **International Unit**
U for Unit	Write the word **Unit**

The **Institute for Safe Medication Practices** (ISMP) has published a list of dangerous abbreviations relating to medication use that it recommends should be explicitly prohibited. This list is available on the ISMP website: **www.ismp.org.**

Abbreviations	Preferred Term
QD for Every Day	Write **Every Day** or **Daily**
Q.O.D. for Every Other Day	Write **Every Other Day**
Leading zero	Use zeros before the decimal point (for example, 0.X instead of .X)
MS & MS04 for morphine	Write **morphine sulfate**
MGS04	Write **Magnesium Sulfate**

Source: Nicole Blackwelder, PharmD, Baptist Medical Center, Beaches, Jacksonville, FL. Reprinted with permission. Adapted from the Joint Commission on Accrediation of Healthcare Organizations "Do Not Use" Abbreviations, www.jcho.org.

PHARMACOKINETICS

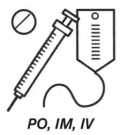

PO, IM, IV

Pharmacology Made Insanely Easy will not review routes or dosages. This information can be found in drug books or pharmacology references.

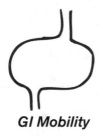

GI Mobility

Alterations in the gastric motility may have effects on how the drugs are absorbed.

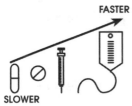

FASTER

SLOWER

Absorption

Absorption can also be affected by route of administration or an impairment in circulation.

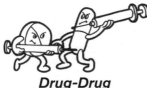

Drug-Drug Interaction

Gut = pH of stomach 4–5. Some drugs require an acidic enviroment for absorption (i.e., tetracycline), raising the pH will alter the absorption.

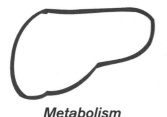

Metabolism

Many drugs pass initially through the liver prior to being available to tissue. Liver disease may ↑ or ↓ action of a drug depending on the metabolism in the body. Infants and elderly have ↓ liver function.

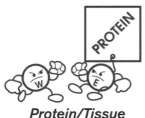

Protein/Tissue Binding

Many drugs bind to protein. When two drugs that are highly protein bound are given together, the one with lesser affinity will be more abundant in its free form. **Warfarin** is an example of a highly protein bound drug. Protein binding is a manner of storage. Highly bound drugs have a longer duration of action (this creates difficulty with toxicity).

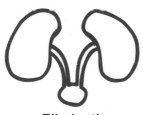

Elimination

Routes of elimination include the kidney, lungs, skin, GI tract, breast milk. Kidney is the major route of excretion. Adequate blood flow to the kidney and renal function are major contributors to drug clearance. If the drug is excreted unchanged such as digoxin or potassium, the renal function must be intact. Elderly have ↓ renal function.

DRUG-DRUG INTERACTIONS

The complexity of modern pharmacology is a growing concern as the list of drug-drug interactions and food-drug interactions continue to grow. "**The Mad War**" on the next page outlines some of the drugs commmonly involved in drug-drug interactions. There are several factors influencing the drug interactions including the absorption of the intestine, competition for plasma protein binding, drug metabolism, action at the receptor site, renal elimination, and electrolyte imbalance.

Absorption of the intestine: Antacids or foods containing aluminum, calcium, or magnesium may bind with tetracycline, decreasing the absorption of the antibiotic. Some drugs require an acidic environment for absorption; increasing the pH will alter the absorption. (pH of stomach is 4–5).

Competition for plasma protein binding: One of the major reasons for drug-drug interactions is the binding of many drugs to proteins, mainly albumin proteins. When 2 drugs that are highly protein bound are administered together, the one with a lesser affinity will be more abundant in its free form. As an individual ages, the number of binding sites on blood proteins is finite. An example of a highly protein bound medication is warfarin.

Drug metabolism: The monoamine oxidase inhibitors prevent the biotransformation of tyramine. Tyramine is present in products such as over-the-counter cold medicines, aged cheese, liver, preserved meats (i.e., bologna, pepperoni, sausage), red wine, tea, colas containing caffeine, chocolate drinks, avocado, figs, pear extracts, etc. This lack of biotransformation of tyramine may result in a hypertensive crisis.

Action at the receptor site: There are many drugs that will intensify or antagonize the action of another drug. For example, alcohol will increase the effects of CNS depressants; antihistamines will decrease the effects of histamine.

Renal elimination: An example of a drug altering renal excretion is probenecid (Benemid) which inhibits the renal clearance of penicillin.

Electrolyte imbalance: Potassium sparing diuretics in combination with ace inhibitors may result in hyperkalemia. An alteration in the sodium level will alter the range of lithium. The use of loop diuretics may result in hypokalemia, which predisposes the client to the potential risk for digitalis toxicity.

DRUG-DRUG INTERACTIONS

T ricyclic antidepressants

H $_2$ Histamine Antagonist
     (Tagamet)

E thanol
  rythromycin

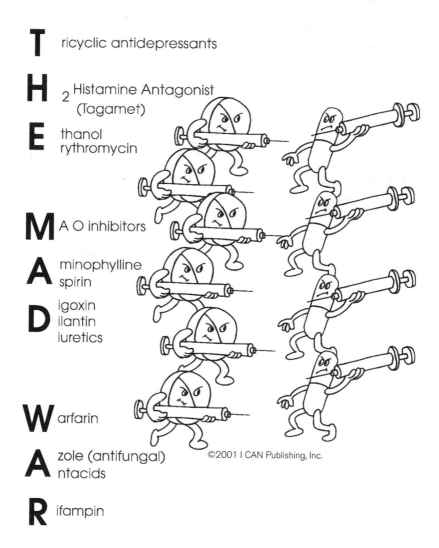

M A O inhibitors

A minophylline
  spirin

D igoxin
  ilantin
  iuretics

W arfarin

A zole (antifungal)
  ntacids

©2001 I CAN Publishing, Inc.

R ifampin

FOOD-DRUG INTERACTIONS

Drug	Foods to Avoid

Antacids
calcium carbonate
(Tums used as calcium
supplement)

bran and whole grain breads

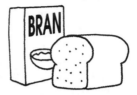

Antibiotics
erythromycin, penicillin

citrus fruit, colas and any food

Tetracycline

calcium

Anticoagulants
warfarin (coumadin)

Vitamin K

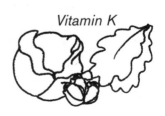

MAO Inhibitors

tyramine

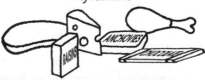

DRUGS THAT CAN CAUSE NEPHROTOXICITY

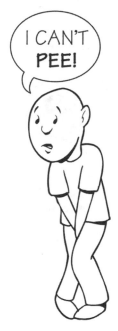

acetaminophen (high doses, acute)

acyclovir, parenteral (Zovirax)

aminoglycosides

amphotericin B, parenteral (Fungizone)

analgesic combinations containing acetaminophen, aspirin or other salicylates in high doses, chronically

ciprofloxacin

cisplatin (Platinol)

methotrexate (high doses)

nonsteroidal anti-inflammatory drugs (NSAIDs)

rifampin

sulfonamides

tetracyclines (exceptions are doxycycline and minocycline)

vancomycin, parenteral (Vancocin)

DRUGS THAT CAN CAUSE HEPATOTOXICITY

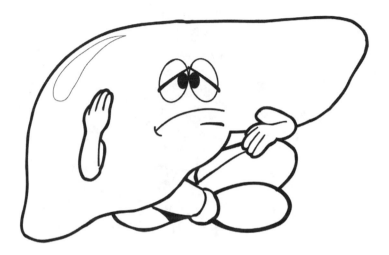

ACE inhibitors
acetaminophen
alcohol
iron overdose
erythromycins
estrogens
fluconazole (Diflucan)
isoniazid (INH)
itraconazole (Sporanox)
ketoconazole (Nizoral)
nonsteroidal anti-inflammatory drugs (NSAIDs)
phenothiazines
phenytoin (Dilantin)
rifampin (Rifadin)
sulfamethooxazole and trimethoprin (Bactrin, Septra)
sulfonamides

DRUGS THAT CAN CAUSE OTOTOXICITY

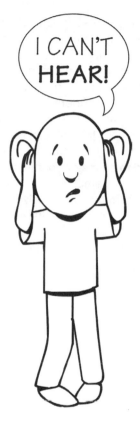

aminoglycosides
bumetanide, parenteral (Bumex)
cisplatin
erythromycin (renal impairment and high doses)
ethacrynic acid (Edecrin)
furosemide (Lasix)
hydroxychloroquine (Plaquenil)
nonsteroidal anti-inflammatory drugs (NSAIDs)
salicylates (chronic high doses, overuse)
vancomycin, parenteral (high doses and renal impairment)

POLYPHARMACY

Polypharmacy is the prescription of numerous medications. Numerous medications may be necessary when a client has several medical disorders, when various medications improve the symptoms of a specific disease, or when one medication improves the action of another. Multiple medication regimens, however, frequently lack rationale for each medication. Elderly clients typically have more than one provider of health care, which may result in poorly coordinated care. The major problem is that medicines administered to relieve nonspecific symptomatology or the undesirable effects of other medicines are believed to be major contributing factors to undesirable effects resulting from polypharmacy.

As you review pharmacology, polypharmacy and drug-drug interactions must always be part of the assessment and planning. While polypharmacy will not be repeated with the categories and individual medication reviews, it is a major part of the management.

POLLY PHARMACY

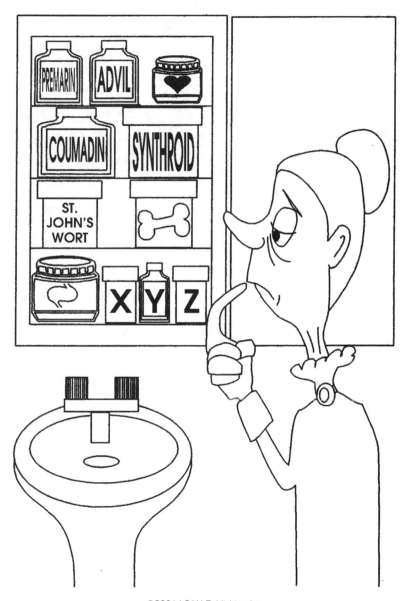

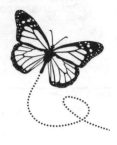

A loving heart is the truest wisdom.

CHARLES DICKENS

Cardiovascular Agents

CHF Drugs

Action: Inhibits the sodium-potassium ATPase, resulting in an increase in cardiac contraction. Decreases heart rate.

Indication: CHF, atrial fibrillation and/or flutter, and paroxysmal atrial contractions.

Warnings: **HIGH ALERT DRUG** Ventricular fibrillation/tachycardia; severe bradycardia; digitalis toxicity; caution with impaired renal or hepatic function; incomplete AV block; elderly; or electrolyte abnormality ($\downarrow$ K$^+$, $\downarrow$ Mg^{++}, $\uparrow$ Ca^{++}), or acute MI.

Undesirable Effects: Anorexia, nausea (*first signs of adult toxicity*), upset stomach (*first sign of toxicity in older child*). Vertigo, headache, depression, muscle weakness, drowsiness, confusion (*may be first sign in the elderly client*). Bradycardia, ECG changes, heart block. Photophobia, yellow-green halos around visual images, flashes of light.

Other Significant Information: $\downarrow$ K$^+$, $\downarrow$ Mg^{++}, and $\uparrow$ Ca^{++} may be associated with digitalis toxicity. Administer separately from antacids (1 to 2 hours apart). Use cautiously with calcium channel blockers or beta blockers. Numerous drug interactions may occur. (Refer to a Drug Handbook for the specifics. This is beyond the scope of this book.) Incompatible with dobutamine.

Interventions: Monitor K$^+$, Mg^{++}, ECG, liver/renal function tests, drug level (therapeutic level 0.5–2.0 ng/ml, toxicity is > 2.0 ng/mL). Before each dose, assess apical pulse for full minute; record and report changes in rate or rhythm. Withhold drug and contact provider if pulse is < 60/minute (adults) or < 90/minute (children) (unless provider has outlined specific parameters). Weigh daily, monitor I & O, and signs of CHF. Antidote: use digoxin immune FAB (Digibind or Digifab) for life-threatening digoxin intoxication (> 10 mg/ml or K$^+$ 7.5 mg/L).

Education: Avoid giving with meals. Teach to take pulse correctly and report if pulse is out of parameter. Weigh every other day and record. Restrict alcohol, sodium, smoking. Consult with provider prior to taking OTC meds. Eat foods rich in potassium. Wear medical alert tag. Emphasize importance of regular checkups. Report N & V or "yellow" vision.

Evaluation: A normal sinus rhythm on ECG. Clinical improvement as evidenced by no S3, edema, etc. Cardiomegaly decreased.

Drugs: digitoxin (Crystodigin); digoxin (Lanoxin)

LIZZY DIGGY

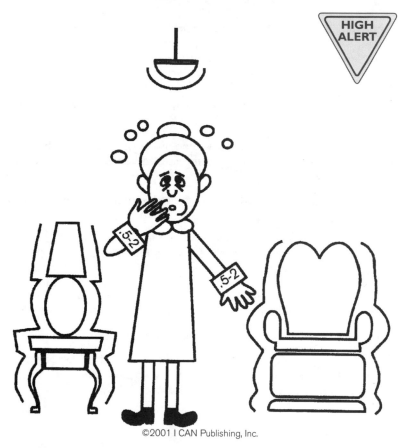

©2001 I CAN Publishing, Inc.

D ig level 2 ng/ml or greater is toxic

I ncreases myocardial contractility

G I or CNS signs indicate adverse effects

Lizzy Diggy is a little old lady that does not do well on DIG. She gets confused, dizzy, nauseated and sees halos and different colored lights.

NATRECOR

Action: Uses DNA technology; human B-type natriuretic peptide binds to the receptor in the vascular smooth muscle and endothelial cells, leading to smooth muscle relaxation.

Indications: Acutely decompensated CHF.

Warnings: Hypersensitivity, cardiogenic shock or BP<90 mm Hg as primary therapy.

Undesirable Effects: Headache, insomnia, hypotension, tachycardia, dysrhythmias, ventricular tachycardia, nausea, vomiting, rash, sweating, pruritus. Increased cough, hemoptysis, apnea.

Other Specific Information: Increased symptomatic hypotension with ACE inhibitors.

Interventions: Assess PCWP, RAP, cardiac index, MPAP, BP, heart rate during treatment until stable. Do not administer nesiritide through a central heparin coated cath. Infuse heparin through a separate line. Prime IV fluid with infusion of 25 ml before connecting to client's vascular accesss port and before bolus dose or IV infusion. Use within 24 hours of reconstitution.

Education: Educate client regarding the purpose of the medication and the expected results.

Evaluation: Client will expect an improvement in the CHF with an improvement in the PCWP, RAP, and MPAP.

Drug: nesiritide (Natrecor)

NATRECOR

As you can see, the heart is relaxing and enjoying nature as a result of natrecor. Natrecor is effective in treating decompensated heart failure.

DOBUTAMINE

Action: Stimulates beta1 adrenergic receptors (myocardial) to increase contractility but with relatively minor effect on heart rate.

Indications: Short-term management of heart failure due to decreased contractility.

Warnings: Hypersensitivity to bisulfites; idiopathic hypertrophic subaortic stenosis; myocardial infarction; atrial fibrillation; pregnancy; lactation; children.

Undesirable effects: ↓ BP, dysrhythmias, tachycardia, headache, angina pectoris, dyspnea, nausea, vomiting.

Other specific information: Beta-adrenergic inhibitors will negate the effects; nitroprusside use has a synergic effect; ↑ risk of dysrhythmias with cyclopropane, halothane, MAO inhibitors, oxytocics, or tricyclic antidepressants.

Interventions: Monitor pulse, blood pressure, respirations, ECG pattern, pulmonary capillary wedge pressure, central venous pressure, cardiac output, urine output, peripheral pulses, and color and temperature of extremities; monitor potassium, electrolytes, BUN, creatinine, and prothrombin time.

Education: Immediately report signs and symptoms of impending myocardial infarction or of worsening of heart failure; notify healthcare provider of pain or discomfort in the site of administration.

Evaluation: ↓ cardiac output; improved hemodynamic parameters; ↑ urine output; improvement in heart failure.

Drugs: dobutamine (Dobutrex)

DOBUTAMINE

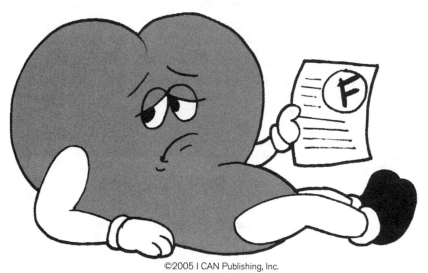

©2005 I CAN Publishing, Inc.

F ailure (heart)

A ngina, arrhythmia—undesirable effect

I ncreases contractility, blood pressure

L ook for an increase in cardiac and urine output

DOPAMINE

Action: Adrenergic. Causes increased cardiac output. Acts on beta 1 and alpha receptors. This results in vasoconstriction in blood vessels; low dose causes renal and mesenteric vasodiation; beta 1 stimulates the production of an inotropic effect with an increased cardiac output.

Indication: Shock; increased perfusion; hypotension. Unlabeled use: COPD, RDS in infants.

Warnings: **HIGH ALERT DRUG** Hypersensitivity. Ventricular fibrillation, tachydysrhythmias, pheochromocytoma. Arterial embolism, peripheral vascular disease.

Undesirable Effects: Headache, Palpitations, tachycardia, hypertension, angina, wide QRS complex, peripheral vasoconstriction. Nausea and vomiting, diarrhea. Necrosis, tissue sloughing with extravasation, gangrene with prolonged use, dyspnea.

Other Specific Information: Do not use within 2 wks of MAOIs, phenytoin; hypertensive crisis may result. Dysrhythmias: general anesthetics. Severe hypertension with ergots. Decreased action of dopamine with beta blockers and alpha blockers. Increased blood pressure with oxytocics. Increased pressor effect with tricyclics, MAOIs.

Interventions: Assess for hypovolemia; if this is a problem correct first. Assess oxygenation and perfusion deficit (check blood pressure, chest pain, dizziness, loss of consciousness). Assess heart failure: S3 gallop, dyspnea, neck vein distention, bibasilar crackles in clients with CHF, cardiomyopathy. I & O, if urine output decreases, without decrease in blood pressure, drug may need to be reduced. ECG during administration continuously; if blood pressure increases, drug should be decreased. B/P and pulse q 5 min after parenteral route. CVP and PWP during infusion if possible. Paresthesias and coldness of extremities; peripheral blood flow may decrease. Injection site: if tissue sloughs administer phentolamine mixed with NS. If overdose occurs, discontinue IV and give a short acting alpha adrenergic blocker.

Education: Instruct the family and client the reason for drug administration.

Staff Education: Do not confuse dopamine with dobutamine. Dopamine is a unique drug and different from the other adrenergic agonists because its actions depends on the dose. Doses of 5 to 10 micorgrams per kg per min. stimulate alpha receptors. Doses of 2–3 micorgrams per kg per min. stimulate dopaminergic receptors, causing dilation of the mesenteric and renal arteries. Dopamine is frequently used to increase blood flow to the kidneys when renal insufficiency is present or to prevent renal failure from shock.

Evaluation: Increased B/P with stabilization; increased urine output.

Drug: dopamine (Dopamine HCl, Intropin)

DO**PAM**INE

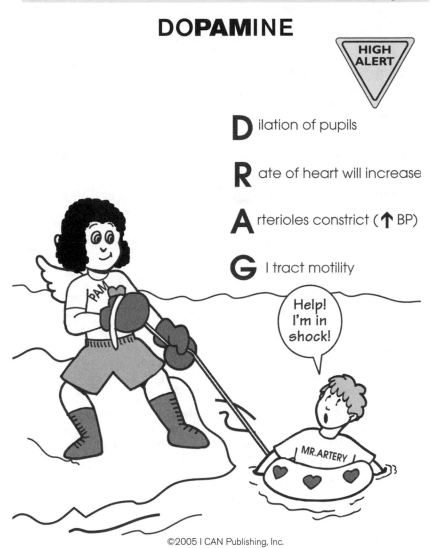

HIGH ALERT

D ilation of pupils

R ate of heart will increase

A rterioles constrict (↑ BP)

G I tract motility

Help! I'm in shock!

MR. ARTERY

©2005 I CAN Publishing, Inc.

"Fight or Flight" angel, PAM, is throwing a life raft to the artery, constricting the artery because it was in shock and over dilated. She will "DRAG" the artery to shore. "DRAG" will assist you in remembering the responses of the alpha and B 1 receptor effects.

EPINEPHRINE

Action: Stimulates alpha- and beta-adrenergic receptors to (1) cause bronchodilation and vasoconstriction, (2) maintain pulse and blood pressure, (3) localize and prolong local and spinal anesthetic, and (4) reverse hypersensitivity reaction.

Indications: Asthma and COPD (maintenance of airway); allergic reactions; cardiac arrest; adjunct to local or spinal anesthesia; antiglaucoma.

Warnings: **HIGH ALERT DRUG** Use with caution in cardiac disease, hypertension, hyperthyroidism, and diabetes mellitus. Elderly persons may require ↓ dosage. Concurrent use with other adrenergic medications will have a synergistic effect. Beta-adrenergic inhibitors may negate the effect of epinephrine. Concurrent use with MAO inhibitors may cause a hypertensive crisis.

Undesirable effects: Nervousness, restlessness, tremors, angina, dysrhythmias, hypertension, tachycardia, headache, insomnia, paradoxical bronchospasm, nausea, vomiting, and hyperglycemia.

Other specific information: Check dosage, concentration, and route of administration carefully prior to administration. During treatment for anaphylactic shock, volume replacement should occur concurrently with epinephrine administration.

Interventions: Monitor pulmonary status before, during, and after bronchodilation treatment; monitor hemodynamic status during and after use for treatment of shock, hypotension, and/or cardiac arrest; treatment may cause ↓ K, ↑ glucose, and ↑ lactic acid.

Education: Take as directed; notify healthcare provider if symptoms are not relieved; discuss with healthcare provider before taking any over-the-counter medication.

Evaluation: Relief or prevention of bronchospasm; easier breathing; prevention of or ↓ frequency of acute asthma attacks; reversal of signs and symptoms of anaphylaxis; ↑ cardiac output and rate in cardiac resuscitation.

Drugs: Adrenalin, Ana-Gard, AsthmaHaler Mist, AsthmaNefrin, Bronitin Mist, Bronkaid Mist, Epifrin, Epinal, EpiPen, Eppy/N, Glaucon, microNefrin, Nephron, Primatene, Racepinephrine, S-2, Sus-Phrine, Vaponefrin.

EPINEPHRINE

N ervousness—undesirable effect

A ngina, arrhythmia—undesirable effect

S ugar↑

C ardiac arrest

A llergic reaction

R espiratory—bronchodialator

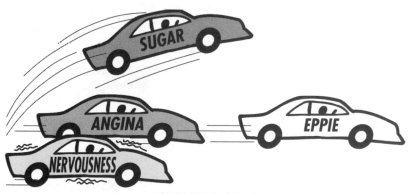

Three of these "NASCARS" experienced collisions (undesirable effects) from epinephrine. Eppie was able to finish the race and achieve desirable outcomes without any collisions (undesirable effects).

NOREPINEPHRINE

Action: Vasopressor; stimulates alpha- and beta-adrenergic receptors to cause vasoconstriction maintaining blood pressure.

Indications: Management of shock.

Warnings: **HIGH ALERT DRUG** Use with MAO inhibitors may result in hypertension; beta-adrenergic blockers may inhibit therapeutic effects; use cautiously in patients with underlying cardiovascular disease, uncorrected dysrhythmias, or hypovolemia due to fluid deficit.

Undesirable effects: Angina, hypertension, tachycardia, dysrhythmias; extravasation may cause severe irritation, necrosis, and sloughing of tissue.

Other specific information: If extravasation occurs, infiltrate area with 10–15 ml of 0.9% NaCl with 5–10 mg of phentolamine.

Interventions: Monitor blood pressure, heart rate, respirations, ECG, and hemodynamic parameters every 5–15 minutes; monitor urine output hourly; administer into a large vein to decrease risk of extravasation; correct hypovolemia before administering drug; administer via infusion pump to ensure precise dosing; titrate to patient response (blood pressure, heart rate, urine output, peripheral perfusion, cardiac output, and presence of ectopic activity).

Education: Immediately report signs and symptoms of chest pain or dyspnea; notify healthcare provider of pain or discomfort in the site of administration.

Evaluation: ↑ blood pressure, ↑ in peripheral circulation, ↑ in urine output.

Drugs: Levophed, Levarternol

NOREPINEPHRINE

HIGH ALERT

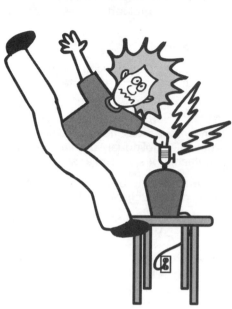

©2005 I CAN Publishing, Inc.

S timulates alpha and beta adrenergic receptors

H ypovolemia—should be corrected before using drug

O utput of urine & cardiac should ↑

C onstriction of blood vessels

K orrect dysrhythmias before using

NITROGLYCERIN

Action: Relaxes the vascular smooth system. ↓ myocardial demand for oxygen. ↓ left ventricular preload by dilating veins, thus indirectly ↓ afterload.

Indications: Angina pectoris.

Warnings: Hypersensitivity. Closed-angle glaucoma, severe anemia, hypotension, early MI, head trauma, ICP, pregnancy, renal or hepatic disease.

Undesirable Effects: Headache (most common), hypotension, postural hypotension, syncope, dizziness, weakness, reflex tachycardia, paradoxical bradycardia. Sublingual: burning, tingling sensation in mouth. Ointment: erythematous, vesicular and pruritic lesions.

Other Specific Information: ↑ effect with alcohol, antihypertensive agents, beta blockers, calcium blockers. ↓ effect of heparin.

Interventions: Record characteristics and precipitating factors of anginal pain. Monitor BP and apical pulse before administration and periodically after dose. Have client sit or lie down if taking drug for the first time. Client must have continuing EKG monitoring for IV administration. Cardioverter/defibrillator must not be discharged through paddle electrode overlying Nitro-Bid ointment or the Transderm-Nitro patch (may cause burns on client). Assist with ambulating if dizzy.

Education: Avoid alcohol. Teach to recognize symptoms of hypotension. Advise to make position changes slowly and to avoid prolonged standing. Teach about the form of nitroglycerin prescribed. Oral: Instruct to take on an empty stomach with a full glass of water. Do not chew tablet. Sublingual: Instruct to take at first sign of anginal pain. May be repeated every 5 minutes to a maximum of 3 doses. If the client doesn't experience relief, advise to seek medical assistance immediately. A stinging or biting sensation may indicate the tablet is fresh. With newer SL nitroglycerin, the biting sensation may not be present. Protect drug from light, moisture, and heat. Instruct to apply Transderm-Nitro patch once a day, usually in the AM. Rotation of sites is necessary. *(Refer to Drug Handbook for detail steps with all forms.)*

Evaluation: The client will report a decrease in frequency and severity of anginal attacks along with an increase in activity tolerance.

Drugs: nitroglycerin **intravenous** (Nitro-Bid IV, Tridil); **sublingual** (Nitrostat); **sustained-release** (Nitroglyn, Nitrong, Nitro-Time); **topical** (Nitro-Bid, Nitrol, Nitrong, Nitrostat); **transdermal** (Minitran, Nitro-Dur, Nitrodisc, Nitro-Derm, Transderm-Nitro); **translingual** (Nitrolingual); **transmucosal** (Nitrogard)

ANDY ANGINA

ACTION

Relaxes vascular smooth muscle

↓ venous return

↓ arterial BP

↓ left ventricular workload

↓ myocardial oxygen consumption

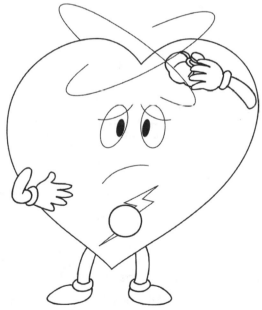

©2001 I CAN Publishing, Inc.

Nitroglycerin is given to decrease Andy's angina. Andy is experiencing some of the undesirable effects from nitroglycerin: headache, syncope, weakness, nausea, and hypotension.

RANEXA

Action: Unknown mechanism of action. Antianginal and anti-ischemic effects. Lowers cardiac oxygen demand resulting with an improvement in exercise tolerance and decrease in pain.

Indications: Used in conjunction with beta-blockers, amlodipine (Norvasc) or an organic nitrate for treatment of chronic stable angina. Used in clients who do not respond to other antianginal therapies.

Warnings: Hypersensitivity; cirrhosis, prolonged QT interval, hypokalemia, severe renal impairment. Avoid use with other drugs that prolong the QT interval (Some Class IA or Class III antidysrhythmics, erythromycin, some antipsychotics).

Undesirable Effects: Severe: Dysrhythmias, Torasades de Pointes, Sudden death, QT prolongation. Common: Dizziness, headache, lightheadedness, nausea, constipation. May cause a reversible increase in BUN, creatinine. May lead to small decrease in hematocrit.

Other Specific Information: Avoid use of potent CYP3A4 inhibitors with this drug (e.g., agents include grapefruit juice, HIV protease inhibitors, azole antifungals, macrolide antibiotics, diltiazem, verapamil). Quinidine and sotalol (Betapace) can further increase QT interval. Concurrent use of digoxin (Lanoxin) and simvastatin (Zocor) increases serum levels of digoxin and simvastatin.

Interventions: Monitor EKG at baseline and periodically. Monitor electrolytes, LFTs, renal function. Monitor digoxin level with concurrent use. Avoid use with liver or renal impairment. Administer as an extended release oral tablet, twice daily. Assess for personal or family history of prolonged QT interval. Elderly may begin therapy at lower doses. Use in combination with beta-blockers, amlodipine, or nitrates.

Education: Take with or without food. Avoid grapefruit products. Swallow tablets whole. Avoid activities requiring mental alertness. Alcohol, exercise, hot weather, fever may increase effects of dizziness. Change positions slowly. Report fainting, palpitations. Do not double doses. If miss a dose, take next dose at scheduled time.

Evaluation: Improvement in status of resistant angina. Prevention of acute anginal attacks.

Drugs: ranolazine (Ranexa)

RANEXA

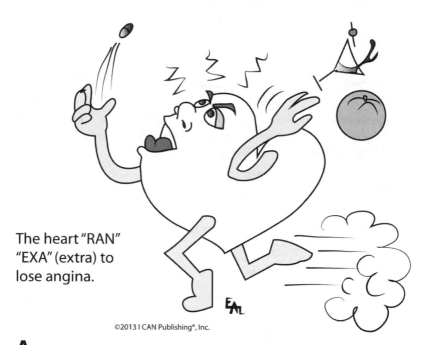

The heart "RAN" "EXA" (extra) to lose angina.

©2013 I CAN Publishing®, Inc.

A ntianginal; assess for dizziness, fainting; no alcohol

N o grapefruit products

G I: nausea, constipation – common; severe: arrhythmias, prolonged QT

I f misses a dose, take next scheduled time.

N ote and monitor EKG at baseline and periodically. Monitor electrolytes, LFTs, renal function.

A void use with liver or renal impairment.

ANTIDYSRHYTHMIC: LIDOCAINE

Action: Decreases cardiac excitability, cardiac conduction is delayed in the ventricle. Decreases automaticity of ventricular cells.

Indications: Ventricular dysrhythmias such as PVCs, ventricular tachycardia, and ventricular fibrillation.

Warnings: **HIGH ALERT DRUG** Advanced atrioventricular blocks, CHF, hepatic disorder, elderly client.

Undesirable Effects: Bradycardia, tachycardia, hypotension, confusion, drowsiness (*1st sign of toxicity*), dizziness, nausea, vomiting, seizures (*severe toxicity*), cardiac arrest.

Other Specific Information: ↑ effects with ranitidine, cimetidine. ↑ risk of toxicity with beta-adrenergic blockers, (LOL's).

Interventions: Monitor EKG, BP, pulse, and rhythm continuously. Monitor serum lidocaine levels throughout therapy; therapeutic range 1.5–5 mcg/mL. Monitor intake and output. Do not mix in same syringe with amphotericin B or cefazolin. Administer Lidocaine IV. In case of circulatory depression, have dopamine available.

Education: Instruct client and family about drug. Recommend client walk with another person due to dizziness and drowsiness.

Evaluation: Client will have a decrease in or will be free of ventricular dysrhythmias.

Drug: lidocaine (Lido Pen Auto injector, Xylocaine HCL IV)

LIDDY LIDOCAINE

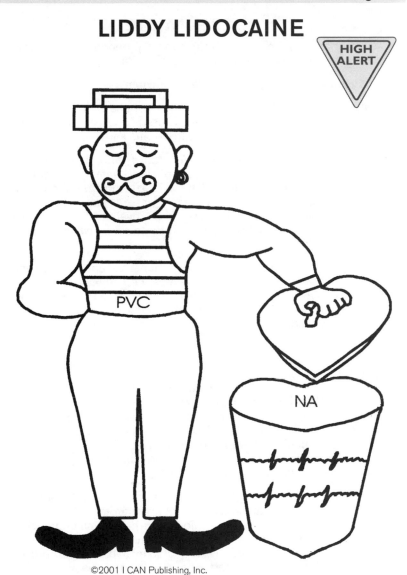

©2001 I CAN Publishing, Inc.

Liddy Lidocaine is the strongman that puts the lid on the sodium trash can of PVCs. This drug reduces sodium permeability, resulting in a decrease in ventricular arrhythmias and cardiac irritability.

Observe for undesirable effects, such as dizziness, drowsiness, and confusion.

PROCAINAMIDE

Action: Antidysrhythmic. Prolongs refractory period of the cardiac conduction system. Decreases myocardial excitability.

Indications: Treatment of ventricular dysrhythmias.

Warnings: Hypersensitivity. Lactation. Do not use with complete AV block, asymptomatic PVCs, history of lupus erythematosus. Large doses may cause AV block. Caution with hepatic and renal dysfunction.

Undesirable Effects: Serious: Ventricular fibrillation, asystole, seizures, thrombocytopenia, neutropenia, hemolytic anemia, lupus erythematosus, agranulocytosis. **Common:** Hypotension, bradycardia, flushing, pruritis, rash, fever, nausea, bitter taste, confusion, depression, vomiting, diarrhea, elevated LFTs, dizziness. Black box warning: Medication may lead to positive ANA titer with or without symptoms of lupus.

Other Specific Information: Antihypertensives and nitrates may potentiate hypotensive effect. Potentiates neuromuscular blocking agents . Additive anticholinergic effects with other drugs possessing anticholinergic properties, including antihistamines, antidepressants, atropine, haloperidol, and phenothiazines. Effects of procainamide may be ↑ by quinidine, cimetidine, or trimethoprim.

Interventions: Monitor ECG, pulse, and blood pressure continuously throughout IV administration. Available: PO/IM/IV. Monitor BP. Place client supine during IV administration. PO administration preferred. IV use in life-threatening situations, IM use when client NPO or with malabsorptive syndromes. Therapeutic drug level 4-8 mcg/mL.Toxic serum levels over 16 mcg/mL. Restrict to use with life-threatening ventricular arrhythmias. May cause blood dyscrasias. Monitor CBC. Monitor ANA periodically during prolonged therapy if symptoms of lupus-like reaction occur.

Education: Take with a full glass of water (lessens GI irritation). Take 1 hour before or 2 hours after meals for ideal absorption. May take with meals if GI symptoms are severe. Monitor HR. Recommend sucking on hard candy or chewing gum can help relieve dry mouth. Administer stool softeners such as docusate sodium (Colace), to prevent constipation. Swallow sustained release preparations whole. May cause dizziness. Caution with activities such driving or other activities that require mental alertness. Report sore throat, fever, rash, chills, diarrhea, increased palpitations. Do not suddenly stop medication. Do not take OTC medications without consulting healthcare provider.

Evaluation: Termination of dysrhythmias. Return of stable rhythm.

Drugs: procainamide (Pronestyl, Apo-procainamide, Procan-SR)

PROCAINAMIDE

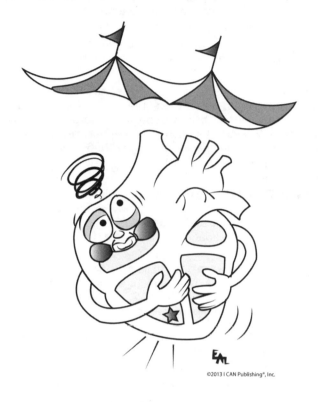

Ventricular rhythm is off stride;
Just like it got off a circus ride.
Please tell the nurse at the bedside,
The importance of giving Procainamide.

PROPAFENONE

Action: Oral antidysrhythmic. Causes a local anesthetic effect on myocardium. Stabilizes cardiac membranes. Slows atrioventricular conduction; has slight beta-adrenergic blocking activity.

Indications: Reduce recurrence of paroxysmal atrial fibrillation/flutter, supraventricular tachycardia; treatment of sustained or life-threatening ventricular arrhythmias.

Warnings: Hypersensitivity, lactation, uncontrolled CHF, cardiogenic shock, sick sinus syndrome, AV block, bradycardia, severe hypotension, electrolyte imbalances, bronchospastic disorders. Caution with MI within past 2 years. Caution with hepatic or renal impairment, pacemaker, myasthenia gravis, poor CYP2D6 metabolizer. Caution with changes in smoking habit. Lower dosage may be required for geriatric clients.

Undesirable Effects: Serious: Dysrhythmias, prolonged QT interval, CHF, agranulocytosis, myasthenia gravis exacerbation. **Common:** Dizziness, nausea, unusual taste changes, dyspnea, fatigue, constipation, edema, headache, bradycardia, first-degree heart block, vomiting, weakness.

Other Specific Information: Black box warning: Medication may lead to positive ANA titer with or without symptoms of lupus. Any inhibitors of CYP2D6, CYP1A2, or CYP3A4 enzymes may ↑ levels , including desipramine, paroxetine, ritonavir, sertraline, ketoconazole, erythromycin. Quinidine is a strong inhibitor of CYP2D6 and significantly ↑ levels of propafenone. Propafenone may slow medication metabolism and cause an increase in the levels of digoxin, oral anticoagulants, and propanolol.

Interventions: Monitor electrolytes and ECG at baseline, then periodically. Monitor for bradycardia and hypotension. Monitor for dizziness and weakness. Monitor LFTs, CBC, electrolytes, renal function. Monitor for anemia, agranulocytosis, leukopenia, thrombocytopenia, altered PT and coagulation times.

Education: Sustained release tablets can be taken with or without food. Do not crush sustained release tablets. Drink plenty of fluids (2-3 Liters/day). Increase fiber and bulk to diet to prevent complication. Report dizziness or unusual taste if interferes mobility or nutritional status. Report signs/symptoms chest pain, SOB, palpitations, unusual bleeding. Reports signs of liver failure (e.g., yellow eyes, skin, dark yellow urine). Record all BP pulse readings for provider to evaluate.

Evaluation: Termination of dysrhythmia. Restoration of stable rhythm. Therapeutic drug level 0.5-3 mcg/mL.

Drugs: propafenone(Rythmol, Rythmol SR)

PROPAFENONE (RYTHMOL)

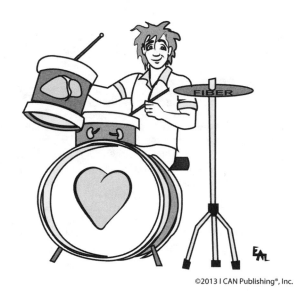

©2013 I CAN Publishing®, Inc.

Rhythm of heart restored

Reduces rate of heart

Renal and Liver function needs to be monitored

Reduce constipation by increasing fiber and bulk in diet

Report dizziness or unusual taste in mouth

Report chest pain, shortness of breath, unusual bleeding

Report significant drop in blood pressure

Restoration of stable rhythm

AMIODARONE (CORDARONE)

Action: Antidysrhythmic (class III). Prolongs duration of action potential and effective refractory period, noncompetitive alpha and beta adrenergic inhibition; increases PR and QT intervals, decreases sinus rate, decreases peripheral vascular resistance.

Indication: Severe ventricular tachycardia, supraventricular tachycardia, (unlabeled use atrial fibrillation), ventricular fibrillation not controlled by first-line agents, cardiac arrest.

Warning: **HIGH ALERT DRUG** 2nd-, 3rd-degree AV block, bradycardia, severe sinus node dysfunction, neonates, infants.

Undesirable Effects: Headache, dizziness, fatigue, malaise, corneal microdeposits, Adult Respiratory Distress Syndrome (ARDS), Pulmonary Fibrosis, CHF, worsening of arrhythmias, bradycardia, hypotension. Liver function abnormalities: anorexia, constipation, nausea and vomiting. Toxic epidermal necrolysis: photosensitivity, hypothyroidism, ataxia, involuntary movements, peripheral neuropathy, poor coordination.

Other Specific Information: If taken with beta blockers or calcium channel blockers bradycardia may occur. Increased levels of digoxin (digoxin should be decreased by 50%), quinidine, procainamide, flecainide, disopyramide, phenytoin, theophylline, cyclosporine, dextromethorphan, methotrexate. Increased anticoagulant effects with warfarin (warfarin should be decreased by 33%–50%). Amiodarone effects may be increased if client is taking aloe, buckthorn bark/berry, cascara sagrada bark, rhubarb root, senna leaf/fruits.

Interventions: Assess I & O ratio: electrolytes (K, Na, Cl); liver function studies: AST, ALT, bilirubin, alk phosphatase. ECG continuously to determine drug effectiveness, measure PR, QRS, QT intervals, check for PVCs, other dysrhythmias, B/P continuously for hypotension, hypertension. Assess for rebound hypertension after 1–2 hr. Assess for ARDS, pulmonary fibrosis. Monitor pulse, respiratory rate, chest pain. Administer with meals if GI symptoms occur. If IV, administer via volumetric pump. Use an in line filter.

Education: Instruct to take drug as directed; avoid missed doses. Use sunscreens or stay out of sun to prevent burns. Report side effects. Advise that skin discoloration usually is reversible. If photophobia occurs, advise to wear sunglasses. Report unusual bleeding or bruising.

Staff Education: Do not confuse amiodarone (cordarone) with amrinone which is now called inamrinone (Inocor).

Evalutation: Client will have a decrease in ventricular tachycardia, supraventricular tachycardia or fibrillation.

Drugs: amiodarone (Cordarone, Pacerone)

CORDARONE

C oumadin must be decreased

O rdered for ventricular arrhythmias

R espiratoy Distress Syndrome (ARDS)—undesirable effect

D igoxin must be decreased

A taxia and dizziness—undesirable effects

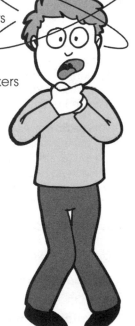

R isk of bradycardia with beta blockers and calcium channel blockers

O ral—administer with meals if GI distress occurs

N ot confuse with amrinone

E valuate ECG for drug effectiveness

ADENOSINE

Action: Slows conduction through AV node, can interrupt reentry pathways through AV node, and can restore normal sinus rhythm in clients with supraventricular tachycardia (SVT).

Indications: SVT, as a diagnostic aid to assess myocardial perfusion defects in CAD.

Warnings: **HIGH ALERT DRUG** Hypersensitivity, 2nd- or 3rd-degree heart block, AV block, sick sinus syndrome, atrial flutter, atrial fibrillation.

Undesirable Effects: Nausea, metallic taste, throat tightness, groin pressure; dyspnea, chest pressure, hyperventilation; lightheadedness, dizziness, arm tingling, numbness, apprehension, blurred vision, headache; chest pain, atrial tachydysrhythmias, sweating, palpitations, hypotension, facial flushing.

Other Specific Information: Increased effects of adenosine with dipyridamole. Decreased activity of adenosine when taken with theophylline or other methylxanthines (caffeine). An increased degree of heart block may occur when taken with carbamazepine. Possible ventricular fibrillation with digoxin. Smoking may increase tachycardia. May increase adenosine effect if taken with aloe, buckthorn bark/berry, cascara sagrada bark, rhubarb root, senna leaf/fruits. Decreased adenosine effect when taken with guarana.

Interventions: Assess I & O ratio, electrolytes (K, Na, Cl). Assess B/P, pulse, respiration, ECG intervals (PR, QRS, QT); check for transient dysrhythmias (PVCs, PACs, sinus tachycardia, AV block). Assess respiratory status: rhythm, rate, breath sounds. Assess for dizziness, confusion, psychosis, paresthesias, seizures. Treat overdose with defibrillation and vasopressor for hypotension.

Education: Advise to report facial flushing, dizziness, sweating, chest pain, or palpitations. Advise to rise slowly for a sitting or standing position to prevent orthostatic hypotension.

Staff Education: Do not confuse Adenocard with adenosine phosphate.

Evaluation: Client will have a normal sinus rhythm.

Drug: adenosine (Adenocard, Adenoscan)

ADENOSINE

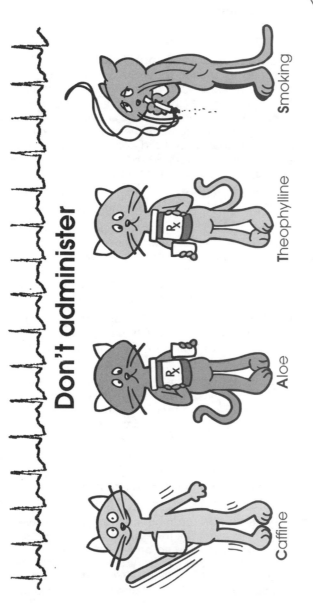

These CATS will help you remember which agents to stay away from when taking these drugs. The first letter of each of these agents spells CATS!

Concept:
ANTIHYPERTENSIVE MEDICATIONS

Pressure (blood) monitor: Monitor blood pressure and pulse closely. A decrease in the blood pressure is an expected outcome, but it can also drop too much which can be unsafe.

Rise slowly to reduce orthostatic hypotension: Since orthostatic hypotension may occur, recommend the client to change positions slowly from recumbent to upright and dangle the feet from the edge of the bed to prevent dizziness. Recommend that the client not stand for long periods of time, not take hot showers, baths, or do strenuous exercise. Operating hazardous machinery or driving is not recommended until the response of the drugs has been determined since dizziness may occur. A Medic Alert bracelet or identification card should be carried in case of an emergency.

Eating must be considered (diet): The nonpharmacologic measure of sodium and fat reduction in the diet are strongly recommended.

Stay on medications: Clients have a tendency to stop a medication when they are feeling better. Instruct client regarding the importance of taking the medicine at the same time every day and taking it as prescribed. Recommend client stay away from over-the-counter cold, cough, or allergy medicines without first discussing with provider. Many are contraindicated with hypertension.

Skipping or stopping is a no-no: Review the importance of continuing drug even if undesirable effects occur; notify provider if effects occur. Abrupt discontinuation of these drugs may result in rebound hypertension.

Undesirable responses: Discuss with client that dizziness, drowsiness, and lightheadedness may occur initially; inform provider of these symptoms. Each antihypertensive drug also has specific undesirable effects and should be reviewed with client. Instruct client to report these effects to provider and not to abruptly stop the drug.

Remind to exercise, no alcohol: Nonpharmacologic management of hypertension is important to emphasize. Regular exercise, weight reduction, behavior modification to promote relaxation, and moderate consumption of alcohol may assist in controlling hypertension.

Eliminate smoking; educate: The importance for smoking cessation should be emphasized to client. Instruct client and family members how to take a blood pressure reading and pulse. A record for the daily pressures should be recorded in a diary. Discuss the implications of hypertension and the long-term effects. Review the importance of periodic follow-up visits, so the blood pressure can be evaluated.

PRESSURE

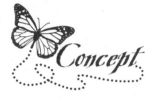

P ressure (blood) monitor

R ise slowly to reduce orthostatic hypotension

E ating must be considered (diet)

S tay on medications

S kipping or stopping is a no-no

U ndesirable responses

R emind to exercise, ↓ alcohol

E liminate smoking; educate

ACE INHIBITORS

Action: Suppresses renin-angiotensin-aldosterone system; blocks conversion of angiotensin I to angiotensin II (a potent vasoconstrictor).

Indications: Hypertension, adjunctive therapy for CHF; reduces development of severe heart failure following MI in clients with impaired left ventricular function; protects against kidney failure in Type II diabetes.

Warnings: Renal or thyroid disease; severe salt/volume depletion; coronary insufficiency; leukemia.

Undesirable Effects: Gastric irritation, headache, dizziness, tachycardia, angioedema, cough, maculopapular rash, pruritus, infection, hyperkalemia.

Other Specific Information: Probenecid ↓ elimination of ace inhibitors. NSAIDs may ↓ hypotensive effects. ↑ hypotensive effects with other antihypertensives. ↑ K+ may occur with potassium-sparing diuretics, potassium supplements, or potassium containing salt substitutes.

Interventions: Obtain baseline and monitor serum/urine protein, BUN, creatinine, glucose, CBC with differential, potassium and sodium levels. First dose syncope may occur in those with CHF. Provide mouth care; alteration in taste may occur. (Refer to **"PRESSURE"**.)

Education: Report any signs of infection, bruising, or bleeding. Captopril, moexipril, quinapril, and ramipril will have reduced absorption if given with food. 'Other ace inhibitors are not affected by food. Instruct not to use potassium supplements or any food or substance containing a large amount of potassium. (i.e., low-sodium milk, salt substitutes, etc.) (Refer to **"PRESSURE"**.)

Evaluation: The blood pressure will return to normal limits without undesirable effects of these drugs.

Drugs: *(These drugs end in "pril".)* benaze**pril** (Lotension); capto**pril** (Capoten); enala**pril** (Vasotec); fosino**pril** (Monopril); lisino**pril** (Prinivil, Zestril); moexi**pril** (Univasc); perindo**pril** (Aceon); quina**pril** (Accupril); rami**pril** (Altace); trandola**pril** (Mavik)

PRIL SISTERS

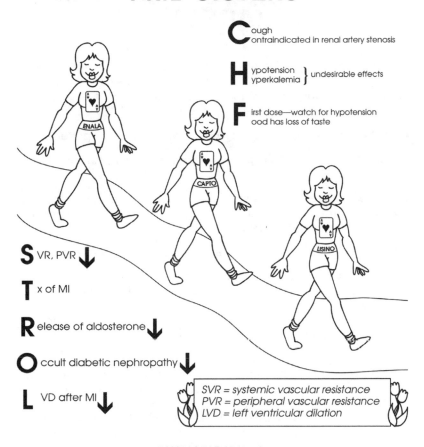

C ough
   ontraindicated in renal artery stenosis

H ypotension } undesirable effects
   yperkalemia

F irst dose—watch for hypotension
   ood has loss of taste

S VR, PVR ↓

T x of MI

R elease of aldosterone ↓

O ccult diabetic nephropathy ↓

L VD after MI ↓

SVR = systemic vascular resistance
PVR = peripheral vascular resistance
LVD = left ventricular dilation

©2001 I CAN Publishing, Inc.

The "Pril" sisters are taking a "strol" through the park to prevent cardiac problems. "STROL" will assist you in remebering the actions of ace inhibitors. "CHF" will help you in remembering some undesirable effects from these drugs.

ANGIOTENSIN II RECEPTOR BLOCKERS (ARBS)

Action: Blocks the binding of angiotensin II to the AT1 receptor found in many tissues *(i.e., adrenal, vascular smooth muscle)*. This blocks the vasoconstriction effect of the renin-angiotensin system as well as the release of aldosterone resulting in a decreased BP.

Indication: Hypertension. Used alone or with other antihypertensives.

Warnings: Renal/hepatic impairment; pregnancy/lactation; potassium supplements.

Undesirable Effects: Occasional–cough, upper respiratory infection, dizziness, diarrhea. Rare–back and leg pain, sinusitis, dyspepsia, insomnia. Overdosage– ↓ BP.

Other Specific Information: Phenobarbital may ↓ effects.

Interventions: Monitor renal function tests. Monitor BP and apical HR prior to each dose and on a regular basis. If hypotension occurs, place client in the supine position with feet slightly elevated. Maintain hydration. Administer without regard to meals. Assess for signs of upper respiratory infection, cough, and diarrhea. Assist with ambulation if dizziness occurs.

Education: Report any signs of an infection. Do not take cold preparations or nasal decongestants. Caution about exercising during hot weather due to potential dehydration and hypotension. Use a barrier method of birth control. Instruct not to use potassium supplements or any food containing large amounts of potassium (i.e., salt substitutes). (Refer to "**PRESSURE**".)

Evaluation: Client's blood pressure will return to normal range with no undesirable effects.

Drugs: *(These drugs end in "sartan".)* cande**sartan** (Atacand); epro**sartan** (Teveten); irbe**sartan** (Avapro); lo**sartan** (Cozaar); olme**sartan** (Benicar); telmi**sartan** (Micardis); val**sartan** (Diovan)

SARTAN SISTERS

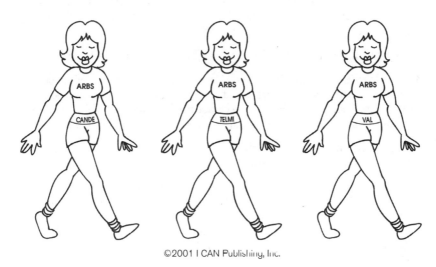

©2001 I CAN Publishing, Inc.

A dminister without regard to meals

R enal function tests—review

B locks vasoconstriction effect of renin—angiotensin system

S alt substitution or potassium supplements—do not use

ALPHA ADRENERGIC BLOCKERS

Action: Blocks alpha1 adrenergic receptors resulting in vasodilation of arteries and veins. ↓ peripheral vascular resistance; relaxes smooth muscle of bladder/prostate.

Indications: Hypertension (terazosin, doxazosin). Prazosin has been used as adjunct therapy for CHF. Doxazosin and terazosin may be used for benign prostatic hyperplasia.

Warnings: Renal disease. Elderly may be more sensitive to drug.

Undesirable Effects: Dizziness, drowsiness, weakness, depression; palpitations, tachycardia, orthostatic hypotension; urinary frequency, dry mouth; impotence. First-dose syncope (hypotension with sudden loss of consciousness) may occur between 2–6 hrs. after initial dose.

Other Specific Information: ↑ hypotensive effect with other antihypertensives, nitrates, alcohol.

Interventions: Monitor BP frequently and protect from falling/injury after the first dose and with each ↑ due to first-dose syncope. If initial dose or ↑ in dose is during the day, client must remain recumbent for 3–4 hours. Assess BP and HR immediately before each dose. Assist with ambulating if client is dizzy. (Refer to **"PRESSURE".**)

Education: Caution that the first-dose syncope may occur, and implement safety precautions. Report if edema is present in the AM. Sugarless gum, sips of tepid water, etc. may relieve dry mouth. (Refer to **"PRESSURE".**)

Evaluation: Client's blood pressure will remain in normal limits with no undesirable effects from the medications.

Drugs: alfuzo**sin** (Uroxatral), doxazosin (Cardura); prazo**sin** (Minipress); terazo**sin** (Hytrin)

MINI'S SINS

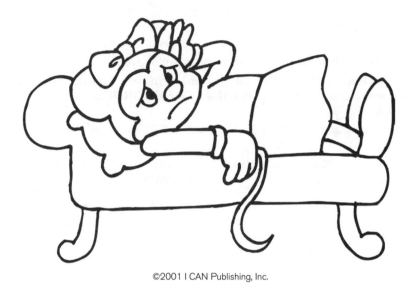

©2001 I CAN Publishing, Inc.

S yncope
exual dysfunction

I ncreased drowsiness, orthostatic hypotension, HR

N eed to be recumbent for 3–4 hours after initial dose

BETA-ADRENERGIC BLOCKERS

Action: Binds to beta 1–(cardiac) and/or beta 2–(lungs) adrenergic receptor sites that prevents the release of catecholamine. Refer to page 58 to assist with this information. The "**LOL**" Team will also assist you in recalling the actions of this category. They include a ↓ in contractility, ↓ renin release, and ↓ in the sympathetic output .

Indications: Hypertension, angina, MI; migraine headaches, situational anxiety; thyrotoxic storm/crisis; upper GI bleed; familial (essential) tremors; and assists in treatment of dysrrhythmias.

Warnings: COPD, asthma, CHF, sinus bradycardia, heart block > first degree; diabetes mellitus. **HIGH ALERT IV DRUGS**: propranolol, metoprolol, labetalol.

Undesirable Effects: Refer to "**BLOCKER**" to assist in recalling these effects (page 53).

Other Specific Information: Anticholinergics ↑ absorption. Antacids ↓ absorption. ↑ risk for bradycardia when used concurrently with cardiac glycosides and calcium channel blockers. ↑ hypotensive effects when given with diuretics. Sudden discontinuing may cause refractory hypertension. *(Refer to a Drug Handbook for reviewing the numerous drug-drug interactions which may occur.)*

Interventions: Monitor blood sugar closely in clients with diabetes. Monitor triglyceride and cholesterol level (LDL). Monitor BP and pulse prior to administering. If pulse is < 60 or SBP < 90, withhold and notify provider of health care. Monitor any change in the cardiac rhythm or any signs of CHF. (Refer to "**PRESSURE**".)

Education: Instruct client regarding self assessment of pulse, character, and rhythm; signs and symptoms of CHF. Avoid heat, excessive exercise, hot showers, baths and hot tubs. (Refer to "**PRESSURE**".)

Evaluation: The blood pressure will return to normal limits. If given for arrhythmias, the ECG will record a normal sinus rhythm.

Drugs: *(These drugs end in "lol".)* **Cardioselective (Beta 1 receptors):** acebuto**lol** (Sectral), ateno**lol** (Tenormin), betaxo**lol** (Kerlone), bisopro**lol** (Zebeta), esmolol (Brevibloc), metopro**lol** (Lopressor, Toprol XL); **Nonselective (Beta 1 and Beta 2 receptors)**: carteo**lol** (Cartrol); carvedi**lol** (Coreg); labeta**lol** (Normodyne); nado**lol** (Corgard); penbuto**lol** (Levotol); pindo**lol** (Visken); pranrano**lol** (Inderal); timo**lol** (Blocadren)

For Beta 2 Selective Drugs see Max Air

THE "LOL" TEAM

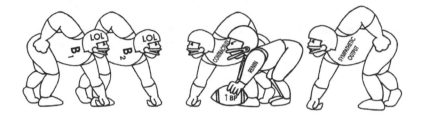

©2001 I CAN Publishing, Inc.

The "**LOL**" team blocks hypertension by "blocking" (decreasing) the contractility in the heart, the renin release from the kidneys, and the sympathetic output from the vasomotor center of the brain.

BETA BLOCKER ACTIONS

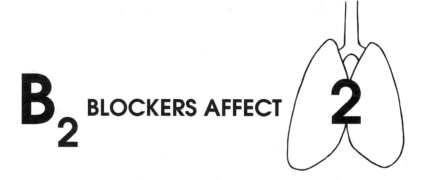

B₁ **BLOCKERS AFFECT 1**

Beta1 Blockers affect the Beta1 receptors in the heart. They ↓ the excitability, cardiac workload, O_2 consumption, renin release and lower blood pressure

B₂ **BLOCKERS AFFECT 2**

Beta₂ Blockers stimulate the beta receptors in the lung, relax bronchial smooth muscle, ↑ vital capacity, and ↓ airway resistance. Higher doses may cause undesirable cardiac effects.

BLOCKER

BRADYCARDIA
BLOOD PRESSURE—TOO LOW
BRONCHIAL CONSTRICTION
BLOOD SUGAR—MASKS LOW
BLOCKS (HEART) > 1st DEGREE

"BLOCKER" outlines undesirable effects of Beta Blockers.

CALCIUM CHANNEL BLOCKERS

Action: Blocks calcium access to the cells causing a ↓ in contractility, ↓ arteriolar constriction, ↓ PVR, and ↓ BP.

Indications: Hypertension; vasospastic angina; classic chronic stable angina; atrial fibrillation or flutter; migraine headaches. **Nimodipine** is selective for cerebral arteries. **Bepridil** prevents coronary artery spasm making it an agent for chronic stable angina. **These 2 medications are not indicated for hypertension.** Research indicates verapamil may slow the progression of diabetes mellitus.

Warnings: Severe CHF; 2nd or 3rd degree AV block; sick sinus syndrome; SBP < 90 mm Hg; bradycardia; aortic stenosis; caution in the elderly client due to long half-life.

Undesirable Effects: Hypotension, headache, dizziness; atrioventricular block; worsens CHF; peripheral edema; constipation. *(Refer to image on next page!)*

Other Specific Information: Beta-adrenergic blockers may ↑ cardiac depression when given with calcium channel blockers. ↑ serum levels of digoxin, carbamazepine, and quinidine result when given with calcium channel blockers. ↑ serum levels when administered with cimetidine or ranitidine. Grapefruit juice and verapamil or diltiazem may lead to toxicity.

Interventions: Monitor hepatic and renal function studies. Monitor ECG and avoid giving when heart blocks are present. During bepridil therapy, periodic K+ levels may be required. Have emergency equipment available with IV administration. Protect drug from light and moisture. Position client to decrease peripheral edema. (Refer to **"PRESSURE".**)

Education: Instruct to ↑ dietary fiber, fluid intake, and exercise. Avoid overexertion when anginal pain is relieved. Encourage to take with meals or milk. Recommend client not to chew or crush sustained-release. Advise to avoid drinking grapefruit juice. (Refer to **"PRESSURE".**)

Evaluation: The blood pressure will be within normal limits. There will be a normal sinus rhythm on the ECG. If administered for angina or headaches, there will be a decrease in the symptoms.

Drugs: amlodi**pine** (Norvasc); amlodi**pine** with benazepril (Lotrel); amlodi**pine** with valsartan (Exforge); bepridil (Vascor); diltiazem (Cardizem, Tiazac); felodi**pine** (Plendil) SR; isradi**pine** (DynaCirc) SR; nicardi**pine** (Cardene, Cleviprex) SR; nifedi**pine** (Adalat, Procardia) SR; nisoldi**pine** (Sular); verapamil (Isoptin, Calan)

SR = Sustained release

CALCIUM CHANNEL BLOCKERS

"DON'T GIVE A FLIP PILLS"

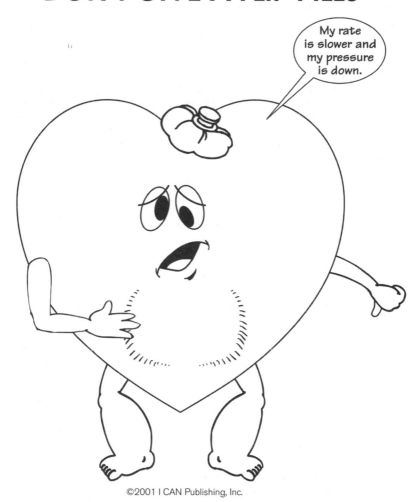

©2001 I CAN Publishing, Inc.

Major undesirable effects of calcium channel blockers include: headache (most common), hypotension, syncope, peripheral edema, bradycardia and constipation. These clients "don't give a flip" at times (syncope) or from just feeling "blah" from the other undesirable effects.

AMLODIPNE/ATORVASTATIN (CADUET)

Action: It is a fixed dose combination drug containing the calcium channel blocker amlodipine and the statin atorvastatin.

Indications: Treatment of hypertension and high cholesterol. Lipitor is also used to lower the risk for heart attack, stroke, certain types of heart surgery, and chest pain in clients who have heart disease of risk factors for heart disease such as: age, smoking, high blood pressure, low HDL-C, heart disease in the family. Lipitor can lower the risk for heart attack or stroke in clients with diabetes and risk factors such as: diabetic eye or kidney problems, smoking, or high blood pressure.

Warnings: Hypersenstivity to either amlodipine and/or the statin. Caduet contains atorvastatin and is therefore contraindicated in clients with active liver disease, which may include unexplained persistent elevations in hepatic transaminase levels. Kidney disease. Pregnancy; lactation.

Undesirable Effects: Allergic reactions; upset stomach, tendon problems. Elevation in the liver enzymes. Dizziness.

Other Specific Information: Refer to Calcium Channel Blockers and the HMG CoA Inhibitors in this book for specific interactions.

Interventions: Monitor BP and Cholesterol. Review necessary health promotion program for client. To reduce risk of dizziness and lightheadedness, get up slowly when rising from a sitting or lying position. Limit alcoholic beverages. Daily use of alcohol may increase risk for liver problems, especially when combined with atorvastatin.

Education: This drug may make client dizzy. Advise not drive, use machinery, or do any activity that requires alertness until cognitive state has been established in order to perform activities safely. Reduce the risk of dizziness and lightheadedness by instructing client to get up slowly when rising from a sitting or lying position. Review importance of not drinking alcohol. Older adults may be more sensitive to the side effects of the drug, especially muscle problems and dizziness. Advise they notify provider of care.

Evaluation: Blood pressure and liver enzymes will remain within normal range, and client will not experience a CVA or heart attack.

Drugs: amlodipine besylate/atorvastatin calcium (Caduet)

CADUET

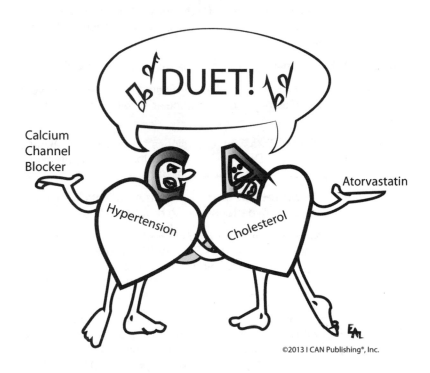

Calcium Channel Blocker

Atorvastatin

©2013 I CAN Publishing®, Inc.

D ecreased B/P and Cholesterol

U ndesirable effects: GI, Tendon problems, and dizziness

E valuate Cholesterol, liver enzymes; must eliminate alcohol

T o decrease dizziness, get up slowly when rising from a sitting position

CENTRAL ALPHA₂ AGONISTS

Action: Decreases the release of adrenergic hormones from the brain, resulting in a ↓ in the peripheral vascular resistance and blood pressure.

Indications: Hypertension (stepped-care approach, step 2 drug).

Warnings: Acute hepatitis; active cirrhosis. Recent MI; severe coronary artery insufficiency; cerebrovascular disease; chronic renal failure.

Undesirable Effects: Transient drowsiness, headache, weakness during initial therapy. Dry mouth, constipation, hypotension, bradycardia, occasional edema, or weight gain.

Other Specific Information: ↓ antihypertensive effects with TCAs (imipramine). Paradoxical hypertension with propranolol.

Interventions: Monitor liver/renal function tests, CBC, baseline BP, P, and weights. Monitor BP and VS every 30 minutes until stable during initial therapy. Rapid ↑ in BP and symptoms of sympathetic over activity (i.e., ↑ pulse, tremor agitation, and anxiety) may occur. Catapres may be given to rapidly ↓ BP in some hypertensive emergencies.

Education: Recommend the last dose of the day be taken at bedtime. Give medication with snack. Thorough effect of oral administration may take 2–3 days. Weigh daily. Notify provider if weight gain > 4 lbs. in 1 week. Drowsiness disappears during continued therapy. Sugarless gum, sips of tepid water may relieve dry mouth. Give diuretic if needed. If need to discontinue, taper dose gradually over more than one week. Urine may darken in color. (Refer to "**PRESSURE**".)

Evaluation: Blood pressure will return to normal limits with no undesirable effects from the medications.

Drugs: clonidine (Catapres); methyldopa (Aldomet)

CATAPRES

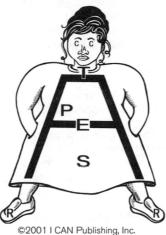

©2001 I CAN Publishing, Inc.

C is at her eyes because the adrenergic hormone is released from the brain.

A is at her nose because the risk factors of hypotension, hepatotoxicity and hemolytic anemia are as clear as the nose on her face.

T is at her chin as it drops with transient drowsiness.

A is "body-wide" because arterial pressure all over the body is lowered.

P indicates paradoxical hypertension with propranolol.

R is at her baseline feet to remind you to record baseline vital signs.

E on her belt may expand because she may have a weight gain; evaluate her liver.

S is tapered down her dress because the drugs should be slowly tapered down and not stopped suddenly.

Catapres, a commonly used antihypertensive drug is the name of our image to review the actions of central alpha$_2$ agonists. Studies show that women of color have increased risk of hypertension. See that the letters in Catapres are placed on her image.

VASODILATORS

Action: Direct relaxation of vascular smooth muscle, producing vasodilation of arterioles which decreases afterload.

Indications: Hypertension.

Warnings: Coronary artery disease, rheumatic heart disease, hydralazine-lupus, pregnancy, impaired renal function, CVA.

Undesirable Effects: Headache, dizziness; anorexia, nausea, vomiting, diarrhea; palpitations, tachycardia, hypotension, occasional postural hypotension; edema and/or weight gain (drugs can cause sodium and water retention); flushing; nasal congestion. Lupus-like reaction (fever, facial rash, muscle and joint ache, splenomegaly).

Other Specific Information: ↑ hypotensive effects with anti-hypertensives, beta blockers, and diuretics.

Interventions: Monitor BP, heart rate, daily weight, CBC, ANA titers, renal function tests, urinalysis. (Refer to "**PRESSURE**".)

Education: Instruct how to take heart rate. If rate is > 20 beats per minute over normal, notify provider. Report a 5 lb. weight gain. Monitor and report muscle and joint aches, fever (lupus-like reaction). Monitor bowel activity. Take with meals; for nausea eat unsalted crackers or dry toast. Report peripheral edema of hands and feet. Lie down if dizzy. (Refer to "**PRESSURE**".)

Evaluation: Client's BP will return to normal range with no undesirable effects.

Drugs: hydralazine (Apresoline); minoxidil (Loniten)

DILLY DILATOR

D irectly acts on vascular smooth muscle, causing vasodilation

I ncreases renal and cerebral blood flow

L upus-like reaction (fever, facial rash, muscle and joint ache, splenomegaly—U E)

A ssess for peripheral edema of hands and feet

T ake with food

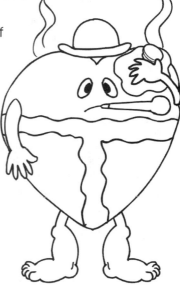

O ther U E—headache, dizziness, anorexla, tachycardia, hypotension

R eview BP

©2001 I CAN Publishing, Inc.

Dilly Dilator's heart vessels are enlarged to allow more O_2 to the heart muscle. If they become too dilated he will have hypotension on rising, headache, and diarrhea. His temperature may rise due to a "lupus-like" reaction.

NITROPRESS

Action: Direct vasodilation of arteries and veins resulting in a rapid decrease in the blood pressure (decrease in both the preload and afterload).

Indications: Hypertensive emergencies

Warnings: Contraindicated in hypersensitivity, pregnancy, and decreased cerebral perfusion. Use cautiously in clients who have liver and kidney disease, fluid and electrolyte imbalance, and in older clients.

Undesirable Effects: Excessive hypotension, dizziness; abdominal pain, nausea. Thiocyanate poisoning. Cyanide poisoning (drowsiness and headache may lead to cardiac arrest).

Other Specific Information: Increase hypotensive effect with ganglionic blocking agents, general anesthetics, and other antihypertensives. Estrogens and sympathomimetics may decrease the response to nitorprusside. Nitroprusside should not be administered in the same infusion as any other medication.

Interventions: Administer slowly due to rapid administration will result in blood pressure decreasing quickly. Monitor the blood pressure and ECG. Risk of cyanide poisoning may be reduced by administering medication at a rate of 5 mcg/kg/min or less, and administering thiosulfate concurrently. DC med if cyanide toxicity occurs. Assess for altered mental status which may indicate thiocyanate poisoning. Avoid prolonged use of nitroprusside. Monitor plasma levels if used for more than 3 days. Maintain level at less than 0.1 mg/mL. Prepare medication by adding to diluents for IV infusion. Note color of solution. Solution may be light brown in color. Discard solution of any other color. Protect tubing and IV container from light. After 24 hours, discard medication. Assess vital signs and ECG continuously.

Education: Review undesirable effects with client and instruct to report to provider of care.

Evaluation: Client will experience a decrease in blood pressure and maintain normotensive blood pressure. The client will have an improvement of heart failure such as ability to participate in activities of daily living. There will be an improvement in renal function and delay of further progression of renal disease.

Drugs: nitroprusside sodium (Nitropress)

NITROPRESS

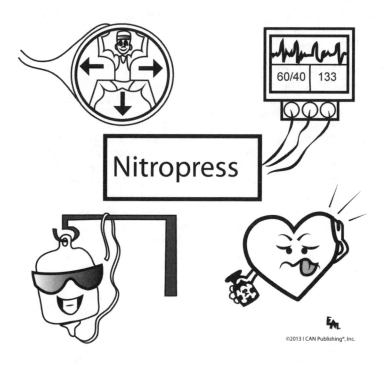

Nitropress

©2013 I CAN Publishing®, Inc.

D ilation of arteries and veins lead to rapid
        decrease in blood pressure (Action)

I ncrease hypotensive effect with general
        anesthetics and other antihypertensives

L ight brown color (solution color);
        Protect tubing and IV container from light

A fter 24 hours, discard medication

T he ECG and vital signs must be monitored

E valuate for cyanide poisoning (drowsiness
        and headache can lead to cardiac arrest)

Concept: DIURETICS

Diet: Instruct client to eat a low sodium diet and a diet rich in potassium. Clients taking potassium-sparing diuretics should not eat a diet rich in potassium!

Intake and Output, daily weight: These are outcomes that can assist in evaluating the effects of the drugs. There should be an increase in the urine output. Hard candy, sips of water, sugarless gum, etc. may be effective if client has a dry mouth.

Undesirable effects: fluid and electrolyte imbalance: Monitor the fluid and electrolytes while a client is taking diuretics and report changes to provider. *Hypovolemia:* ↑ HR with weak pulse, ↑ respirations, ↓ B/P, and ↓ output. *Hypokalemia:* abnormal ECG, orthostatic hypotension, flaccid paralysis, and weakness. *Hyperkalemia:* nausea, diarrhea, abnormal ECG, confusion, muscle weakness, tingling in the extremities, paresthesia, dyspnea, and fatigue. (concern with potassium-sparing diuretic) (Therapeutic: 3.5–5.0 mEq/L). *Hyponatremia:* lethargy, disorientation, muscle tenseness, seizures, coma (Therapeutic: 135–145mEq/L)

Review HR and BP: Due to potential hypovolemia, monitor the HR and BP. If client is taking digoxin, evaluate for signs of hypokalemia due to risk of digoxin toxicity.

Elderly–CAREFUL: Due to physiological changes in this population, an accurate assessment of fluid, electrolytes, and BP is important. Evaluate adequate renal function by checking the creatinine clearance in the elderly.

Take with or after meals and in AM: Instruct client to take with or after meals if GI distress occurs. Nausea and vomiting may be a result of electrolyte disturbance. Administering the diuretics early in the day will help avoid nocturia.

Increase risk of orthostatic hypotension: Due to this risk, instruct client to change positions slowly especially when rising.

Cancel alcohol: Alcohol products need to be canceled due to the diuresing effect and the risk of decreasing the blood pressure too much.

DIURETIC

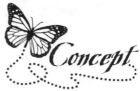

D iet— ↑ K+ for all except aldactone

I ntake & output, daily weight

U ndesirable effects: fluid & electrolyte imbalance

R eview HR, BP, and electrolytes

E LDERLY—careful

T ake with or after meals and in AM

I ncrease risk of orthostatic hypotension; move slowly

C ancel alcohol

LOOP DIURETICS

Action: Inhibits sodium, chloride, and water reabsorption in the proximal portion of the ascending loop of Henle.

Indications: Edema associated with congestive heart failure, cirrhosis with ascites, or renal dysfunction. Furosemide for hypertension or in combination with other antihypertensive medications.

Warnings: Hypokalemia, hypersensitivity to sulfonamides or loop diuretics; renal/hepatic dysfunction; gout; diabetes.

Undesirable Effects: Hyponatremia, hypokalemia, hypocalcemia, hypomag-nesemia, hypochloremic alkalosis, hyperglycemia, and hyperuricemia. *(Remember everything is decreased except the glucose and uric acid!)* Hypotension; blurred vision, headaches, dizziness, lightheadedness; anorexia, nausea, diarrhea; dehydration, muscle cramp, ototoxicity. Furosemide and ethacrynic acid may cause leukopenia and photosensitivity.

Other Specific Information: ↑ in digitalis and lithium toxicity. ↓ K⁺ with corticosteroids, and some penicillins. ↓ effects of antiocoagulants. Avoid amphotericin B, nephrotoxic, or other ototoxic medications.

Interventions: Monitor serum glucose, and electrolytes. (Refer to **"DIURETIC"**.)

Education: Report changes in hearing, irritability, vomiting, anorexia, nausea, diarrhea, twitching, or tetany. (Refer to **"DIURETIC"**.)

Evaluation: Client's blood pressure and edema will decrease and remain within normal range.

Drugs: bumetanide (Bumex); ethacrynic acid (Edecrin); furosemide (Lasix); torsemide (Demadex)

LOU LA BELL

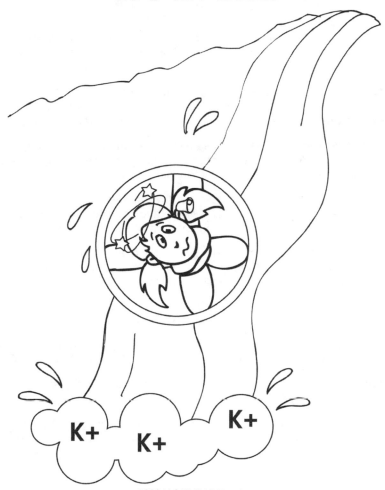

Lou La Bell goes spinning over the falls because she has lost so much fluid from diuresing. Her ears are ringing and she is dizzy from a decrease in her blood pressure. She has lost potassium in the falls. Loop diuretics act in the ascending loop of Henle and one common drug is Lasix.

Remember, Thiazides at the distal tubule (major differences between undesirable effects between Thiazides and Loops is that Loops may cause ototoxicity and hypocalcemia).

THIAZIDES

Action: Increases urine output by inhibiting reabsorption of sodium, chloride, and water in the distal portion of the ascending Loop of Henle.

Indications: Edema associated with congestive heart failure, cirrhosis with ascites, and some types of renal impairment *(i.e., acute glomerulonephritis, and nephrotic syndrome)*. Hypertension.

Warnings: Hypokalemia; hypersensitivity to sulfonamides or thiazide diuretics; renal/hepatic dysfunction. Caution with the elderly, clients with diabetes mellitus, gout, or history of lupus erythematosus.

Undesirable effects: Hypokalemia; hyponatremia; hyperuricemia; hypercalcemia; hyperglycemia. Orthostatic hypotension, syncope; anorexia, nausea, or vomiting; dehydration; photosensitivity.

Other Specific Information: ↑ risk of digitalis (if hypokalemia present) and lithium toxicity. ↑ loss of potassium when taking corticosteroids and some penicillins. ↓ effects of antidiabetic agents.

Interventions: Check for allergies to sulfonamides. Monitor serum glucose, and K+ levels. (Refer to "**DIURETIC**".)

Education: Instruct to discontinue thiazides prior to parathyroid function tests due to the altered calcium levels. (Refer to "**DIURETIC**".)

Evaluation: Client's blood pressure and edema will be ↓ and remain within normal range.

Drugs: chlorothiazide (Diuril); chlorthalidone (Hygroton); hydrochlorothiazide (Esidrix, HCTZ, HydroDiuril); indapamide (Lozol); metolazone (Zaroxolyn)

THIAZIDE DIURETICS
"LOU LA BELL"

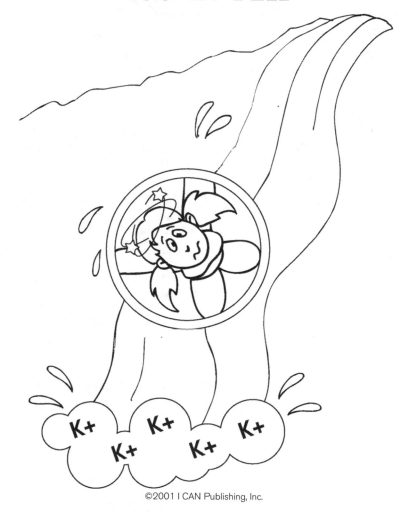

Lou La Bell is experiencing syncope, dehydration (from all the diuresing "waterfall"), electrolyte imbalance (hypokalemia) and orthostatic hypotension from the thiazide diuretics.

Thiazides act in the distal tubule. Major differences from the loop diuretics are calcium may be high (rhymes with thigh[azide]) and the client experiences no ototoxicity with thiazide diuretics.

POTASSIUM SPARING DIURETICS

Action: Promotes excretion of sodium and water, but retains potassium in the distal renal tubule.

Indications: Used with loop or thiazide diuretics in treating CHF and hypertension. Diuretic induced hypokalemia. Steroid-induced edema. Hyperaldosteronism.

Warnings: Impaired renal functions; PIH; hyperkalemia; diabetes mellitus.

Undesirable Effects: Nausea, diarrhea, dizziness, headache, dry mouth, rash, photosensitivity. ↑ K^+ levels result in peaked T waves on ECG.

Other Specific Information: ↑ digitalis and lithium toxicity. ↑ K^+ levels when taken with ACE inhibitors, potassium containing medications, or potassium supplements. ↓ anticoagulant effects.

Interventions: Monitor K^+ and digitalis levels. (Refer to **"DIURETIC".**)

Education: Inform client that maximum hypotensive effect may not be seen for 2 weeks. Counsel client to avoid citrus juices, colas, milk low in sodium, some salt substitutes, or other potassium supplements. Monitor for ↑ K^+ during blood transfusion. (Refer to **"DIURETIC".**)

Evaluation: Client's blood pressure and serum potassium will remain within normal limits; edema will decrease.

Drugs: spironolactone (Aldactone), amiloride (Midamor), triamterene (Dyrenium)

ALAN ALDACTONE

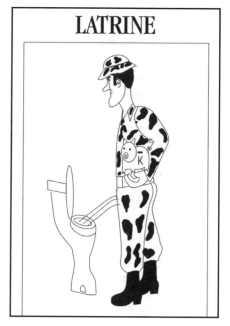

LATRINE

©2001 I CAN Publishing, Inc.

L ow Na$^+$

E levated T waves from ↑K$^+$

A granulocytosis with triamterene

K $^+$ level must be monitored

Alan Aldactone is at the latrine taking a leak and getting rid of the extra volume that's increasing his blood pressure. Alan is holding his piggy bank with K$^+$ on it, as aldactone helps in saving potassium.

OSMOTIC DIURETICS

Action: Increases osmotic pressure of glomerular filtrate, thus preventing reabsorption of water. Increases excretion of sodium and chloride.

Indications: Oliguria, edema, increased intracranial pressure; increased intracocular pressure; treat certain drug toxicities.

Warnings: Heart failure, renal failure, hypertension, pulmonary edema due to transient increase in blood pressure; intracranial hemorrhage; severe dehydration. Serum osmolality > 310–320 mOsm/kg is contraindicated.

Undesirable Effects: Dry mouth, thirst, nausea, vomiting, blurred vision, headache, dizziness. Cellular dehydration; fluid and electrolyte imbalance; pulmonary edema.

Other Specific Information: May ↑ Digitalis toxicity.

Interventions: Monitor renal function tests, serum and urine K⁺ and Na⁺ levels, CVP, and vital signs. Watch for rapid ↑ in BP and symptoms of sympathetic overactivity (i.e., ↑ heart rate, tremor, and agitation). Solutions given IV only via an in line filter. IV solution may crystallize; re-dissolve before infusing by warming bottle. Never give solutions with undissolved crystals. (Refer to **"DIURETIC".**)

Education: Advise client that glycerin and isosorbide are for the reduction of intraocular pressure and should be monitored by the provider of care frequently. (Refer to **"DIURETIC".**)

Evaluation: Intracranial or intraocular pressure should be reduced. If given for renal failure, diuresing should occur with an improvement in the BUN and serum creatinie values.

Drugs: glycerin (Osmoglyn); isosorbide (Ismotic); mannitol (Osmitrol); urea (Ureaphil)

BUSTER BRAIN MAN

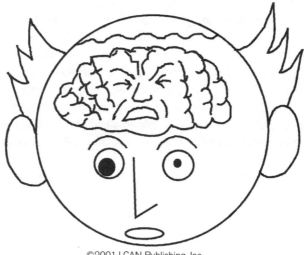

©2001 I CAN Publishing, Inc.

O liguira, edema, ↑ ICP—indications

S tops reabsorption of water

M annitol

O utput of urine, electrolytes—monitor

T issue dehydration—U E

I ncreased frequency/volume of urination

C irculatory overload—U E

Buster Brain Man is feeling the squeeze from too much fluid in the brain. He can't think, he can't blink, and he may sink without an osmotic diuretic. Mannitol will reduce this cerebral edema.

73

Concept: ANTICOAGULANTS

This category is commonly referred to as anticoagulants or "blood thinners". While they do not actually **"thin"** the blood, they work on different factors in the blood to decrease its ability to clot. This decrease in clotting prevents harmful clots from forming in the vessels. They also can interfere or inhibit platelet aggregation which in turn prevents the clots from forming or attaching to the vessels. Despite the type of action they have, all blood viscosity reducing agents are considered **HIGH ALERT** medications and safeguards at practice sites should be adopted.

ANTICOAGULANTS

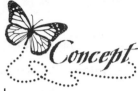

T hese belong to class of meds called anticoagulants

H ospitalization required for IV Heparin

I nform other physicians (dentists, surgeons, etc.) that client is taking these meds

N ote an increase in bruising or bleeding tendencies

B eware of mixing with herbal supplements

L ook for nose bleeds—this may be the first sign that dose is too high

O ral drugs require frequent blood test to monitor

O ften prescribed with heart valve replacements

D on't take in large amounts of vitamin K (fish, liver, spinach, cabbage, etc.)

WARFARIN

Action: Interferes with the hepatic synthesis of vitamin K-clotting factors (II, VII, IX, and X).

Indications: Prevents or slows extension of a blood clot.

Undesirable Effects: Anorexia, nausea, diarrhea; rash; bleeding, hematuria, thrombocytopenia, hemorrhage.

Warnings: **HIGH ALERT DRUG** Pregnancy; hemorrhagic tendencies such as hemophilia, thrombocytopenia purpura, leukemia; peptic ulcer; cerebral vascular accident (CVA); severe renal or hepatic disease.

Other Specific Information: Foods–↑ risk for bleeding when taken with warfarin include: (i.e., asparagus, cabbage, cauliflower, turnip greens, and other green leafy vegetables). Drugs–↑ risk for bleeding include: **G**lucocorticosteroids, **A**lcohol, **S**alicylate (**GAS**). Drugs ↓ effectiveness: **R**ifampin, **O**ral contraceptives, **P**henytoin, **E**strogen (**ROPE**). ↑ risk of bleeding with chamomile, garlic, ginger, ginkgo, and ginseng therapy. There are numerous interactions. *(Refer to a Drug Handbook.)*

Interventions: "CORA" on the next page will help you remember 4 major interventions. Anticoagulant effects may be reversed by vitamin K injections. Check all drugs for potential drug-drug interactions.

Education: Evaluation of PT/INR will be required to regulate dosage; report any unusual bleeding. Review a diet low in vitamin K. Wear a medical identification card or jewelry (Medic Alert). Always advise other providers (i.e., dentists, surgeon, etc.) of medication; no strenuous activities (skydiving, long distance running, football); no OTC medication without provider approval.

Evaluation: PT will have a value of 1.5 to 2.5 times the control value in seconds; the INR will be 2–3. The client will have no signs or symptoms of bleeding.

Drug: warfarin (Coumadin)

CORA COUMADIN

HIGH ALERT

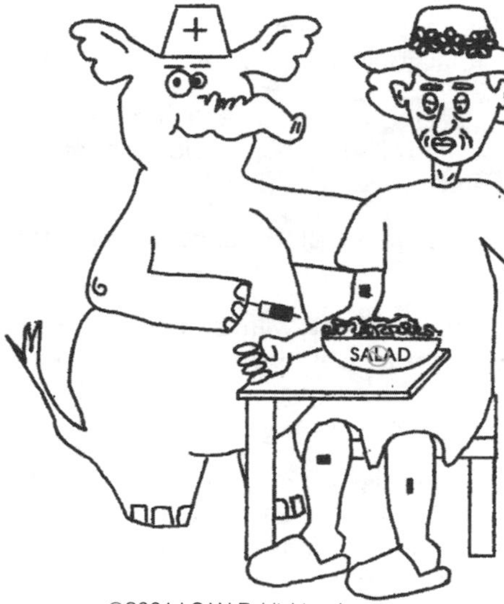

©2001 I CAN Publishing, Inc.

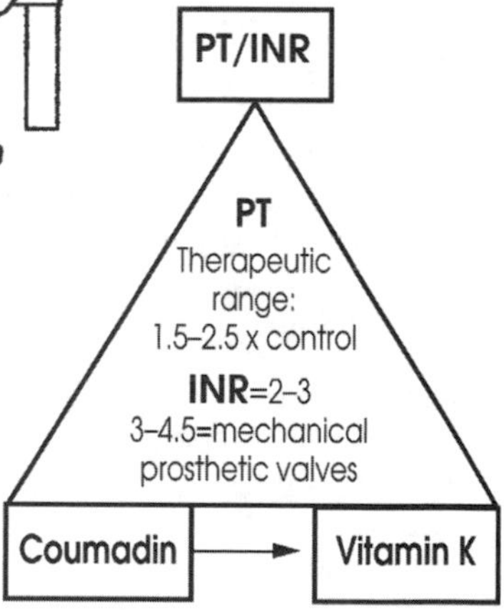

Check VS, platelet count, PT

Observe for bleeding

Review bleeding protocol (i.e., electric razors, soft toothbrushes, etc.)

Avoid ASA, may use acetaminophen

PT/INR

PT
Therapeutic range:
1.5–2.5 x control
INR=2–3
3–4.5=mechanical prosthetic valves

| Coumadin | → | Vitamin K |

Cora Coumadin is having her blood drawn for coagulation levels. If her PT is > 1.5–2.5 x the control, she may experience excessive bruising and have bloody stools. Foods high in vitamin K (such as green leafy vegetables) should be avoided since they will increase the risk of clotting.

HEPARIN SODIUM

Action: Combines with antithrombin III to retard thrombin activity. Low-molecular-weight heparin blocks factor Xa, factor IIa.

Indications: Thrombosis. Reduces risk of myocardial infarction (MI), CVA, clots associated with atrial fibrillation; pulmonary embolism.

Warnings: **HIGH ALERT DRUG** Hypersensitivity to heparin; severe thrombocytopenia; uncontrolled bleeding; ulcers or any risk of hemorrhage; liver or renal disease.

Undesirable Effects: Hemorrhagic tendencies: hematuria, bleeding gums, frank hemorrhage.

Other Specific Information: ↑ effect with aspirin, alcohol, and antibiotics. ↓ effect with digoxin (Lanoxin), antihistamines, and nitroglycerin products. ↑ risk of bleeding with chamomile, garlic, ginger, ginkgo, and ginseng therapy.

Interventions: Monitor PTT (usually 1.5–2.5 times control values) and platelet count. Monitor for signs of unusual bleeding (petechiae, hematuria, GI bleeding, gum bleeding). Initiate bleeding protocol measures (use electric razors, hold pressure for 5 minutes with venipunctures, soft toothbrushes). Monitor IV site carefully. Heparin has short half life, therefore, with discontinuation, PTT will usually return to baseline within 1–2 hours. Have protamine sulfate available as an antidote.

Education: Explain bleeding protocol precautions; explain the need for several PTT evaluations; teach signs of unusual bleeding; avoid activities with risk of injury; caution with sharp utensils while cooking or eating. Avoid salicylates or any OTC medication without approval from provider. Wear identification that notes anticoagulant therapy. Inform provider of therapy prior to surgical procedure.

Evaluation: The client's PTT will show values 1.5–2.5 times the control value in seconds, and there will be no signs or symptoms of bleeding or thrombus formation.

Drugs: He**parin** Sodium (He**parin**); **Low-Molecular-Weight Heparins:** arde**parin** (Normiflo); dalte**parin** (Fragmin); enoxa**parin** (Lovenox)

HARRY HEPARIN

HIGH ALERT

©2001 I CAN Publishing, Inc.

PTT
Therapeutic range:
1.5–2.5 x control

Heparin → **Protamine Sulfate**

Harry Heparin is getting his anticoagulant IV or SubQ in the abdomen. His soft toothbrush will help keep gums from bleeding and his electric razor will keep him from bleeding when he shaves. Even the band-aid when pulled off his arm may cause a big bruise. If Harry's PTT is > 1.5–2.5 x control, he may bruise and bleed too freely.

LOW MOLECULAR WEIGHT HEPARIN

Action: Anticoagulant, antithrombotic. Prevents conversion of fibrinogen to fibrin and prothrombin to thrombin by enhancing inhibitory effects of antithrombin III; produces higher ratio of anti-factor Xa to IIa

Indications: Prevention of deep-vein thrombosis, pulmonary emboli in hip and knee replacement

Warnings: `HIGH ALERT DRUG` Hypersensitivity to drug, heparin, or pork; hemophilia, leukemia with bleeding, peptic ulcer disease, thrombocytopenic purpura, heparin-induced thrombocytopenia, clients with prosthetic heart valves.

Undesirable Effects: Fever, confusion, nausea, edema, hypochromic anemia, thrombocytopenia, bleeding, cardiac toxicity, ecchymosis.

Other Specific Information: Increased action of enoxaparin: anticoagulants, salicylates, NSAIDs, antiplatelets. Increased hypo-prothrombinemia: plicamycin, valproic acid. **DO NOT MIX WITH OTHER DRUGS OR INFUSION FLUIDS.** Increased risk of bleeding when taken with bromelain, cinchona bark, garlic ginger, ginkgo, and ginseng.

Interventions: Assess blood studies (i.e., Hct, CBC, coagulation studies, platelets, occult blood in stools), anti-factor Xa; thrombo-cytopenia may occur. Assess for bleeding: gums, petechiae, ecchymosis, black tarry stools, hematuria; notify prescriber. Assess for neurologic symptoms in clients who have received spinal anesthesia. Administer only after screening for bleeding disorders. **SC only (do not aspirate or massage); do not give IM**, begin 2 hrs prior to surgery, do not aspirate, rotate sites, do not expel bubble from syringe prior to administration. Insert whole length of needle into skin fold held with thumb and forefinger. Administer only this drug when ordered; not interchangeable with heparin. Leave vascular access sheath in place for 6 hr after dose, then give next dose 6 hr after sheath removal. Avoid all IM injections that my cause bleeding. Treatment of overdose should be Protamine Sulfate; dose should equal dose of enoxaparin.

Education: Instruct client to use soft-bristle toothbrush to avoid bleeding gums, to use electric razor. Report any signs of bleeding: gums, under skin, urine, stools. Avoid over the counter drugs containing aspirin.

Staff Education: Do not confuse enoxaparin with enoxacin or Lovenox with Lotronex.

Evaluation: Client will not experience any deep vein thrombosis and will have a therapeutic response.

Drugs: *(These drugs end in "parin".)* dalte**parin** (Fragmin); enoxa**parin** (Lovenox); tinza**parin** (Innohep)

ENOXAPARIN
"LOVENOX"

L ow molecular weight

O rthopedic surgeries

D **V** T prophylaxis, immobility, stints, cardiac surgeries
—indicators

L **E** ave bubble in syringe

N ever by IM, only subcutaneous—give within 2 hours
of preop abdominal surgery and 12 hours of
knee surgery

N **O** rubbing after administered, no aspiration, no mixing with
other drugs

X out for pork allergies,
heparin allergies; PUD;
leukemia

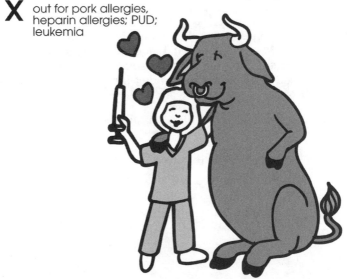

©2005 I CAN Publishing, Inc.

"Love an ox" by initiating bleeding protocols, having protamine sulfate
on hand for antidote and monitoring coagulation studies.

PRADAXA

Action: Stops the formation of thrombin so fibrinogen cannot be made into fibrin. Prevents the formation of a clot. Used especially to prevent cerebral vascular accident (CVA)

Indications: Currently only for use to prevent thrombus formation in clients with atrial fibrillation.

Warnings: **HIGH ALERT DRUG** Bleeding!

Undesirable Effects: Bleeding, especially GI bleeds, stomach pain, indigestion

Other Specific Information: Do not stop the medication unless advised by healthcare provider. Do not take with the antibiotic, Rifampin (used for MRSA infections and Tuberculosis). Rifampin decreases the effectiveness of Pradaxa.

Interventions: Monitor hemoglobin and Hematocrit; watch for s/s of GI bleed (coffee ground emesis, black tarry stools, hypovolemia). Hold medication if any active bleeding. Labor and Delivery increases risk of severe bleeding. Careful use in older adults. Clients > 75 years old have more incidence of major bleeding episodes.

Education: Report bleeding that cannot be controlled with pressure x 10 minutes. Report s/s of GI bleed identified above. Advise to use a soft bristled tooth brush and electric razor. Does NOT require repeated blood tests or changes in diet *(an advantage over warfarin (Coumadin).*

Evaluation: Prevention of CVA in clients with atrial fibrillation. Prevention of clots.

Drugs: dabigatran etexilate (Pradaxa)

THE ABC'S FOR PRADAXA

HIGH ALERT

Atrial fibrillation: Used to prevent thrombus formation

Bleeding is a major RISK!

Contraindicated for any complications involving BLEEDING! Labor and Delivery ↑ bleeding risk

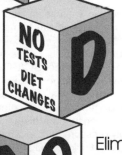

NO TESTS DIET CHANGES

Does not require blood tests or diet changes (a major advantage over Coumadin)

RIFAMPIN

Eliminate Rifampin when taking Pradaxa. Elderly clients >75 years old ↑ bleeding risk

FONDAPARINUX (ARIXTRA)

Action: Anticoagulant, antithrombin. Binds selectively to antithrombin III, potentiating neutralization of Factor Xa and inhibiting formation of thrombin.

Indications: DVT prophylaxis. Treatment of acute DVT or PE.

Warnings: **HIGH ALERT DRUG** Hypersensitivity. Hypersensitivity to latex. CrCl < 30 (severe renal impairment). Thrombocytopenia. Use is not advised in anticoagulated clients. Black Box Warning: Risk of epidural or spinal hematoma after spinal puncture in anticoagulated clients. Spinal hematoma may lead to permanent paralysis. Risk is increased with indwelling epidural catheter use. Avoid use with anticoagulants, antiplatelets, NSAIDS, thrombolytics. Active bleeding or risk for bleeding. Caution with history of GI bleed or hemorrhagic stroke. Recent surgery or trauma. Uncontrolled HTN. Elderly. Risk of hemorrhage increases with renal impairment.

Undesirable Effects: Serious: Hemorrhage, anemia, thrombocytopenia, heparin-induced thrombocytopenia, epidural/spinal hematoma, paralysis. Common: Bleeding complications, injection site bleeding, pruritis or rash at site, elevated PTT.

Other Specific Information: Unit dosage cannot be used interchangeably with heparin or other LMW heparins. Anti-platelet agents such as aspirin, NSAIDs, and other anticoagulants may increase risk for bleeding.

Interventions: Monitor vital signs. No IM administration. Monitor creatinine clearance at baseline and periodically, CBC, platelets (discontinue if less than 100,000 mm^3), potassium, LFTs, anti-F Xa, stool for occult blood. May increase LFTs. May cause hypokalemia. Administer SubQ in fatty tissue. Discontinue and contact provider if bleeding occurs. If client had a spinal or epidural anesthesia, assess insertion site for swelling. Monitor sensation and movement of lower extremities. Notify provider of care regarding abnormal findings.

Education: Report signs and symptoms of bleeding such as an increase in the heart rate, decrease in the blood pressure, bruising, petechiae, hematomas, etc. Report changes in LOC, confusion, headaches, dizziness, chest pain, nose bleeds, shortness of breath, blood in urine, abdominal pain, coffee-ground emesis, tarry stools, excessive bruising, paleness. Teach proper SC/SQ/subQ administration. Rotate site of administration. Review the importance of using a 20 to 22 gauge needle to withdraw medication from the vial. Then, change to a small needle (gauge 25 or 26, 1/2 to 5/8 in length). Deep subcutaneous injections should be administered in the abdomen, ensuring a distance of 2 inches from the umbilicus. Do not aspirate. Apply pressure for 1 to 2 min after the injection. Rotate and record injection sites. Avoid using OTC agents such as aspirin or NSAIDs without physician approval. Review importance to take precautionary measures to avoid injury.

Evaluation: Prevention of DVT or client will have no worsening in status of acute DVT or PE.

Drugs: Fondaparinux (Arixtra)

FONDAPARINUX (ARIXTRA)

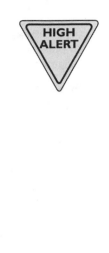

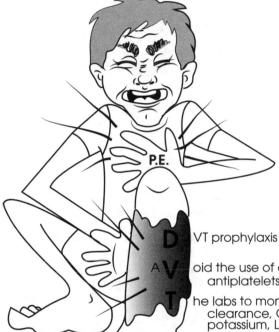

VT prophylaxis

oid the use of anticoagulants,
antiplatelets, NSAIDS

he labs to monitor are creatinine
clearance, CBC, platelets,
potassium, LFTs

©2013 I CAN Publishing®, Inc.

ANTIPLATELET: ASPIRIN

Action: Platelet aggregation inhibitor; inhibits platelet synthesis of thromboxane A2, a vasoconstrictor and inducer of platelet aggregation. This occurs at low doses and lasts for 8 days (life of the platelet).

Indications: TIAs; CVAs with a history of TIA due to fibrin platelet emboli. Reduces risk of death from MI in clients with a history of infarction or unstable angina. (Refer to **NSAIDs.**)

Warnings: Allergy to salicylates or NSAIDs. Bleeding disorders, renal or hepatic disorders,chickenpox, influenza (risk of Reye's Syndrome in children), pregnancy, lactation.

Undesirable Effects: GI discomfort, bleeding, dizziness, tinnitus. (Refer to NSAIDs.)

Other Specific Information: ↑risk of bleeding with anticoagulants, thrombolytics. ↑risk of GI ulceration with alcohol, NSAIDs, phenyl-butazone, steroids.

Interventions: Monitor liver and renal function tests, CBC, clotting times, stool guaiac, blood drug levels, and vital signs.

Education: Instruct to take drug with food and a full glass of water. Do not crush and do not chew sustained-release preparations. Use only as recommended. Review undesirable effects and the importance of reporting them to the provider. Initiate safety precautions to keep out of children's reach since it can be very dangerous. (Refer to **NSAIDs.**)

Evaluation: Client will experience no thrombotic episodes, such as a stroke.

Drugs: aspirin (Bayer, Bufferin, Ecotrin); Other antiplatelet drugs are listed below; however, there are numerous differences between each drug. (*Refer to Drug Handbook.*) abciximab (ReoPro); cilostazol (Pletal); clopidogrel (Plavix); dipyridamole (Persantine); eptifibatide (Integrilin)

ANNIE ASPIRIN

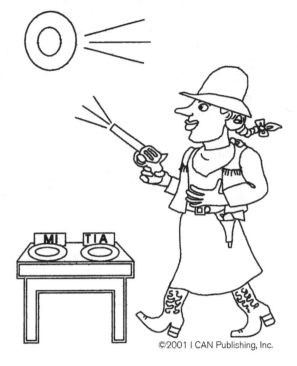

©2001 I CAN Publishing, Inc.

F ever

I nflammation

R educes TIAs due to fibrin platelet embolus

E liminates (reduces) death with hx of MI

Annie (git yer gun) Aspirin is busy "firing" at platelets to reduce the blood coagulation in her body, especially with myocardial infarction or transient ischemic attack. She is holding her stomach as this med can cause stomach irritation. "FIRE" reviews other indications for prescribing aspirin.

AGGRENOX

Action: Prevents blood clots from forming by interfering with the tendency of blood platelets to clump together. Putting the two ingredients together is more effective than one ingredient alone for preventing strokes (aspirin and extended-release dipyridamole).

Indications: For clients who have had a transient ischemic attack "mini-stroke" or a full stroke due which was caused from a blood clot blocking an artery in the brain.

Warnings: This drug should not be taken by clients who are allergic to aspirin or aspirin containing drugs and any other nonsteroidal anti-inflammatory drugs (Advil, Naprosyn, and Motrin). Risk of Reye's Syndrome. Clients who consume alcohol are at risk for bleeding. This drug should be used with caution by clients with a recent heart attack, chest pain, and even heart disease.

Undesirable Effects: Abdominal pain, back pain, headache, nausea, bleeding, diarrhea. Headache was most notable in the first month of treatment.

Other Specific Information: Alcohol and aggrenox may result in bleeding.

Interventions: Monitor clotting time, BUN, bleeding time, GI side effects, Hepatic enzymes, blood urea nitrogen and serum creatinine, hyperkalemia, proteinuria.

Education: This drug may be taken with or without food. If a dose is missed, take as soon as you remember. Check with pharmacist. Check with your provider of care or pharmacist for the numerous drug-drug interactions.

Evaluation: Client will not experience a stroke and will have no complications with bleeding.

Drug: aspirin and extended-release dipyridamole (Aggrenox)

ANNIE AND THE OX

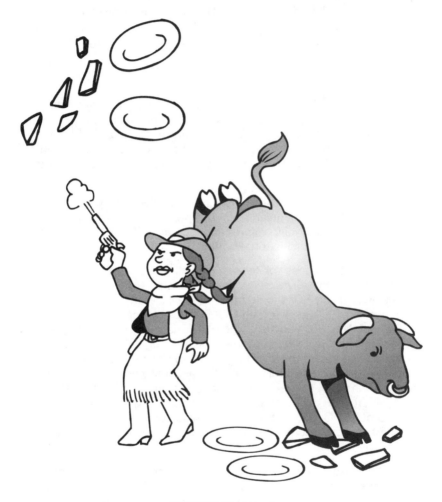

We are destroying these platelets, so they can't be used for clotting.

GLYCOPROTEIN IIB/IIIA INHIBITORS

Action: Antiplatelet action. Platelet glycoprotein antagonist. This agent reversibly prevents fibrinogen, von Willebrand's factor from binding to the glycoprotein IIb/IIIa receptor, inhibiting platelett aggregation.

Indications: Acute coronary syndrome including those with PCI (percutaneous coronary intervention)

Warnings: **HIGH ALERT DRUG** Hypersensitivity, active internal bleeding; history of bleeding. CVA within 1 month. Major surgery with severe trauma, severe hypotension, history of intracranial bleeding, intracranial neoplasm, arteriovenous malformation/aneurysm, aortic dissection, dependence on renal dialysis. Severe uncontrolled hypertension.

Other Specific Information: Increased bleeding with aspirin, heparin, NSAIDs, anticoagulants, ticlopidine, clopidogrel, dipyridamole, thrombolytics, plicamycin, valproate, abciximab. Do not administer with platelet receptor inhibitors IIb, IIIa.

Interventions: Assess platelets, Hgb, Hct, creatinine, PT/APTT baseline INR within 6 hr of loading dose and every day thereafter. Clients undergoing PCI should have ACT evaluated; the APTT should be between 50–70 sec. unless PCI is to be performed; during PCI, ACT should be 300–350 sec; if plateletts drop < 100,000/mm^3, review additional platelet count; discontinue drug if thrombocytopenia is confirmed and also draw a Hct, Hgb, and serum creatinine. Assess for bleeding (i.e., gums, bruising, petechiae, ecchymosis; GI, GU tract, cardiac cath sites, or IM injection sites). Aspirin and heparin may be given with this drug. D/C heparin prior to removing any femoral artery sheaths after PCI. Do not administer discolored solutions or those with particulates, discard unused amount. Discontinue drug prior to CABG.

Education: Review reason for taking the medication. Instruct the importance of reporting bruising, bleeding and chest pain. Half-life is 2.5 hr, steady state 4–6 hr, metabolism limited, excretion via kidneys. Creatinine clearance will be calculated prior to starting medication.

Evaluation: Client will experience therapeutic effects from the medication with no undesirable effects.

Drugs: eptifibatide (Integrilin), tirofiban (Aggrastat), Reopro

EPTIFIBATIDE (INTEGRILIN)

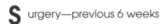

S urgery—previous 6 weeks

P lanned administration of parenteral GP II b/IIIa

R enal dialysis

U ncontrolled hypertension

C VA within 30 days of hemorrhagic CVA

E vidence of a bleeding disorder
valuate creatinine clearance

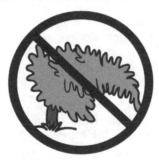

If serum creatinine more than 2 mg/dl or estimated CrCl less than 50 mL/min., reduce continuous infusion rate to 1 mcg/Kg/min.

To estimate CrCl, use the following formula
(calulation to be verified by two people)

CrCl - $\dfrac{(140 - age) (Weight\ in\ Kg)}{72\ (serum\ creatinine)}$ Multiply by 0.85 if female

CrCl = _____ mL/min

Remember, the "SPRUCE" tree is falling down. If "SPRUCE" is present, do not administer Integrilin.

CLOPIDOGREL (PLAVIX)

Action: Platelet aggregation inhibitor by inhibiting the first and second phases of ADP-induced effects in platelet aggregation.

Indications: Reduces atherosclerotic events such as a stroke, MI, vascular death, or peripheral vascular disease

Warnings: Hypersensitivity, pathologic bleeding (i.e., peptic ulcers, intracranial hemorrhage), lactation

Undesirable Effects: Depression, dizziness, fatigue, headache, epistaxis, cough, chest pain, hypertension, GI BLEEDING, abdominal pain, diarrhea, dyspepsia, gastritis, pruritus, purpura, rash, BLEEDING, NEUTROPEINA, THROMBOCYTOPENIC PURPURA, hypercholesterolemia, arthralgia, back pain, Hypersensitivity reactions including ANGIOEDEMA, ANAPHYLACTOID REACTIONS, BRONCHOSPASM

Other Specific Information: Concurrent abciximab, eptifibatide, tirofiban, aspirin, NSAIDs, heparin, heparinoids, thrombolytic agents, ticlopidine, or warfarin may increase bleeding. Plavix may decrease metabolism and increase effects of phenytoin, tolbutamide, tamoxifen, torsemide, fluvastatin, warfarin, and many NSAIDs.

Interventions: Assess for symptoms of stroke, MI during treatment. Liver function studies: AST, ALT, bilirubin, creatinine (long-term therapy). Blood studies: CBC, Hct, Hgb, PT, cholesterol (long-term therapy)

Education: Educate client that blood work will be necessary during treatment. Report any unusual bruising or bleeding. Recommend taking with food or just after eating to minimize GI discomfort. Report diarrhea, skin rashes, chills, fever, sore throat, or subcutaneous bleeding. All health care providers must be told that clopidogrel is being used.

Staff Education: Do not confuse Plavix with Paxil or Elavil.

Evaluation: Client will not experience any occurrence of atherosclerotic events.

Drugs: clopidogrel (Plavix)

PLAVIX

B leeding, bronchospasms—undesirable effects

L owers risk of atherosclerotic events

E valuate bruising

E valuate liver function and blood studies

D rug/drug interactions are many!

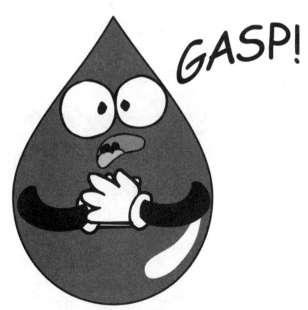

©2005 I CAN Publishing, Inc.

"BLEED" will help you remember some important facts regarding Plavix.

THROMBOLYTIC AGENTS

Action: Barinds with plasminogen causing conversion to plasmin, which dissolves blood clots.

Indications: Dissolves blood clots due to coronary artery thrombi, deep vien thrombosis, pulmonary embolism.

Warnings: **HIGH ALERT DRUG** Active internal bleeding; recent CVA; aneurysm; hypertension; anticoagulant therapy; ulcerative colitis. Severe allergic reactions to either anistreplase or streptokinase. Caution: Alphabet Soup names = high error risk. TNK is weight-based. TPA is the only thrombolytic approved for use in non-hemorrhagic stroke.

Undesirable Effects: Hemorrhage, headache, nausea, rash, fever, bleeding, allergic reaction, hypotension.

Other Specific Information: Client's risk of bleeding is increased. Amino-caproic acid inhibits streptokinase and cannot be used to reverse its fibri-nolytic effects. Effects of drug disappear within a few hours after discontinuing, but the systemic effect of coagulation and the risk of bleeding may persist for 24 hours. Increase in risk for bleeding with heparin, oral anticoagulants, antiplatelet drugs, and NASIDs.

Interventions: Monitor CBC especially hgb/hct, coagulation tests. Evaluate bleeding at a sutured wound, arterial site, central line. Monitor vital signs during and after infusion; monitor EKG for re-perfusion dysrhythmias. Watch for unusual bleeding disturbance (GI, GU); initiate bleeding protocol measures for several hours (e.g., no venipunctures, repetitive manual blood pressure, or removal of IV lines or catheters).

Education: Explain the treatment to client and family. Explain need for frequent VS and other assessments. Instruct client to report any undesirable effects.

Evaluation: The client's clot has dissolved and there are no signs and symptoms of active bleeding or other undesirable effects.

Drugs: alteplase (Activase, tPA); anistreplace (APSAC, Eminase); streptokinase (Streptase); urokinase (Abbokinase); reteplase (rRA); tenecteplase (TNK)

ADAM ASE

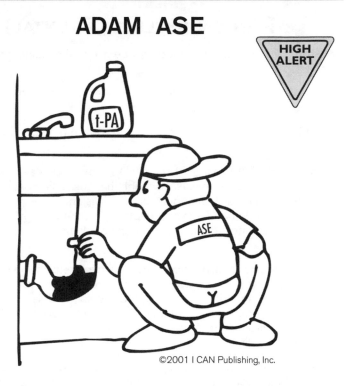

HIGH
ALERT

©2001 I CAN Publishing, Inc.

C BC, hgb, hct—monitor

L ook for dysrhythmias

O bserve for bleeding

T he vital signs must be monitored

Adam **"ASE"** will dissolve the clog in this sink just as he dissolves the "CLOT" in a blood vessel. He will use t-PA or another thrombolytic agent that ends in **"ASE"**.

PENTOXIFYLLINE (TRENTAL)

Action: Blood viscosity reducing agent by stimulating prostacyclin formation.

Indications: Intermittent claudicaton. Related to chronic occlusive vascular disease.

Warnings: Hypersensitivity to this drug or xanthines; retinal/cerebral hemorrhage.

Undesirable Effects: Epistaxis, flu like symptoms, nasal congestion, laryngitis, leukopenia, malaise, weight changes, agitation, drowsiness, dizziness, nervous, insomnia, blurred vision, dyspnea, angina, arrhythmias, edema, flushing, hypotension, abdominal discomfort, belching, bloating, diarrhea, dyspepsia, flatus, nausea, vomiting, tremor.

Other Specific Information: Additive hypotension may occur with antihypertensives and nitrates. May increase the risk of bleeding with warfarin, heparin, aspirin, NSAIDs, cefamandole, cefoperazone, cefotetan, plicamycin, valproic acid, clopigogrel, ticlopidine, eptifibatide, tirofiban, or other thrombolytic agents. May increase the risk of theophylline toxicity.

Interventions: Assess blood pressure, respirations of client. If GI and CNS undesirable effects occur, decrease dose to twice daily; discontinue if effects continue. May cause dizziness and blurred vision; caution client to avoid driving and other activities requiring alertness until response to medication is determined. Administer with meals to prevent GI upset. Do not break, crush, or chew ext. released tabs.

Education: Advise client to avoid smoking due to nicotine constricting blood vessels. Instruct client to notify provider of care if nausea, vomiting, GI upset, drowsiness, dizziness, or headache persists. Advise client that it may take 2–4 weeks to maintain a therapeutic response. Decreased fats and cholesterol, increased exercise, decreased smoking are necessary to correct condition. Observe feet for arterial insufficiency. Use cotton socks, well-fitted shoes; not to go barefoot. Observe for bleeding, bruises, epistaxis. Avoid smoking to prevent blood vessel constriction.

Evaluation: Client will experience a decrease in pain and cramping and will have an increase in the ability to ambulate.

Drug: pentoxifylline (Trental)

TRENTAL

T aken 1x daily

R educes RBC aggregation and hyperviscosity

H **E** lps with signs and symptoms of Intermittent Claudication

N on-labeled FDA use for diabetic complications, acute alcoholic hepatitis

T oxic drug/drug effects with theophylline and other "xanthines"

A lways ask about recent surgeries, recent bleeding even retinal or cerebral

L ike client to take with meals or food

©2005 I CAN Publishing, Inc.

TRENT will be **ALL** better when his intermittent claudication subsides. The medication TRENTAL is used to decrease this medical condition.

BILE ACID SEQUESTRANT

Action: Combines with bile acids in the intestine resulting in excretion in the feces. Cholesterol is oxidized in the liver to replace the lost bile acids; serum cholesterol and LDL are decreased.

Indications: Hypercholesterolemia when dietary management does not lower cholesterol.

Warnings: Complete biliary obstruction, abnormal function of the intestine; hepatic or renal dysfunction; pregnancy, lactation; elderly client.

Undesirable Effects: Constipation, indigestion, nausea, vomiting, or GI bleeding; headache, syncope; increased bleeding tendencies due to vitamin K malabsorption; rash; muscle pain.

Other Specific Information: ↓ absorption of warfarin. ↓ absorption of digoxin, thiazides, propranolol, penicillin, tetracyclines, vancomycin, folic acid, and thyroid hormones. ↓ absorption of fat soluble vitamins (A, D, E, K).

Interventions: Monitor serum cholesterol, triacylglycerol levels, and PT in relation to baseline at regular intervals. Monitor appropriate drug levels based on current drug intake. Monitor I & O and bowel status.

Education: Take other meds 1 hour before or 4 to 6 hours after choles-tyramines or colestipol. Diet low in fats, cholesterol, and sugars; high in fiber. Follow directions in mixing; never take as a dry powder. (Incomplete mixing may result in mucosal irritation!) Mix with 3–6 oz. water, milk, fruit juice, or soup. Take before meals and drink several glasses of water between meals. Instruct that a laxative or stool softener may assist in preventing constipation. Report unusual bleeding or bruising.

Evaluation: Serum cholesterol and low-density lipoprotein (LDL) levels will decrease and remain within the normal range.

Drugs: cholestyramine (Questran); colestipol (Colestid)

BILE ACID SEQUESTRANT

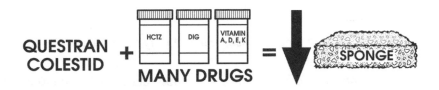

©2001 I CAN Publishing, Inc.

L DL is ↓15–30%

I ncrease fluids and fiber

P T monitoring

I ncrease in GI distress—constipation

D ecreases absorption of many meds

FIBRIC ACID

Action: Increases activity of lipoprotein lipase, promoting VLDL and triacylglycerols catabolism. Promotes transfer of cholesterol to HDL. The reduction of triacylglycerols is significant.

Indications: Hyperlipidemia.

Warnings: Liver or renal disease, primary biliary cirrhosis, gallbladder disease, peptic ulcer disease.

Undesirable Effects: GI effects include abdominal distention, constipation, diarrhea, flatulence, nausea, vomiting; cholelithiasis; myositis; headache, dizziness, blurred vision with gemfibrozil; rash, urticaria; neutropenia, leuko-penia, anemia, or agranulocytosis.

Other Specific Information: May ↑ effect of warfarin, sulfonyureas, and insulin. Concomitant use of probenecid ↑ clofibrate levels. If gemfibrozil is administered with lovastatin, an ↑ risk of rhabdomyolysis and myoglobinuria may result in acute renal failure.

Interventions: Monitor liver/renal function tests, cholesterol, and triacylglycerol levels in relation to baseline and at regular intervals. Monitor serum glucose (if on antidiabetics), uric acid, and CBC. Monitor PT if client is taking oral anticoagulants. Monitor GI response and urine output.

Education: Attempt dietary corrections before meds. Encourage a diet low in fats, cholesterol, and/or sugars. Restrict alcohol. Instruct to take med before meals. Encourage weight reduction and physical exercise. Instruct that a paradoxic rise in levels may occur in the initial 2 or 3 months, but decrease after this period. Instruct regarding the importance of keeping clinical appointments for laboratory studies and reevaluation by the provider.

Evaluation: Serum cholesterol and triacylglycerol levels will be reduced to normal limits.

Drugs: clofibrate (Atromid-S); gemfibrozil (Lopid)

FIBRIC ACID

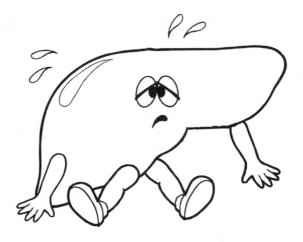

L iver or renal disease—WARNING

I ncreases effect of warfarin or sulfonlyureas

V LDL, LDL, triacylglycerols and cholesterol—monitor

E ncourage diet ↓ in fat, cholesterol and sugars

R estrict alcohol

HMG CoA INHIBITORS

Action: The "statins" are competitive inhibitors of HMG-CoA reductase, an enzyme necessary for cholesterol biosynthesis in the intestine and liver.

Indications: Hypercholesterolemia; ↓ low-density lipoprotein (LDL); ↑ high-density lipoprotein (HDL).

Warnings: Active liver disease; unexplained, persistent elevations in liver function tests. Caution: alcoholism; acute infections; metabolic disorders; electrolyte imbalance; hypotension.

Undesirable Effects: GI distress: (dyspepsia, diarrhea, constipation, gas); headache; blurred vision with lovastatin. Rare: liver dysfunction, myalgia, myopathy, or myositis.

Other Specific Information: ↑ effect of warfarin. Bile acid binding acids may ↓ availability of "statin". Digoxin ↑ "statin" levels. Concomitant use of ACE inhibitors may result in ↑ K^+. Concomitant use of erythromycin, fibric acid derivatives, immunosuppressive drugs, and niacin may ↑ rhabdomyolysis.

Interventions: Monitor serum cholesterol and triacylglycerol levels, serum creatine kinase (CK), and LFT in relation to baseline and at regular intervals. Discontinue "statins" if LFT ↑ > 3 times normal. Prior to initiating drug therapy, encourage appropriate diet, exercise, and weight reduction.

Education: Drink 2–3 liters of fluid daily. Take with food and at bedtime; reduce cholesterol, fats, and sugar; diet high in fiber (whole grain cereals, fruits, and vegetables). Exercise and weight reduction should also be encouraged for obese clients along with therapy. It may take several weeks before blood lipid levels decrease. If taking lovastatin, report changes in vision and have an annual eye exam.

Evaluation: Serum cholesterol and triacylglycerol levels will decrease and return to the normal limits. The HDL serum level will have a modest increase.

Drugs: *(These drugs end in "statin".)* atorva**statin** (Lipitor); ceriva**statin** (Baycol); fluva**statin** (Lescol); lova**statin** (Mevacor); prava**statin** (Pravachol); rosuva**statin** (Crestor); simva**statin** (Zocor)

L. L. STATIN

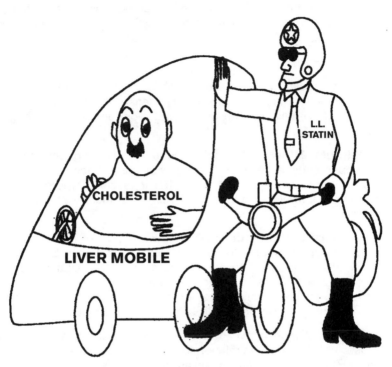

©2001 I CAN Publishing, Inc.

Officer "L. L. (lipid lowering) Statin" has stopped the liver mobile and its driver, Cholesterol. These drugs lower cholesterol and can be highly toxic to the liver. Drugs that are in this group end in **"statin"**.

NIACIN

Action: Inhibits free fatty acid release from adipose tissue by inhibiting accumulation of cAMP stimulated by lipolytic hormones. Increases rate of triacylglycerol removal from the plasma.

Indication: Hyperlipidemia.

Warnings: Acute MI, heart failure; diabetes mellitus; gout; hepatic/ renal dysfunction; active peptic ulcer disease; concomitant HMG-CoA reductase inhibitors; severe hypotension; arterial hemorrhage; pregnancy.

Undesirable Effects: Headache, GI upset, flushing and itching over upper body (face, neck, arms) with raised rash appearance (resolves approximately 1/2–1 hour after ingestion), hyperglycemia, hyperuricemia, myalgia, cardiac dysrhythmias in those with coronary artery disease.

Other Specific Information: Most severe cases of hepatotoxicity have been reported with SR forms. Flushing is ↓ with SR preps, but GI effects are ↑. Lovastatin, pravastatin, simvastatin may ↑ risk of rhabdomyolysis and acute renal failure. ↑ effectiveness of antihypertensives, vasoactive drugs. ↑ risk of bleeding with anticoagulants. ↓ absorption with bile acid sequestrants.

Interventions: Monitor liver function tests, serum uric acid, serum glucose, and cholesterol in relation to baseline and at regular intervals. Monitor PT and platelets if taking an anticoagulant. Monitor for flushing, discomfort after medicating (i.e., headache, dizziness, blurred vision), or orthostatic hypotension.

Education: Take with food and at bedtime. Avoid alcohol and take bile acid sequestrant (if prescribed) 4–6 hours apart. Pretreatment with 325 mg ASA may ↓ undesirable effect of vasodilation. Follow diet regimen-low cholesterol and low saturated fats. If dizziness occurs, change position slowly. Undesirable effects are typically transient and will usually subside with continued therapy. Review importance for follow-up evaluation during long-term therapy.

Evaluation: LDL and triacylglycerol levels will decrease and return to normal limits. HDL will increase.

Drug: niacin (Niaspan)

NIACIN

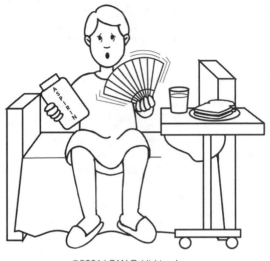

©2001 I CAN Publishing, Inc.

N ote liver function tests—regular intervals

I tching and flushing—U E

A spirin before Niacin may ⬇ U E of vasodilation

C ontraindications: hepatic disease, pregnancy

I nstruct to take with food and at bedtime

N o high cholesterol foods

ANTILIPEMIC: ZETIA

Action: Inhibits absorption of cholesterol by the small intestine.

Indications: Hypercholesterolemia, homozygous familial hypercholesterolemia, homozygous sitosterolemia.

Warnings: Hypersensitivity, severe hepatic disease.

Undesirable Effects: Fatigue, dizziness. Nausea, diarrhea, abdominal pain. Chest pain. Myalgias, arthralgias, back pain. Pharyngitis, sinusitis, cough.

Other Specific Information: Toxicity: cyclosporine. Decreased action of ezetimibe with antacids, cholestyramine. Increased action of ezetimibe with fibric acid derivatives.

Interventions: Assess lipid levels, LFTs baseline and periodically during treatment. Administer without regard to meals.

Education: Advise the importance for compliance. Review the importance of decreasing risk factors: high-fat diet, smoking, alcohol consumption, absence of exercise. Notify provider if suspect pregnancy.

Evaluation: Decrease in the cholesterol.

Drug: ezetimibe (Zetia)

ZETIA

Z Di**Z**zines, respiratory, HA, diarrhea may be side effects

E ncourage use of contraceptive barriers if used with "STATINS"

T aken without regard to food

I nhibits absorption of dietary cholesterol

A djunct to diet & exercise

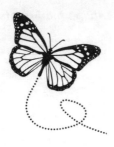

Life's not the breaths you take.
But the moments that take your breath away.

UNKNOWN

Respiratory
Agents

Concept: BRONCHODILATORS

Breathing and coughing techniques: This will facilitate the removal of respiratory secretions and optimize oxygen exchange.

Relaxation techniques: Since anxiety may result in respiratory difficulty, review ways to alleviate anxiety such as music and relaxation techniques.

Evaluate heart rate and BP: Teach client to monitor heart rate and BP since an undesirable effect of these medications may be tachycardia, cardiac arrhythmias, and a change in blood pressure. (Beta2 Adrenergic Agonists can cause hypertension; methylxanthines can cause hypotension at theophylline levels > 30-35 mcg/ml.)

Arm identification: Recommend clients having asthmatic attacks to wear an ID bracelet or tag.

Tremors: Evaluate client for tremors from these medications.

Have 8 or more glasses of fluids: Fluid will assist in decreasing the viscosity of the respiratory secretions.

Emphasize no smoking: Encourage the client to stop smoking under medical supervision.

BRONCHODILATORS

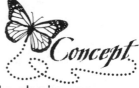

Concept

B reathing and coughing techniques

R elaxation techniques

E valuate heart rate and blood pressure

A rm identification

T remors

H ave 8 or more glasses of fluids

E mphasize no smoking

ANTIHISTAMINES

Action: Blocks histamine release at H1 receptors.

Indications: Upper respiratory allergic disorders; anaphylactic reactions; blood transfusion reactions; acute urticaria; motion sickness.

Warnings: Allergies, acute asthmatic attack, lower respiratory disease, hepatic disorder, narrow-angle glaucoma, symptomatic prostatic hypertrophy, pregnancy, lactation.

Undesirable Effects: Depression, sedation, dry mouth, GI upset, bronchospasm, thickening of secretions, (anticholinergic effects), arrhythmias.

Other Specific Information: Alcohol, CNS depressants may ↑ CNS depressant effect. Ketoconazole may alter metabolism of antihistamine. ↑ levels and possible toxicity with ketoconazole, erythromycin when given with fexofenadine. Avoid MAO inhibitors

Interventions: Monitor vital signs, intake and output. If secretions are thick, use a humidifier.

Education: Instruct client to take with food; drink a minimum of 8 glasses of fluid per day. Advise to do frequent mouth care; may use sugarless gum, lozenges, or candy. Notify provider if confusion or other undesirable effects occur. Instruct client not to drive or operate machinery if drowsiness occurs or until response to drug has been determined. For prophylaxis of motion sickness, recommend taking 30–60 minutes before traveling. Avoid alcohol and other CNS depressants.

Evaluation: Client will have improvement of histamine-associated (i.e., rhinitis, conjunctivitis, motion sickness, etc.) with no undesirable effects from the medication.

Drugs: azatadine (Optimine); azelastine (Astelin); brompheniramine (Dimetapp); buclizine (Bucladin-S); cetirizine (Zyrtec); chlorpheniramine (Chlor-Trimeton); clemastine (Tavist); cyclizine (Mazerine); cyproheptadine (Periactin); dexchlorpheniramine (Polaramine); dimenhydrinate (Dramamine); diphenhydramine (Benadryl); fexofenadine (Allegra); hydroxyzine (Atarax, Vistaril); loratidine (Claritin); meclizine (Antivert); promethazine (Phenergan)

ANTIHISTAMINES

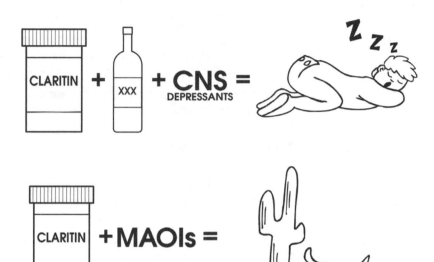

Antihistamines (Claritin) combined with alcohol and CNS depressant may result in sleep. Antihistamines and MAOIs may result in dryness.

BETA₂ ADRENERGIC AGONISTS

Action: Stimulates beta receptors in lung. Relaxes bronchial smooth muscle. Increases vital capacity; decreases airway resistance.

Indications: Asthma, bronchitis, emphysema, relief of bronchospasm occurring during anesthesia, exercised-induced bronchospasm.

Warnings: Hypersensitivity, angina, tachycardia, cardiac arrhythmias, hypertension, cardiac disease, narrow-angle glaucoma, hepatic disease.

Undesirable Effects: Nervousness, tremors, restlessness, insomnia, headache; nausea, vomiting; tachycardia, irregular heart beat, hypertension, cardiac dysrhythmia.

Other Specific Information: ↑ effects with other sympathomimetics. ↓ with beta blockers.

Interventions: Monitor breath sounds; sensorium levels for confusion and restlessness due to hypoxia; and vital signs (pulse and blood pressure can increase greatly). Check for cardiac dysrhythmias.

Education: Caution against overuse. Notify provider before taking other meds or if symptoms are not relieved. Demonstrate correct use of inhalers or nebulizers. Teach about metered-dose inhalers (MDI). When two puffs are needed, 1–3 minutes should lapse between the two puffs. A spacer may be used to increase the delivery of the medication. If a glucocorticoid inhalant is to be used with a bronchodilator, wait 5–15 minutes before using the inhaler containing the steroid for the bronchodilator effect. Assist client in identifying the cause of the acute bronchial attack. (Refer to "**BREATHE**".)

Evaluation: Client will be able to breathe without wheezing and without undesirable effects of the drug. Client will be able to participate in activities of daily living without dyspnea.

Drugs: *(Nonselective Adrenergic):* epinephrine (Adrenalin); *(Nonselective Beta-Adrenergic):* isoproterenol (Isuprel); (Selective B₂): albuterol (Proventil, Ventolin); bitolterol (Tornalate); isoetharine (Bronkosol); metaproterenol (Alupent); pirbuterol (Maxair); salmeterol (Serevent); terbutaline (Brethine, Bricanyl)

MAX AIR

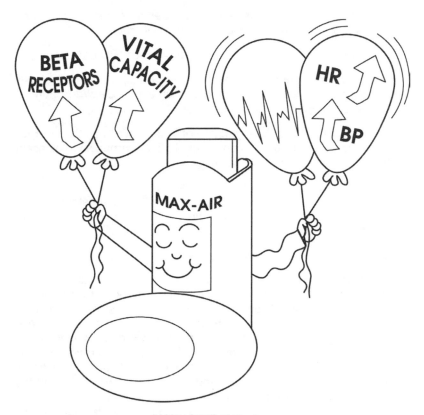

Max Air is smiling because he has been able to relieve bronchospasms from asthma and other respiratory diseases. He has plenty of air to breathe and blow up the balloons in the right hand. His left hand is shaky and weak. His heart is beating fast and his blood pressure is up from undesirable effects of his medication.

CORTICOSTEROID INHALERS

Action: Decreases inflammation and edema in respiratory tract. Reduces bronchoconstriction and secretion of mucus.

Indications: Chronic asthma; exacerbation of COPD or CAL.

Warnings: Bronchiectasis; Systemic fungal infections; persistently positive sputum culture for candida albicans. *Caution:* adrenal insufficiency; pregnancy/lactation.

Undesirable Effects: Usually does not induce systemic toxicity. Risk of oral candida albicans infection (thrush). Sore throat, an unpleasant taste in mouth, or dysphonia may occur.

Other Specific Information: Mild suppression of the pituitary-adrenal axis may occur with prolonged use. Decreased steroid levels with barbiturates, phenytoin, rifampin. Decreased effectiveness of salicylates.

Interventions: Monitor respiratory status on an ongoing basis.

Education: Instruct not to use for acute attacks. If taking bronchodilators, instruct client to use bronchodilator before corticosteroid aerosol. After inhaling, the client should hold the inhaled drug for a few seconds before exhaling. Allow 1–3 minutes to elapse between each inhalation. Rinse mouth with water after inhalations. A spacer is particularly important for client inhaling corticosteroids. It will reduce risk of steroid-associated oropharyngeal candidiasis. Keep inhaler clean and unobstructed. Wash in warm water and dry thoroughly. Notify provider if sore throat or sore mouth occurs; do not stop abruptly. Must taper off gradually under provider supervision. Encourage the use of a diary to record administration of meds and the clinical response.

Evaluation: The client will experience fewer asthmatic episodes of lesser severity without undesirable effects.

Drugs: beclomethasone (Beclovent, QVAR, Vanceril); budesonide (Pulmicort Flexhaler); flunisolide (AeroBid, AeroBid-M, Aerospan); fluticasone (Flovent, Flovent HFA); mometasone (Asmanex, Nasonex); triamcinolone (Azmacort)

ASTHMA

A ction = decreased respiratory track edema

S pacer use recommended

T hrush

H ave client use bronchodilator first

M ust taper off gradually

A sthma control—not acute attacks

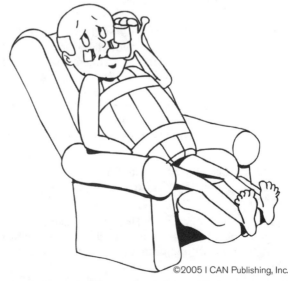

CORTICOSTEROIDS (NASAL)

Action: Potent, locally acting anti-inflammatory and immune modifier. Decreases symptoms of allergic or nonallergic rhinitis. Decrease in symptoms of nasal polyps.

Indications: Nonallergic rhinitis (fluticasone). Treatment of nasal polyps. Allergic rhinitis.

Warnings: Active untreated infections. Diabetes, glaucoma; underlying immunosuppression. Do not abruptly stop systemic corticosteroid therapy when initiating intranasal therapy. Recent nasal trauma, septic ulcers, or surgery.

Undesirable Effects: Dizziness, headache; epistaxis, nasal burning, nasal congestion/irritation, rhinorrhea, tearing eyes; dry mouth, nausea, vomiting; adrenal suppression (increased dose, long-therapy only); cough, bronchospasm.

Other Specific Information: Ketoconzaole increases effect of budesonide, ciclesonide, and fluticasone. Ritonavir increases effects of fluticasone (concomitant use not recommended).

Interventions: Assess degree of nasal stuffiness, amount and color of nasal discharge. Periodic otolaryngologic examinations for clients on long term therapy. Monitor growth rate in children receiving chronic therapy. Periodic adrenal function test may be ordered to assess degree of hypothalamic-pituitary-adrenal (HPA) axis suppresssion for long therapy. Decrease dose to lowest amount after desired clinical effect has been obtained.

Education: Advise client to take medication as ordered. Clients also taking a nasal decongestant should be administered decongestant 5–15 minutes prior to corticosteroid nasal spray. Instruct client to blow nose gently in advance of medication. Keep head upright. Breathe in through nose during administration. Sniff hard for a few minutes after administration. Shake well prior to use. Explain that temporary nasal stinging may occur. Notify provider of care if symptoms do not improve within 1 month, if symptoms get worse, or if nasal irritation or sneezing occur.

Evaluation: Client's nasal stuffiness, discharge, and sneezing in seasonal or perennial allergic rhinitis or nonallergic rhinitis will be relieved.

Drugs: beclomethasone (Beconase, Vancenase), budesonide (Rhinocort), ciclesonide (Omnaris), flunisolide (Nasalide), fluticasone (Flonase, Veramyst), mometasone (Furoate, Nasonex), triamcinolone (Nasacort)

CORTICOSTEROIDS (NASAL)

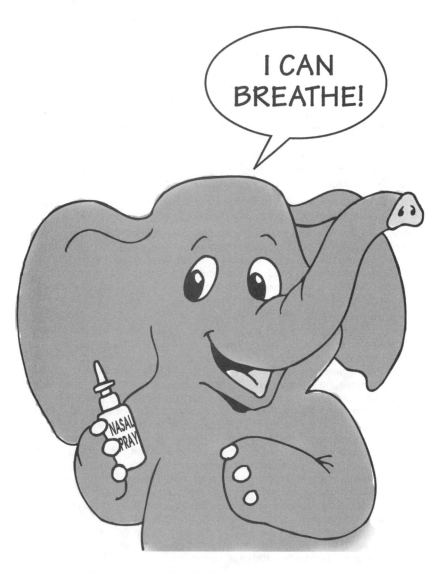

ANTICHOLINERGIC INHALER

Action: Acts as an anticholinergic by selectively and reversibly inhibiting M3 receptors in smooth muscle of airways.

Therapeutic Effects: Decreased severity and incidence of bronchospasm.

Indications: Long-term maintenance treatment of bronchospasm due to COPD.

Warnings: Contraindicated in hypersensitivity to tiotropium, atropine of their derivatives. Concurrent ipratropium. Use cautiously in angle-closure glaucoma, prostatic hyperplasia, bladder neck obstruction (may worsen condition); CCr < 50 ml/min (monitor closely); Pregnancy, lactation or children (safety not established).

Undesirable Effects: Glaucoma; paradoxical bronchospasm, tachycardia; dry mouth, constipation; urinary difficulty, urinary retention, hypersensitivity reactions including **ANGIODEMA**.

Other Specific Information: Do not use concurrently with ipratropium (Atrovent) due to risk of additive anticholinergic effects.

Interventions: Assess respiratory status (rate, breath sounds, pulse, degree of dyspnea) prior to administration and at peak of medication. Consult healthcare provider/physician about alternative medication if severe bronchospasm is present. Onset of action is too slow for a client in acute distress. If paradoxical bronchospasm (wheezing) is present, withhold med and notify healthcare provider.

Education: Instruct client not to swallow capsules; used only for inhalation. Take missed doses as soon as remembered unless it is close for time of next dose. While tiotropium may be continued during an acute exacerbation, it is not to be used for acute bronchospasms. Teach how to clean the Handihaler inhaler properly. Store capsules in sealed blisters; remove only immediately prior to use. If capsule is removed prior to this time, the effectiveness of the capsule will be reduced. If a capsule is inadvertently exposed to air, discard it. Do not use with other medications in the Handihaler. Tiotropium should be administered only via the Handihaler. When discarding after use, a tiny amount of powder left in the capsule is normal. Review the importance of rinsing mouth after use of inhaler, good oral hygiene, and sugarless gum or candy may decrease the dry mouth. Review the importance of notifying healthcare provider immediately if signs of glaucoma (e.g., eye pain or discomfort, blurred vision, visual halos, colored images in association with red eyes from conjunctival congestion) occur. Caution with spraying medication, so it does not go into the eyes; may result in blurring of the vision and dilation of the pupils. Discuss the importance of consulting with the healthcare provider prior to taking any additional drugs.

Evaluation: Client will experience decreased dyspnea with improved breath sounds.

Drugs: tiotropium (Spiriva)

TIOTROPIUM (SPIRIVA)

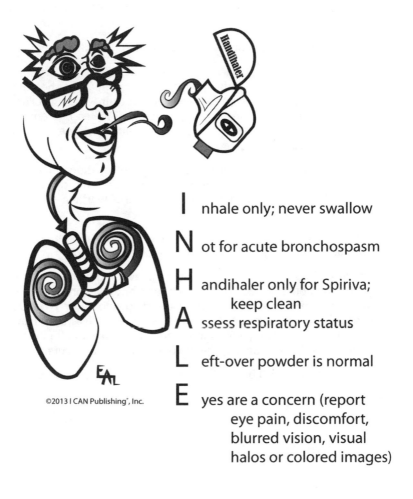

©2013 I CAN Publishing®, Inc.

I nhale only; never swallow

N ot for acute bronchospasm

H andihaler only for Spiriva; keep clean

A ssess respiratory status

L eft-over powder is normal

E yes are a concern (report eye pain, discomfort, blurred vision, visual halos or colored images)

LEUKOTRIENE RECEPTOR ANTAGONIST

Action: Blocks the receptor that inhibits leukotriene formation, preventing many of the signs of asthma.

Indications: Prophylaxis and chronic treatment of asthma in adults and children > 6yrs. old.

Warnings: Hypersensitivity; acute asthmatic attacks; pregnancy/lactation.

Undesirable Effects: Headache, dizziness; nausea, diarrhea; nasal congestion. More serious undesirable effects can occur if client is taking zafirlukast (*i.e., Churg-Strauss syndrome, which presents with eosinophilia, vasculitic rash, cardiac and pulmonary complications*) when oral steroid dose is decreased.

Other Specific Information: ↓ effects if taking montelukast with phenobarbital, rifampin. Numerous interactions may occur when taking zafirlukast. Propranolol, theophylline, and warfarin levels may have ↑ effects when given with zileuton.

Intereventions: Monitor breath sounds and for gastric distress. Monitor liver function tests when client is taking zieleuton.

Education: Recommend taking drug in the evening without regard to food. Not effective for acute asthma attack or acute bronchospasm. Instruct regarding the importance of avoiding aspirin or NSAIDs in clients with hypersensitivities while they are taking this drug. Review the importance of having alternative medication available for an acute asthma attack. Review safety precautions if dizziness occurs.

Evaluation: Client will be free from signs and symptoms of asthma.

Drugs: montelukast (Singulair); zafirlukast (Accolate); zileuton (Zyflo)

LOOK, A TRAIN!

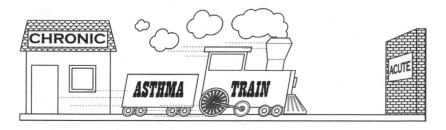

©2001 I CAN Publishing, Inc.

It is okay to board the train in the town of Chronic, but it is too late by the time the train gets to the town of Acute (asthma).

DECONGESTANTS

Action: Stimulates alpha 1 and beta-adrenergic receptors. Produces vasoconstriction in the respiratory tract mucosa (alpha-adrenergic stimulation) and possibly bronchodilation (beta$_2$-adrenergic stiumlation). Reduces nasal congestion, hyperemia, and swelling in nasal passages.

Indications: Symptomatic management of nasal congestion associated with acute viral upper respiratory tract infections.

Warnings: Contraindicated in clients who have chronic rhinitis; hypersensitive to sympathomimetic amines; hypertension, severe coronary artery disease; concurrent MAO inhibitor therapy; known alcohol intolerance. Use cautiously in hyperthyroidism; diabetes mellitus; prostatic hyperplasia; ischemic heart disease; glaucoma.

Undesirable Effects: Anxiety, nervousness, dizziness, drowsiness, excitability; palpitations, hypertension, tachycardia; anorexia

Other Specific Information: Concurrent use with MAO inhibitors may cause hypertensive crisis; concurrent use with beta blockers may result in ↑ BP or ↓ HR. Drugs that alkalinize the urine (sodium bicarbonate, high-dose antacid therapy) may intensify effectiveness.

Interventions: Assess congestion (nasal, sinus, etc.) before and during therapy. Assess HR and BP before and during therapy. Assess lung sounds and evaluate secretions. Encourage fluid intake of 1500-2000 mL/day to decrease thickness of secretions. Administer pseudoefedrine at least 2 hr prior to bedtime to decrease insomnia. Extended-release tablets and capsules should be swallowed whole; do not crush, break, or chew. Contents of the capsule can be mixed with jelly or jam and swallowed without chewing for clients with difficulty swallowing.

Education: Instruct client to take as directed and not to take more than recommended. When administering nasal drops, instruct clients to be in the lateral, head low position to increase the desired effect and to prevent swallowing the medication. Drops are preferred for children since they can be administered precisely and toxicity can be avoided. Educate that topical agents are typically more effective and work faster. Vasoconstriction and CNS stimulation are uncommon with topical agents, but are a concern with oral agents. Oral agents do not lead to rebound congestion. Advise the use of topical decongestants for no longer than 3 to 5 days to avoid rebound congestion. Take missed doses within 1 hour if remember. Instruct client to notify HCP if nervousness occurs or experiences slow or fast HR, difficulty breathing, hallucinations, or seizures occur, since these symptoms may indicate overdose. If symptoms do not improve within 7 days or if fever is present notify HCP.

Evaluation: Decreased nasal, sinus, or eustachian tube congestion

Drugs: pseudoephedrine (Pedia-Care Infants' Decongestant Drops, Pediatric Nasal Decongestant, Sudafed, Sudodrin, Triaminic Allergy Congestion Softchews, Unifed)

DECONGESTANTS

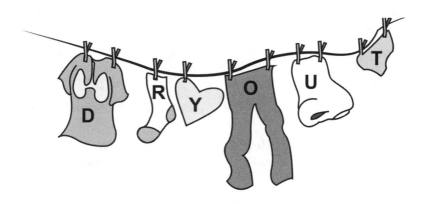

D econgestants "DRY" you "OUT"

R espiratory tract mucosa vasoconstriction and bronchodilation

Y ucky congestion is reduced

O ffer pseudoephedrine at least 2 hrs before bedtime to decrease insomnia

U pper respiratory tract infections

T achycardia, palpitations, anxiety, excitability, hypertension, nervousness, dizziness, drowsiness - UE

MUCOLYTICS

Action: Mucolytics enhance the flow of secretions in the respiratory passages.

Indications: Acute and chronic pulmonary disorders; cystic fibrosis; antidote for acetaminophen poisoning.

Warnings: Contraindicated in clients at risk for GI hemorrhage. Use cautiously in clients who have peptic ulcer disease, esophageal varices, and severe liver disease.

Undesirable Effects: Aspiration and bronchospasm when administered orally.

Other Specific Information: Drug stability and safety of Mucomyst (acetylcysteine) when mixed with other drugs in a nebulizer have not been established.

Interventions: Monitor clients for signs of aspiration and bronchspasm. Stop med immediately and notify HCP. Acetylcysteine is administered by inhalation to liquefy nasal and bronchial secretions and facilitate coughing. For acetaminophen overdose, the medication is administered orally or IV. Oral doses are mixed with fruit juice, cola drinks, or water. Doses are administered every 4 to 72 hours. Have suction available if client aspirates with oral administration.

Education: Review with client that acetylcysteine has an odor that smells like rotten eggs.

Evaluation: If therapeutic intent is to decrease secretions, then the outcome would be an improvement of symptoms as demonstrated by regular respiratory rate, clear lung sounds, and increased ease of expectoration. If intent is for acetaminophen overdose, then the client would present with no signs of overdose.

Drugs: acetylcysteine (Mucomyst, Acetadote)

MUCOLYTICS (MUCOMYST)

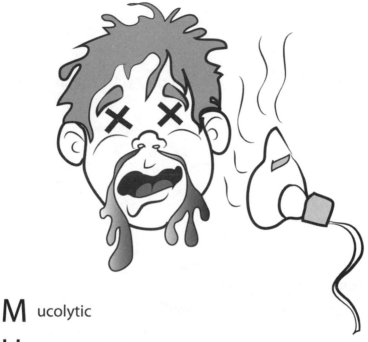

M ucolytic

U sed as antidote for Acetaminophen O.D.

C hronic and acute pulmonary disorders

U npleasant odor (rotten eggs)

S top med if aspiration or bronchospasm occur

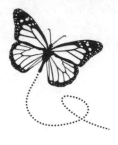

Your real influence is measured by your treatment of yourself.

A. BRONSON ALCOTT

The Greatest Gift You Will Ever
Receive is the Gift of Loving and
Believing in Yourself. Guard this
Gift with Your Life. It is the Only
Thing That Will Ever Truly be Yours!

TIFFANY LOREN ROWE

Anti-Infective Agents

Concept: ANTIBIOTICS

Monitor superinfections: Monitor for a secondary infection (bacterial or fungal growth) due to drug therapy. Assess for signs and symptoms of stomatitis (mouth ulcers), furry black tongue; genital discharge (vaginitis); and anal or genital itching. Elderly clients, children, and clients with a depressed immune system should be monitored carefully.

Evaluate renal/liver functions: Since many antibiotics are metabolized in the liver and excreted via the kidneys, it is of paramount importance to have adequate functioning of these two systems. Evaluate laboratory tests for liver and kidney function; these include liver enzymes, BUN, and serum creatinine.

Diarrhea: Recommend that client eat yogurt to prevent this undesirable effect.

Inform provider prior to taking other meds: Due to the possibility of drug-drug interactions it important that the client understands the reason to discuss this with the provider. It is also important to evaluate the current medications the client is taking for potential interactions.

Cultures prior to initial dose: Prior to the initial dose, obtain and send blood cultures to the laboratory to identify the organism and antibiotic sensitivity.

Alcohol is out; ask about allergy: Instruct client to drink no alcohol. If there has been a previous problem with an allergic reaction, do not administer the medicine. The most serious allergic reaction is anaphylaxis. It begins with diffuse flushing, itching, and a general warm feeling. Hives may be present on the client's face, neck, and chest. As this progresses, generalized edema develops. As the face becomes involved, there is a concern with upper airway edema, with potential respiratory difficulty and impending obstruction. This may result in respiratory wheezing, stridor, and shortness of breath.

Take full course of pills: An ineffective course of antibiotics will allow the bacteria to mutate and develop resistance to the antibiotic. It is important that the medicines are not shared with friends and family due to the risk of allergies and may not be appropriate for the specific bacterial growth. Review the importance of not taking medicines that have been in the cabinet for a while since some medicines may become toxic as they degenerate past the date of expiration.

Evaluate cultures, WBC, temperature, blood dyscrasias, and serum electrolytes: A positive response to the therapy is evaluated by negative cultures, WBCs and body temperature within normal range. Since some antibiotics such as penicillin can cause neutropenia or thrombocytopenia, clients must be monitored for blood dyscrasias. The undesirable effect of diarrhea may result in hypokalemia. Hypernatremia may also occur in clients receiving prolonged treatment with intravenous antibiotics.

ANTIBIOTICS

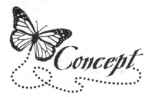

M onitor superinfections

E valuate renal/liver functions

D iarrhea—take yogurt

I nform provider prior to taking other meds

C ultures prior to initial dose

A lcohol is out, ask about allergy

T ake full course (of pills)

E valuate cultures, WBC, temperature, blood

AMINOGLYCOSIDES

Action: Bactericidal. Binds with 30s or 50s ribosomal subunit, thus inhibiting protein synthesis.

Indications: Serious infections caused by gram-negative infections (i.e., Enterobacter, Escherichia coli, Klebsiella, Proteus, Pseudomonas, and Serratia). Streptomycin is one of the drugs primarily used for tuberculosis.

Warnings: Hypersensitivity; renal impairment; vestibular/cochlear impairment; decreased neuromuscular transmission (i.e., myasthenia gravis, Parkinson's disease); heart failure; elderly.

Undesirable Effects: Anorexia, nausea, tremors, tinnitus, photo-sensitivity, superinfection, or agranulocytosis. Significant potential for neurotoxicity, nephrotoxicity, and ototoxicity with high levels for extended periods. Aminoglycoside nephrotoxicity is usually seen as a gradual increase in creatinine over several days. Acute, large changes in creatinine should be investigated for other causes.

Other Specific Information: Loop diuretics may ↑ ototoxic potential when given with this class. Penicillins, vancomycin, amphotericin B, and furosemide may ↑ nephrotoxicity.

Interventions: BUN/creatinine, audiograms, and vestibular function studies should also be monitored periodically during an extended high dose therapy over 10 days. Adjust for renal insufficiency. Monitor vital signs and peak and trough serum levels routinely. For IV administration, dilute and administer slowly over 60 minutes to prevent toxicity. Monitor I & O; hydrate well before and during therapy. If prescribed oral drug, take full course and drink plenty of fluids. If anorexia or nausea occurs, provide small, frequent meals. Establish plan for safety if vestibular nerve effects occur. (Refer to "**MEDICATE**".) Ensure levels are drawn per hospital policy.

Education: Administer other antibiotics 1 hour before/after oral aminoglycosides. Recommend using sun block and protective clothing when exposed to the sun. (Refer to "**MEDICATE**".)

Evaluation: Client's body temperature, WBC count, and cultures will return to normal range.

Drugs: amikacin (Amikin); gentamicin (Garamycin, Jenamicin); kanamycin (Kantrex, Klebcil); neomycin (Mycifradin, Neobiotic); streptomycin (Streptomycin); tobramycin (Nebcin)

AMINO MICE
Genta**myc**in
Amikacin
Kana**myc**in
Neo**myc**in
Strepto**myc**in
Tobra**myc**in

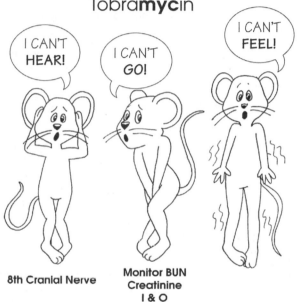

8th Cranial Nerve

Monitor BUN
Creatinine
I & O

©2001 I CAN Publishing, Inc.

Three Amino Mice
(sung to the tune of "Three Blind Mice")

One can't feel,	Vestibular function and audiograms
One can't hear.	Should always be studied in patient care plans
One can't pee—	[or "as part of your plan"]
They're toxic mice, all three.	Grab BUNs and creatinine as quick as you can,
	Yes! Three amino mice.

Our 3 "Amino Mice" will assist you in remembering 3 major undesirable effects of this category of drugs: "ototoxicity", "nephrotoxicity", and "neurotoxicity".

BACTROBAN

Action: Inhibits bacterial protein synthesis.

Indications: Impetigo. Secondarily infected traumatic skin lesions (up to 10 cm in length or 100 cm2 area) caused by Staphylococcus aureus and Streptococcus pyogenes. Intranasal: Eradicates nasal colonization with methicillin-resistant S. aureus.

Warnings: Hypersensitivity to mupirocin or polyethylene glycol. Impaired renal failure.

Undesirable Effects: Nasal only—Headache, cough, itching, pharyngitis, rhinitis, altered taste. Topical only—Burning, itching, pain stinging.

Other Specific Information: Nasal mupirocin should not be used concurrently with other nasal products.

Interventions: Assess lesions before and daily during therapy. Wash affected area with soap and water and dry thoroughly. Apply a small amount of mupirocin to the affected area TID and rub in gently. Treated area may be covered with gauze if desired. **Nasal:** Apply one half of the ointment from the single-use tube to each nostril BID (AM and PM) for 5 days. After application, close nostrils by pressing together and releasing sides of the nose repeatedly for 1 minute.

Education: Instruct client on the correct application of mupirocin. Advise client to apply medication exactly as directed for the full course of therapy. If dose is missed, apply as soon as possible, unless it is time for the next dose. Avoid contact with eyes. Topical: Instruct client and family hygienic measures to prevent spread of impetigo. Instruct parents to notify the school nurse for screening and prevention of transmission. If symptoms have not improved in 3-5 days, then consult provider of care.

Evaluation: Skin lesions will be healed. Methicillin-resistant S. aureus carrier state in clients and health care workers during an institutional outbreak will be eradicated.

Drug: mupirocin (Bactroban, Bactroban Nasal)

BACTROBAN

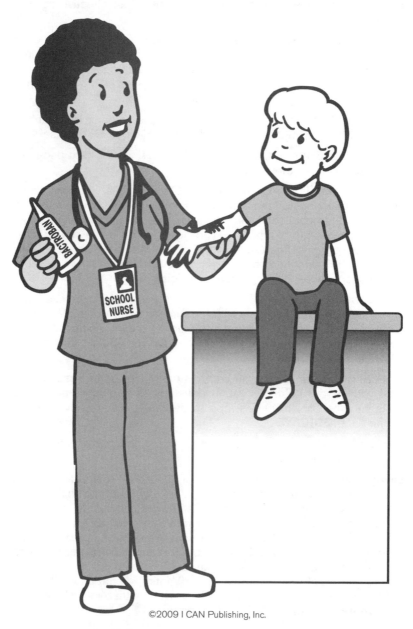

CEPHALOSPORINS

Action: Inhibits bacterial cell wall synthesis. Most effective against rapidly growing organisms.

Indications: 1st generation: Often used in clients allergic to penicillin. Gram-positive organisms and moderate activity against gram-negative organisms. **2nd generation:** Gram-negative organisms. **3rd generation:** Mostly gram-negative organisms. **4th generation:** Gram-negative and gram-positive organisms.

Warnings: Hypersensitivity to cephalosporins or penicillin. Caution with renal/hepatic impairment, bleeding disorders, or GI disease.

Undesirable Effects: Our friend the "**GIANT**" on the next page will help you remember these effects.

Other Specific Information: Cefamandole, cefmetazole, cefoperazone, or cefotetan may result in a disulfiram (Antabuse)–type reaction with alcohol consumption, or an ↑risk of bleeding when given with anticoagulants, or thrombolytic agents. The same drugs (with the exception of cefmetazole) when given with NSAIDs, especially aspirin, ↑ the risk of hemorrhaging. Probenecid may ↑ serum levels of cephalosporins resulting in potential toxicity.

Interventions: Monitor WBC counts, cultures, and PT. Assess BUN and creatinine levels in clients with renal impairment. Monitor VS, I & O, and undesirable effects. If client is a diabetic, monitor glucose levels. For IV administration, refer to drug circular for specific procedure. (Refer to "**MEDICATE**".)

Education: Administer on an empty stomach for better results. May take with food if gastric irritation develops. Use glucose-enzymatic tests such as Clinistix or Tes-Tape to decrease false-positive results. (Refer to "**MEDICATE**".)

Evaluation: Negative cultures. WBC count and body temperature will be within normal range.

Drugs: First generation: cefadroxil (Duricef); cefazolin (Ancef, Kefzol); cephalexin (Keflex); cephapirin (Cefadyl); cephradine (Velosef); **Second generation:** cefaclor (Ceclor); cefamandole (Mandol); cefditoren pivoxil (Spectracef); cefmetazole (Zefazone); cefonicid (Monocid); cefotetan (Cefotan); cefoxitin (Mefoxin); cefprozil (Cefzil); cefuroxime (Ceftin, Zinacef); loracarbef (Lorabid); **Third generation:** cefdinir (Omnicef); cefixime (Suprax); cefoperazone (Cefobid); cefotaxime (Claforan); cefpodoxime (Vantin); ceftazidime (Fortaz); ceftibuten (Cedax), ceftizoxime (Cefizox); ceftriaxone (Rocephin); **Fourth generation:** cefepime (Maxipime)

CEF THE GIANT

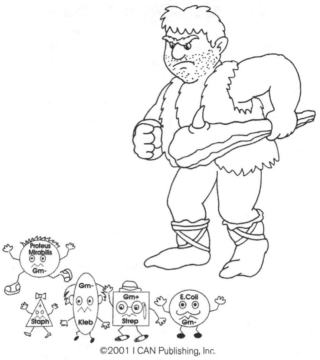

©2001 I CAN Publishing, Inc.

GI: nausea, vomiting, diarrhea

Increase in glucose values

Anaphylaxis may occur; alcohol may cause vomiting

Nephrotoxicity

Thrombocytopenia

Cef/Ceph, the "GIANT" is a powerful antibiotic that can destroy several types of bacteria and represents the 1st generation of cephalosporins. He can also produce "GIANT" undesirable effects.

FLUOROQUINOLONES

Action: Bactericidal. Inhibits bacterial DNA synthesis via inhibition of DNA gyrase.

Indications: Broad spectrum. Wide range of susceptible gram-negative and gram-positive organisms. (i.e., E. coli, P. Pseudomonas aeruginosa). Used for urinary tract infections UTIs), bronchitis, sexually transmitted diseases, bone or joint, or ophthalmic infections. Individual fluoroquinolones vary in their spectrum of activity. All are indicated for UTIs, but only ciprofloxacin is approved for bone cancer and joint infections. *(It is beyond the scope of this book to review every individual drug indications. We refer you to current references.)*

Warnings: Hypersensitivity in children < 18 years of age. Children, pregnancy, lactation; hepatic or renal impairment; CNS disorders, or seizures.

Undesirable Effects: Hypersensitivity. Nausea, vomiting, diarrhea, headache, dizziness, photosensitivity. Rare effects include confusion, hallucinations, psychosis, and tremors.

Other Specific Information: Antacids, iron, sucralfate may ↓ absorption of drug up to 98%. May ↑effects of theophylline and warfarin. ↑ risk of photosensitivity reactions with St. John's Wort therapy.

Interventions: Monitor temperature, WBC counts, cultures, symptoms of infection, BUN, and serum creatinine levels. Monitor I & O and vital signs. Maintain a urinary output of at least 1200 to 1500 ml daily. Slowly infuse IV ciprofloxacin and ofloxacin into a large vein over 1 hour to minimize vein irritation. Refer to drug circular for procedure. (Refer to "**MEDICATE**".)

Education: Instruct to take 2 hours after meals or 2 hours before or after antacids or iron. If GI distress occurs, take with food. Administer with full glass of water. Drink 6–8 glasses (8 oz.) of fluid daily. Protect against sunlight. Advise client to avoid hazardous activities that require alertness until the CNS response has been determined. (Refer to "**MEDICATE**".)

Evaluation: Negative cultures. Body temperature and WBC count within normal range.

Drugs: *(Many of these drugs end in "floxacin")* cipro**floxacin** (Ciloxan, Cipro); enoxacin (Penetrex); gati**floxacin** (Tequin); levo**floxacin** (Levaquin); lome**floxacin** (Maxaquin); moxi**floxacin** (Avelox); nor**floxacin** (Noroxin); o**floxacin** (Floxin, Ocuflox); spar**floxacin** (Zagam); trova**floxacin** (Trovan)

T. T. FLOXACIN

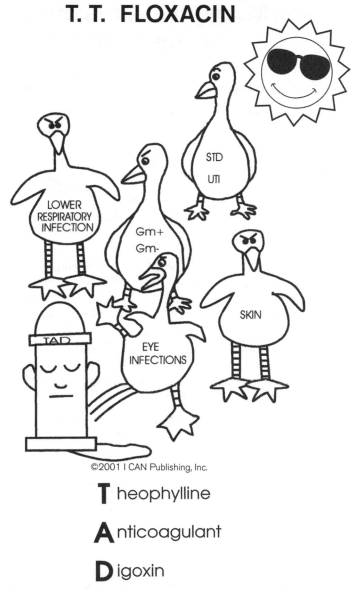

©2001 I CAN Publishing, Inc.

T heophylline

A nticoagulant

D igoxin

T. T. Floxacin and his flock are relieving themselves on TAD the fire hydrant. **T**heophylline, **A**nticoagulants, and **D**ig may result in drug toxicity when taken with the fluoroquinolones. This group of drugs ends in **floxacin** and is used to treat urinary tract infections as well as a wide range of Gm- and Gm+ infections.

MACROLIDE ANTIBIOTIC: ERYTHROMYCIN

Action: Bacteriostatic. Inhibits synthesis of protein in bacteria.

Indications: Clients who are allergic to penicillin. Gram-positive and some gram-negative organisms.

Warnings: Hepatic dysfunction, lactation.

Undesirable Effects: Low rate of undesirable effects. Anorexia, nausea, vomiting, diarrhea (usually dose related); tinnitus; rash.

Other Specific Information: ↑ effect of digoxin, carbamazepine, cyclosporine, theophylline, triazolam, warfarin. ↓ effect of clindamycin, penicillins.

Interventions: Periodic hepatic function studies for high-doses or prolonged IV therapy. Monitor bleeding times if taking warfarin. If administered IV, dilute in an appropriate amount of solution as outlined in the drug book or circular. (Refer to **"MEDICATE".**)

Education: Instruct client to take erythromycin 1 hour before or 2 hours after meals. Take with a full glass of water and not fruit juice. (Acids in fruit juices decrease the activity of the drug.) If GI upset occurs, client may take with food. Chewable tablets should be chewed and not swallowed. Report undesirable effects. (Refer to **"MEDICATE".**)

Evaluation: Negative cultures. Body temperature and WBC count will be within normal range.

Drugs: erythromycin (E-Mycin, Erytab, Eryc, PCE, Ilotycin, Ilosone, EES, EryPed, Erythrocin)

MACROLIDE GIRL

GI disturbances—undesirable effect

I V site—✔ for irritation

R educes activity of med if given with acids (fruit juices) or food.

L iver function tests

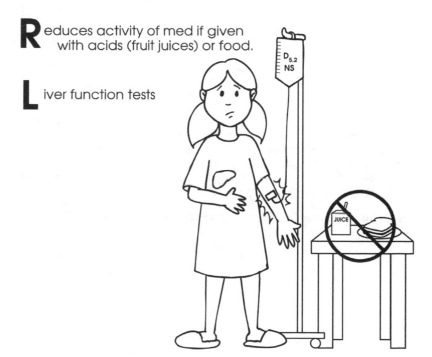

©2001 I CAN Publishing, Inc.

MACROLIDES

Action: Inhibits bacterial protein synthesis.

Indications: Gram positive bacteria with limited gram negative coverage. Uses include respiratory, gastrointestinal tract, skin and soft tissue infections when beta-lactam antibiotics are contraindicated.

Warnings: Hypersensitivity; hepatic/renal dysfunction.

Undesirable Effects: GI upset occurs in 20-30% of clients.

Other Specific Information: Theophyline, digoxin, carbamazepine, phenytoin, methylprednisolone, and warfarin can have ↑effects when taken with these macrolides. ↓ absorption with antacids. ↓ effect of clindamycin.

Interventions: Monitor liver function tests, vital signs, I & O. Maintain good hydration. Evaluate for blood dyscrasias (platelets) especially in long term use of azithromycin. (Refer to **"MEDICATE"**.)

Education: Notify provider of rash or diarrhea. Drink fluids liberally. Azithromycin—take at least one hour prior to or 2 hours after a meal. Avoid giving with food. Avoid simultaneous administration of magnesium or aluminum—containing antacids. Clarithromycin—take without regard to meals. May take with milk. Do not refrigerate the suspension form. Dirithromycin—take with food or within 1 hour of eating. (Refer to **"MEDICATE"**.)

Evaluation: Negative cultures. Body temperature, and WBC count will be within normal range.

Drugs: azithromycin (Zithromax); clarithromycin (Biaxin); dirithromycin (Dynabec); erythromycin (Refer to erythromycin)

ZEB

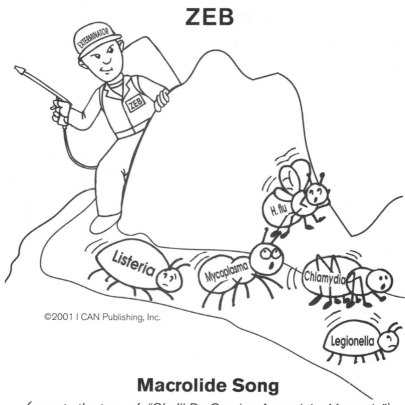

©2001 I CAN Publishing, Inc.

Macrolide Song

(sung to the tune of "She'll Be Coming Around the Mountain")

Chorus
One good bug exterminator–Macrolide
Zithromax, EES, Biaxin are the types.
But if used improperly
Major problems you might see
Always check your text and give it properly.

Verse 1
Contraindicated drugs with Macrolides
Dilantin toxicity, so don't you dare provide
And your blood will soon become too thin
If you take it with your Coumadin
So don't you mix these drugs and you'll
　　survive.

Verse 2
Erythromycin and Biaxin Macrolides
Cause increased levels with carbamaze-
pine
Hold Theophylline and Dig
Cause toxic affects will run real big
Solu Medrol is another risk besides.

Verse 3
If your poop runs and smells real bad
　　on Macrolides
And girls taking these are scratching at
　　their hides.
Or a black tongue that is furry
Call your provider in a hurry.
'Cuz a superinfection these are all the signs.

"ZEB" (Zithromax, Erythromycin, Biaxin) is one good bug exterminator.

PENICILLINS

Action: Bactericidal. Inhibits the enzyme in cell wall synthesis.

Indications: Most gram-positive and gram-negative cocci and bacilli. Pneumonia, respiratory disease, urinary tract infection, syphilis, gonorrhea, meningitis, skin infections, some bone and joint infections, catheter infections. Gram-negative organisms affecting gastrointestinal tract: Salmonella and Shigella.

Warnings: Hypersensitivity to penicillin or cephalosporins. Caution with renal failure, GI disease, bleeding disorders, or hepatic disorders.

Undesirable Effects: Nausea, vomiting, diarrhea, rash, stomatitis. Hypersensitivity ranging from rash, urticaria, pruritus to full anaphylaxis. Superinfection–signs and symptoms include black, furry tongue, thrush, and vaginal discharge. Hematologic effects and neurotoxicity may present in select drugs.

Other Specific Information: Decreased effect with tetracycline and erythromycin.

Interventions: Monitor WBCs, culture/sensitivity reports, I & O, renal function tests, liver enzymes, and temperature. (Sudden increase in temperature may indicate drug fever.) Benadryl may be given for mild reactions. Check for bleeding if high doses of penicillin are being given. Monitor for seizures in clients with renal disease. Dilute medicine for IV use in appropriate amount of solution. Refer to drug circular. (Refer to "**MEDICATE**".)

Education: Call provider immediately if rash, fever, chills, diarrhea, or bleeding occur. For best results take 1–2 hours before or 2–3 hours after meals. May take with food if problems occur with GI upset. Encourage client to increase fluids. Wear a med identification necklace or bracelet if any allergies.(Refer to "**MEDICATE**".)

Evaluation: Negative cultures. Body temperature and CBC, especially WBC count will be within normal range.

Drugs: *Broad spectrum:* amoxicillin (Amoxil, Polymax, Trimox, Wymox); amoxicillin/clavulanate (Augmentin); ampicillin (Omnipen, Polycillin); ampicillin/sulbactam (Unasyn); aztreonam (Azactam), bacampicillin (Spectrobid); ***Extended spectrum:*** carbenicillin (Geocillin); mezlocillin (Mezlin); piperacillin (Pipracil); piperacillin/tazobactum (Zosyn); ticarcillin (Ticar); ticarcillin/calvulanate (Timentin); ***Naturals:*** penicillin G benzathine (Bicillin, Permapen); penicillin G postassium (Pentids, Pfizerpen); penicillin G procaine (Crysticillin, A.S. Wycillin); penicillin V potassium (Pen-Vee K, V-Cillin K, Veetids); ***Penicillinase resistant:*** cloxacillin (Cloxapen, Tegopen); dicloxacillin (Dynapen, Pathocil); methicillin (Staphcillin); nafcillin (Nafcil, Unipen); oxacillin (Bactocill, Prostaphilin)

PENICILLIN

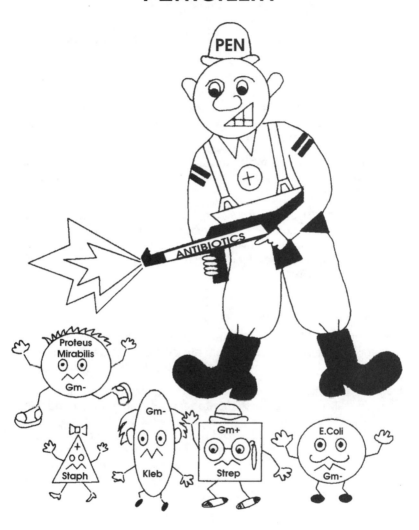

PEN the antibiotic has his "destroyer laser" aimed at several types of bacteria. He is a broad spectrum antibiotic.

SULFONAMIDES

Action: Bacteriostatic. Interferes with bacterial growth by blocking folic acid synthesis in the cell.

Indications: Broad spectrum agents effective against gram-negative and gram-positive organisms. Urinary tract infection; respiratory infection; Pneumocystis carinii pneumonitis; acute otitis media; sinusitis; prostatitis; and gastrointestinal infections such as shigellosis, traveler's diarrhea prophylaxis.

Warnings: Hypersensitivity to trimethoprim or any sulfonamides. Megaloblastic anemia due to folate deficiency. Caution with elderly or renal/hepatic impairment.

Undesirable Effects: Anorexia, nausea/vomiting; rash; photosensitivity; acute hemolytic anemia and other blood dyscrasias; hepatic/renal toxicity; Steven-Johnson Syndrome (blistering and peeling of skin, arthralgia). Increased risk for bone marrow depression with the elderly client.

Other Specific Information: May ↑ effects of warfarin. Antacids ↓ absorption.

Interventions: Baseline hepatic, renal, and hematologic studies. Monitor I & O and vital signs at least twice a day. Adjust fluid intake to maintain output at least 1500 ml in 24 hours. (Refer to "**MEDICATE**".)

Education: Take orally with 8 oz. water; drink several extra glasses of fluids daily (unless contraindicated for renal or cardiac conditions). Administer 1 hour before or 2 hours after meals. If nausea and vomiting occur, administer with food. Avoid direct skin exposure to sun. Instruct clients with diabetes that sulfonamides may result in false-positive urine sugar and ketone test results. Report skin rash, cough, sore throat, sores in mouth, fever, bruising, or bleeding (early signs of blood dyscrasia). (Refer to "**MEDICATE**".)

Evaluation: Negative cultures. Body temperatue and WBC count will be within normal range.

Drugs: sulfadiazine (generic); sulfisoxazole (Gantrisin); trimethoprim-sulfamethoxazole (Bactrim, Septra)

SULFA

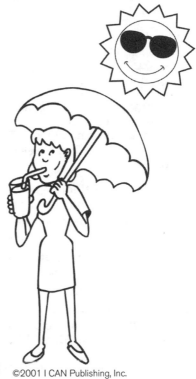

S unlight sensitivity—U E

U ndesirable effects—rash, renal toxicity

L ook for urine output, fever, sore throat and bleeding

F luids galore!

A norexia, anemia—U E

©2001 I CAN Publishing, Inc.

TETRACYCLINES

Action: Bacteriostatic. Inhibits protein synthesis by binding to ribosomes.

Indications: Gram-negative and gram-positive aerobes and anaerobes. Useful in treating skin infections, chlamydia, gonorrhea, syphilis, and atypical diseases such as Borrelia burghdorferi (Lyme disease), rickettsial diseases (Rocky Mountain Spotted Fever).

Warnings: Renal or hepatic dysfunction. Pregnant/breastfeeding women, and children less than 8 years of age due to permanent mottling and staining of teeth. The fetus or child may also experience a decrease in the linear skeletal growth rate. Caution with sun light exposure.

Undesirable Effects: Nausea, vomiting, diarrhea, dysphagia, abdominal cramping; rash; photosensitivity; nephrotoxicity (not as frequently with doxycycline); dental staining; superinfection (especially fungal).

Other Specific Information: Absorption impaired by milk, antacids, and iron. Tetracyclines may ↓ effectiveness of oral contraceptives. May alter effects of anticoagulants.

Interventions: Monitor liver enzymes, BUN, and serum creatinine. Monitor VS and urine output. Assess for rash and pattern of bowel activity. (Refer to **"MEDICATE"**.)

Education: Instruct client to store medicine out of light and heat. Avoid excessive exposure to sunlight; photosensitivity may persist for some time after the drug has been discontinued. Take oral dose on empty stomach (1 hour before or 2 hours after food/beverage); drink full glass of water and avoid bedtime dose. Avoid antacids, dairy, and iron products. Advise that stools may be green or yellow. Topical application may cause skin to turn yellow. Recommend additional contraceptives and not to rely on oral contraceptives. (Refer to **"MEDICATE"**.)

Evaluation: Client's body temperature, WBC count, and cultures will return to normal range.

Drugs: *(These drugs end in "cycline".)* democlo**cycline** (Declomycin); doxy**cycline** (Vibramycin); mino**cycline** (Minocin); oxytetra**cycline** (Terramycin); tetra**cycline** (Achromycin)

TETRA "CYCLINES"

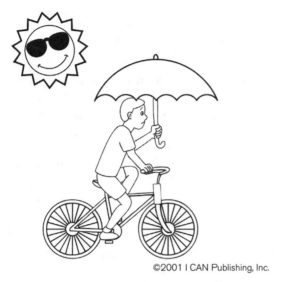

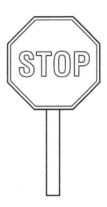

©2001 I CAN Publishing, Inc.

S unlight sensitivity

T ake with full glass of water

Ø antacid, iron, milk

P ut drug into empty stomach

"Trey" the cycler needs to STOP and go protect himself from the sun. "Stop" will help you remember how to safely take tetracyclines.

VANCOMYCIN HYDROCHLORIDE

Action: Bactericidal. Inhibits bacterial cell wall synthesis by binding to a cell wall precursor.

Indications: Antibiotic-associated pseudomembranous caused by Clostridium difficile and staphylococcal enterocolitis. Potentially life-threatening infections not responding to other less toxic antibiotics (parenteral).

Warnings: Renal failure, hearing loss, and concurrent use of other nephrotoxic/ototoxic drugs.

Undesirable effects: Nausea, vomiting, or taste alterations. Dose-related toxicity include tinnitus, high tone deafness, hearing loss, and nephrotoxicity. Rapid IV infusion can produce "red-neck or red man syndrome" resulting in histamine release and chills, fever, tachycardia, profound fall in BP, pruritus, or red face/neck/arms/back.

Other Specific Information: Aminoglycosides, amphotericin, aspirin, and furosemide may ↑ ototoxicity and/or nephrotoxicity.

Interventions: Check baseline hearing. Monitor blood pressure during administration. Monitor renal function tests and I & O. Monitor peak and trough levels. Draw trough level 30 minutes before the third dose is given. Monitor for "red-neck" syndrome. Stop infusion and report to provider of health care. Slowing the infusion or increasing the diluent volume may reduce "redneck" effect. Evaluate IV site for phlebitis. Avoid extravasation. (Refer to "**MEDICATE**.")

Education: Report ringing in ears or hearing loss, fever, and sore throat. Instruct that lab reports are a necessary part of the treatment. (Refer to "**MEDICATE**.")

Evaluation: Client's body temperature, WBC count, and cultures will return to normal range.

Drugs: vancomycin hydrochloride (Vancocin, Vancoled)

RUDOLPH
THE RED-NECK REINDEER

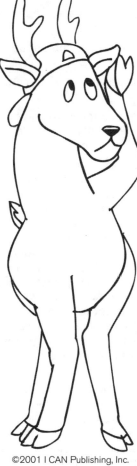

Rudolph the red-neck reindeer

Had an adverse side effect

From the drug Vancomycin,

Must keep all his labs in check.

Caution with renal failure,

Hearing loss and allergies,

Take a temp and blood cultures,

Especially that CBC!!!

CLINDAMYCIN

Action: Anti-infective. Binds to 50S subunit of bacterial ribosomes, suppresses protein synthesis.

Indications: Skin, skin structure, respiratory tract, intra-abdominal and gynecologic infections, septicemia, osteomyelitis, endocarditis prophylaxis, severe acne. Infections caused by staphylococci, streptococci, Rickettsia, Fusobacterium, Actinomyces, Peptococcus, Bacteroides, Pneumocystitis carinii.

Warnings: Hypersensitivity, history of pseudomembranous colitis, severe liver impairment, diarrhea.

Undesirable Effects: Arrhythmias, hypotension, pseudomembranous colitis, diarrhea, bitter taste (IV only).

Other Specific: Decreased absorption when taken with kaolin. May block clindamycin effect when taken with erythromycin. Increased neuromuscular blockade with neuromuscular blockers.

Interventions: Monitor GI status, diarrhea, abdominal cramping, fever, and bloody stools. These may be a sign of pseudomembranous colitis and should be reported immediately. Pseudomembranous colitis may begin up to several weeks following the cessation of therapy. Instruct client to finish the drug completely as directed, even if feeling better. Monitor liver studies, blood studies. Discontinue drug if bone marrow depression occurs. C&S prior to beginning medication. Monitor B/P, pulse in client receiving drug parenterally. Assess for skin irritation, dermatitis after administration. Assess respiratory status. Review potential allergies prior to beginning therapy. Administer with a glass of water; may be given with meals. IM–Do not administer >600 mg in a single IM injection. Intermittent Infusion: Rate: administer each 300 mg over a minimum of 10 min. If experiences an allergic reaction, withdraw drug immediately, maintain airway; administer epinephrine, aminophylline, O_2, IV corticosteroids.

Education: Advise to take po med with a full glass of water. May give with food to reduce GI symptoms. Discuss the importance of taking full course of medication. Report sore throat, fever, fatigue which may indicate a superinfection. Do not break, crush, or chew caps. Drug must be taken in equal intervals around the clock to maintain appropriate blood levels. Report any undesirable effects.

Evaluation: Client will have a normal temperature and a negative C&S.

Drug: clindamycin phosphate (Cleocin Phosphate, Dalacin C, Dalacin C Phosphate), clindamycin HCL (Cleocin HCl), clindamycin palmitate (Cleocin Pediatric, Dalacin C Palmitate)

CLINDAMYCIN

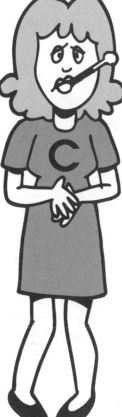

C olitis is a dangerous & life-threatening side effect

L iver function tests—monitor

I M injection limited to 600 mg, inject deep into large muscle to avoid problems

N euromuscular blockade increased with neuromuscular blockers

©2005 I CAN Publishing, Inc.

D iscontinue drug if bone marrow depression occurs

A rrhythmias—undesirable effects

"C LINDA" is sick and needs her **CLINDAMYCIN** to get well.

OXAZOLIDIN: ZYVOX

Action: Binds to bacterial 235 ribosomal RNA of the 50S subunit preventing formation of the bacterial translation process.

Indications: Vancomycin-resistant Enterococcus faecium infections, noscomial pneumonia, uncomplicated or complicated skin and skin structure infections, community-acquired pneumonia.

Warnings: Hypersensitivity. Thrombocytopenia.

Undesirable Effects: Headache, dizziness; nausea, diarrhea, increased ALT, AST, vomiting, taste change, tongue color change; vaginal moniliasis, fungal infection, oral moniliasis; myelosuppression.

Other Specific Information: May decrease the effects of MAOIs; increased effects of adrenergic agents, serotonergic agents.

Interventions: Assess CBC weekly, assess for myelosuppression (anemias, leukopenia, pancytopenia, thrombocytopenia). Assess for CNS symptoms such as headaches, dizziness; liver function tests: AST, ALT; allergic reactions; pseudomembranous colitis.

Education: Advise if dizziness occurs to ambulate, perform activities with assistance. Complete full course of med. Notify provider for any undesirable effects. Avoid large amounts of high-tyramine foods.

Evaluation: Decreased symptoms of infection, blood cultures negative.

Drug: linezolid (Zyvox)

ZYVOX

Z ero drug additives to IV line

T**Y** ramine foods to be avoided

V RE and MRSA effective drug

O ral & IV use same dosages

O**X** azolidin antibiotic

CARBAPENEMS

Action: Beta-lactam antibiotics that destroy bacterial cell walls, resulting in the destruction of micro-organisms.

Indications: Broad antimicrobial spectrum is effective for serious infections such as peritonitis, pneumonia, and urinary tract infections caused by gram-positive cocci, gram-negative cocci, and anaerobic bacteria. If imipem is used alone to treat Pseudomonas aeruginosa, resistance may develop.

Warnings: Contraindicated in clients who experience cross-sensitivity with penicillins and cephalosporins. Use cautiously in client who have renal impairment; seizures, head injury, tumor.

Undesirable Effects: Allergy, hypersensitivity; hypotension; GI symptoms (i.e., nausea, vomiting, diarrhea); superinfection; fever, chills, body aches, flu like symptoms; fast or pounding heartbeats; confusion, tremors, hallucinations, seizures; feeling light-headed, fainting.

Other Specific Information: Do not admix with aminoglycosides (inactivation may occur). Probenecid ↓ renal excretion and ↑ blood levels. ↑ risk of seizures with ganciclovir or cyclosporine (avoid concurrent use of ganciclovir).

Interventions: Assess for infections (vital signs; appearance of wound, urine, sputum, stool; WBC) at beginning and during therapy. Assess previous allergic reactions to penicillins. Persons with a negative history of penicillin sensitivity may still have an allergic response. Obtain specimens for culture and sensitivity prior to initiating therapy. Assess client for signs and symptoms of anaphylaxis (rash, pruritus, laryngeal edema, wheezing). Discontinue the drug and notify the healthcare provider immediately if these occur. Have epinephrine, an antihistamine, and resuscitative equipment close by in the event of an anaphylactic reaction. Assess for GI symptoms (nausea, vomiting, diarrhea) – Notify HCP; monitor the client's I & O. Monitor for colitis (diarrhea, oral thrush, and/or vaginal yeast infection). Monitor BUN, AST, ALT, LDH, serum alkaline phosphatase, bilirubin, and creatinine may be transiently ↑. Hemoglobin and hematocrit concentrations may be ↓.

Education: Advise client to report the signs of superinfection (black, furry overgrowth on the tongue; vaginal itching or discharge; looser foul-smelling stools) and allergy. Consult healthcare professional prior to treating with antidiarrheals. Caution client to notify healthcare provider if fever and diarrhea occur, especially if stool contains blood, pus, or mucus. Advise not to treat diarrhea without consulting health care provider. May occur up to several weeks after discontinuation of medication.

Evaluation: Negative cultures. Body temperature and WBC count within normal range.

Drugs: imipenem/cilastatin (Primaxin), meropenem (Merrem IV)

CARBAPENEMS

B lack furry tongue

I tching vagina and discharge

G I symptoms (N/V/D)

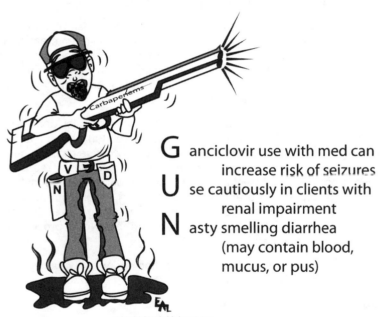

G anciclovir use with med can increase risk of seizures

U se cautiously in clients with renal impairment

N asty smelling diarrhea (may contain blood, mucus, or pus)

©2013 I CAN Publishing®, Inc.

"BIG-GUN" antibiotic (wide-spectrum antibiotic)

ANTITUBERCULAR: ISONIAZID

Action: Interferes with DNA synthesis.

Indications: Tuberculosis; prophylactic drug against tuberculosis.

Warnings: Alcoholism; renal or hepatic disease; diabetic retinopathy; pregnancy, lactation.

Undesirable Effects: Peripheral neuropathy; nausea, vomiting, hepatotoxicity.

Other Specific Information: ↑ risk of isoniazid-related hepatitis with alcohol, rifampin. ↑ drug levels of phenytoin, carbamazepine.

Interventions: Collect specimens for culture and sensitivity; sputum analysis; monitor hepatic function results, BUN, and serum creatinine. Assess for symptoms of peripheral neuropathy, such as tingling or numbness of the extremities. Administer pyridoxine (vitamin B6) to any client who is high risk for developing peripheral neuropathy, such as malnourished, elderly, diabetic, or alcoholics.

Education: Take 1 hour before or 2 hours after meals; don't skip doses; take full length of therapy. Avoid sauerkraut, tuna, aged cheese, smoked fish (foods containing tyramine) that may cause reaction such as pounding heart, dizziness, clammy feeling, headache, red skin. Advise client not to drink alcohol and take meds without consulting provider. Recommend no antacids while taking drug. Instruct client regarding the importance of routine office visits for ongoing evaluation. Review plans for safety with machinery or driving. Notify provider of any undesirable effects.

Evaluation: Client will be free from infection and will have a negative sputum specimen for acid-fast bacilli.

Drugs: isoniazid (INH, Laniazid, Nydrazid)

INA TUBERCULOSIS

L iver enzymes—must be monitored

U se cautiously with renal dysfunction

N o alcohol

G ive pyridoxine (B_6)—prevent peripheral neuropathy

S hould take on empty stomach, screen vision

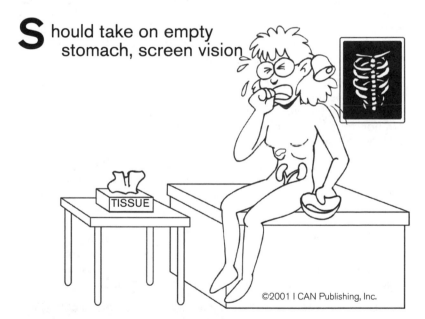

©2001 I CAN Publishing, Inc.

In some communities, Isoniazid (INH) has been nicknamed "INA". INA Tuberculosis has undesirable effects from INH. She is nauseated, has an enlarged liver, and tingling in her feet (peripheral neuropathy). "LUNGS" will help you recall some interventions.

ANTITUBERCULAR: RIFAMPIN

Action: Impairs RNA synthesis.

Indications: Treatment of pulmonary tuberculosis with at least one other antitubercular agent and for asymptomatic meningococcal carriers of Neisseria meningitidis.

Warnings: Hypersensitivity; hepatic dysfunction; active or treated alcoholism; children < than 5 years of age; pregnancy, lactation.

Undesirable Effects: Headache, drowsiness, dizziness; epigastric distress, heartburn, elevations of liver enzymes, hepatitis; rash and "flu-like syndrome" (chills, general discomfort, fever); blood dyscrasias; red-orange color to tears, saliva, sweat, urine, sputum. Soft contact lenses may be permanently stained.

Other Specific Information: When administered in combination with isoniazid, ↑ incidence of rifampin-related hepatitis. ↓ effectiveness of rifampin with ketoconazole. ↓ effectiveness of corticosteroids, metoprolol, propranolol, oral contraceptives, oral sulfonylureas, digitoxin, warfarin, etc. *(It is beyond the scope of this book to review all of the interactions. Refer to Drug Handbook.)*

Interventions: Monitor hepatic and renal function tests, CBC, cultures, sputum analysis, and urinalysis. Monitor CBC results for dyscrasias and observe for infection, hemorrhaging, or unusual fatigue. Arrange for a follow up with an ophthalmologist. If client is unable to swallow, recommend a suspension.

Education: Instruct not to skip dose; do not stop this drug without consulting with provider of care. Advise to take on empty stomach 1 hr. before or 2 hrs. after meals. Advise no alcohol or other meds without consulting provider. Take rifampin at least one hour before antacid. Advise client that urine and secretions may turn red-orange; do not wear soft contact lenses while taking this drug. Notify provider of any undesirable effects. If taking oral contraceptives, recommend alternative birth control. Recommend that client avoid activities that require alertness until response has been determined.

Evaluation: Client will be free of infection with no undesirable effects from the medicine.

Drug: rifampin (Rifadin, Rimactane)

REDMAN RIFAMPIN

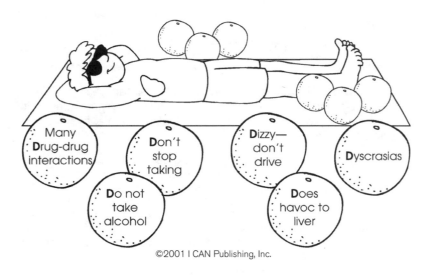

Many **D**rug-drug interactions

Don't stop taking

Dizzy— don't drive

Dyscrasias

Do not take alcohol

Does havoc to liver

©2001 I CAN Publishing, Inc.

Meet Mr. Redman Rifampin. He is taking some r & r (rest and relaxation) and is at the beach eating many oranges. He has had so many oranges his pee and tears are orange. Rifampin is hard on the liver, so it has gotten larger. The oranges will help you recall the 6 D's of rifampin.

ANTIFUNGAL: AMPHOTERICIN B

Action: Alters fungal cell permeability

Indications: Systemic fungal infections such as histoplasmosis or coccidioidomycosis.

Warnings: `HIGH ALERT DRUG` Hypersensitivity. Renal impairment, in combination with antineoplastic therapy. Pregnancy/Lactation.

Undesirable Effects: Very toxic. Infusion-related reaction (fever, chills, nausea, vomiting, headache, hypotension); drying effect with skin, pruritus; nephrotoxicity; thrombophlebtis; anemia; hypokalemia; ventricular fibrillation.

Other Specific Information: Steroids may ↑risk of severe hypokalemia. May ↑digoxin toxicity. Bone marrow depressants may ↑anemia. Nephrotoxic drugs may ↑nephrotoxicity.

Intervention: Monitor I & O, renal function tests for nephrotoxicity, and hepatic function test results. Evaluate potassium and magnesium levels, and hematologic results. Monitor vital signs and assess for undesirable effects q 15 min x 2, then q 30 min for 4 hrs. of initial infusion. Administer Tylenol and Benedryl 1 hour before infusion. Add hydrocortisone to infusion. Observe for signs of hypokalemia (muscle cramps, irregular pulse, and weakness). Large doses of potassium may be needed. Evaluate IV site for phlebitis. If client experiences GI symptoms, a pleasant and relaxed atmosphere for mealtimes along with small, frequent feedings of high-protein, high-calorie foods should be encouraged.

Education: Review oral hygiene such as using soft toothbrushes and floss. Avoid toothpicks. Advise client to notify staff at the first sign of pain at IV site. Report undesirable effects immediately to staff.

Evaluation: The client's infection will be eradicated without undesirable effects from the medication.

Drug: amphotericin B

AMPHOTERRIBLE

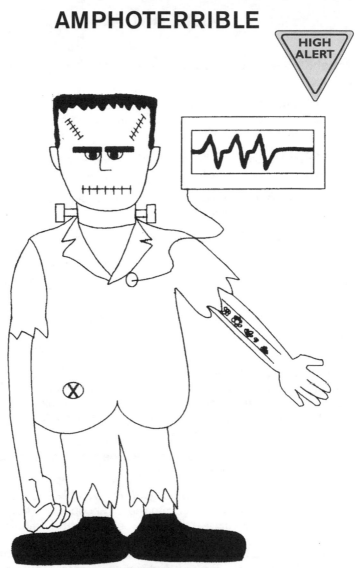

©2001 I CAN Publishing, Inc.

Ampho**terrible** is a monster. He treats monster infections such as histoplasmosis and other life threatening fungal infections. He has a terrible habit of creating irregularities in the heart (arrhythmias). The X marks the spot of the kidney since 80% of clients receiving this drug may develop some nephrotoxicity.

ANTIFUNGALS

Action: Increases permeability of the fungal cell membrane causing cell death.

Indications: Fungal infections: candidiasis, coccidioidomycosis, histoplasmosis, ringworm infections of the skin, tinea corporis, tinea cruris, onchomycosis of nails.

Warnings: Hypersensitivity to any antifungal, liver failure, pregnancy, lactation.

Undesired Effects: Headache, dizziness; nausea, vomiting, pruritus, irritation with topical application.

Other Specific Information: ↓ blood levels with rifampin. ↑ risk of toxicity of cyclosporine with antifungals. ↑ length of suppression of the adrenal cortex when corticosteroids or methylprednisolone are taken with antifungals. Risk of arrhythmias and even death when given with antihistamines.

Interventions: Evaluate liver function tests, CBC and differential, and culture the area prior to starting therapy; LFT may be done monthly. If a severe allergic reaction occurs, have epinephrine available.

Education: Instruct client to take medication with food; provide small frequent meals if GI upset is present. Review importance of taking the full course of medication. If no improvement within 2 wks, notify provider. Discuss hygiene measures to control reinfection. Review safety precautions if dizziness occurs.

Evaluation: Client's fungal infection will be resolved as indicated by a decrease in pruritus, redness, and rawness.

Drugs: *(Many of these drugs end in "zole".)* amphotericin B; flucona**zole** (Diflucan); flucystosine (Ancobon); itracona**zole** (Sporanox); ketocona**zole** (Nizoral); micona**zole** (Monistat IV); nystatin (Nilstat, Nystex); *Vaginal suppositories, topical:* micona**zole** (Micatin, Monistat 3, Monistat 7, Monistat-Derm, Monistat Dual Pak); nystatin (Mycostatin); *Topical:* butenafine (Mentax); butocona**zole** (Femstat 3); ciclopirox (Penlac); clotrima**zole** (Lotrimin, Mycelex); econa**zole** (Spectazole); gentian violet; nafitine (Naftin); oxicona**zole** (Oxistat); terbinafine (Lamisil); tolnaftate (Aftate, Genaspor, Tinactin, Ting)

ZOLE

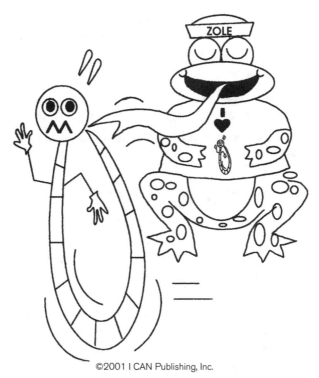

©2001 I CAN Publishing, Inc.

Z OLE—many drug interactions can occur

O bserve hygiene measures to control infectio

L iver Function Tests—monitor

E ducate to take with food

Meet "ZOLE" the toad who destroys fungal infections, such as ringworm. "ZOLE" will help you remember some key points with these drugs. It will also help you remember the medication used for these infections, since they have the letters **zole** in them.

ANTIPROTOZOAL, AMEBICIDE: FLAGYL

Action: Inhibits DNA synthesis in specific anaerobes resulting in cell death. Antiprotozoal-trichomonacidal; amebicidal.

Indications: Trichomoniasis; Gardnerella vaginalis; amebic liver abscess; intestinal amebiasis.

Warnings: Hypersensitivity, blood dyscrasias, CNS diseases, candidiasis, hepatic disease, pregnancy, lactation.

Undesirable Effects: Headache, dizziness, ataxia; anorexia, nausea, vomiting, diarrhea, unpleasant metallic taste; dryness and burning skin; superinfection (candidiasis); disulfiram-like interaction with alcohol.

Other Specific Information: ↓ effectiveness with barbiturates. ↑ bleeding tendencies with oral anticoagulants. If taken with alcohol, client will experience flushing, nausea, increased vomiting, and tachycardia.

Interventions: Monitor CBC and liver function tests.

Education: Instruct to take full course of medication; take with food. Encourage mouth care, sugarless candies, etc. to assist with dry mouth. No alcohol or preparation containing alcohol during therapy and for at least 48 hours afterward. Inform that brown urine may occur. No intercourse unless partner wears a condom. Review undesirable effects and the importance of reporting them to provider. For the topical application, recommend cleaning area and waiting 15 to 20 minutes before applying drug. Avoid eye contact. Cosmetics may be used after applying drug.

Evaluation: Client will maintain an infection free state with no undesirable effects from the drug.

Drugs: metronidazole (Flagyl, Flagyl ER, Flagyl IV, MetroGel)

FLAGYL

F lushing

A LCOHOL will cause these effects

I ncreased vomiting

N ausea

T achycardia

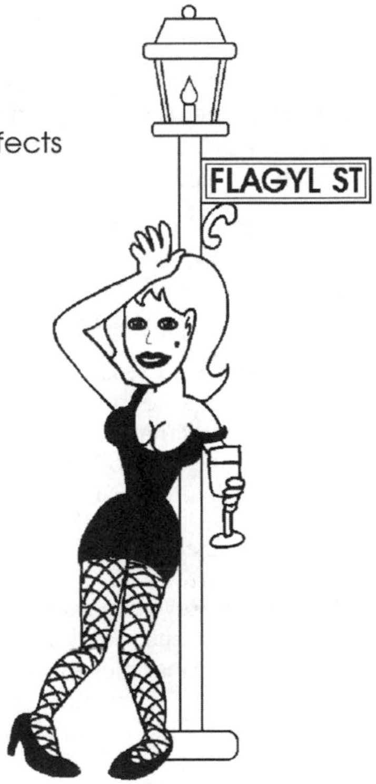

FLAGYL ST

©2001 I CAN Publishing, Inc.

As you can see, this lady has been doing her tricks on Flagyl Street. She evidently had alcohol while on this street. If Flagyl is mixed with alcohol, there will be a disulfiram-like reaction, and that is why this lady feels "FAINT".

ANTIVIRALS

Action: Interfere with DNA synthesis and replication of virus. Virustatic.

Indications: Herpes simplex I, genital herpes II.

Warnings: Hypersensitivity to any component of product. Caution with pregnancy/lactation, renal/hepatic impairment.

Undesirable Effects: Anorexia, nausea, vomiting; light-headedness, headaches, tremors; rash, pruritus. Increased bleeding time; phlebitis at IV site. Acyclovir–(Serious) nephrotoxicity, neuropathy, bone marrow depression.

Other Specific Information: Probenecid may ↑ acyclovir and valacyclovir levels. Increase nephroneurotoxicity when amino-glycosides, probenecid, and interferon are adminstered with acyclovir. None significant for famciclovir.

Interventions: Monitor renal/liver function tests, CBC, I & O, and vital signs (especially blood pressure). Acyclovir may cause orthostatic hyptension. Evaluate for superinfection due to high dose and prolonged use of an antiviral drug. If giving acyclovir IV, never give as a bolus. Refer to drug circular for specific guidelines. Provide analgesics and comfort measures to elderly with shingles. Keep fingernails short and clean.

Education: Review importance of fluid intake. Notify provider if condition worsens. Review ways to control spread. Teach to use finger cot or rubber glove when applying ointment to prevent spread of lesions. These meds do not cure herpes; they only shorten the episode. Pap smears should be done at least annually due to increased risk of cervical cancer in women with genital herpes. Avoid sexual intercourse during treatment for genital herpes.

Evaluation: Client will experience a decrease in the symptoms of the virus with no undesirable effects from the medications.

Drugs: *(end in "vir")* acyclo**vir** (Zovirax); famciclo**vir** (Famvir); valacyclo**vir** (Valtrex)

THE VIR HOUSE OF SHINGLES

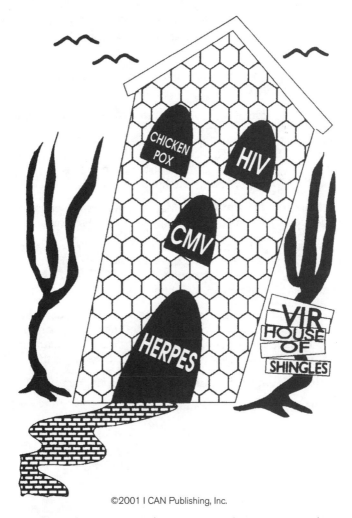

©2001 I CAN Publishing, Inc.

The haunted house of shingles (herpes zoster), chicken pox (varicella zoster), herpes simplex, and the cytomegaly virus is most often repaired with drugs that include **VIR** in them. Acyclo**vir** (Zo**vir**ax), famciclo**vir** (Fam**vir**), and valacyclo**vir** (Valtrex) are a few of these drugs.

The house is haunted and shaky because the recipient of these drugs may experience a headache and shakes from chills. It's enough to make you throw up!

URINARY ANALGESIC: PYRIDIUM

Action: Exact mechanism is not understood. Produces a topical analgesic effect on the urinary tract mucosa from the azo dye that is excreted.

Indications: Symptomatic relief of pain, burning, frequency related to irritation from a UTI.

Warnings: Hypersensitivity to phenazopyridine; renal insufficiency; pregnancy, lactation.

Undesirable Effects: Refer to "**GUSH**". **G**I disturbances, **U**rine may have a yellow-orange discoloration, **S**clera or skin may have a yellowish tinge, **H**emolytic anemia, headache.

Other Specific Information: May interfere with urinalysis color reactions, urinary ketones, glucose, proteins, and steroids.

Interventions: With long-term therapy, assess liver function tests. Do not administer longer than 2 days if given with antibacterial agent for the treatment of UTI. Discontinue drug if sclera or skin become yellowish; this indicates accumulation of drug.

Education: Instruct client to take after meals to decrease gastric irritation. Advise client that urine may be reddish-orange and may stain fabric. Report signs of yellowing of skin or sclera, headache, clay-colored stools, unusual bleeding or bruising, fever, sore throat.

Evaluation: Client will be free of pain from urinary tract in 3 days.

Drug: phenazopyridine (Pyridium)

MR. P. O.

GI disturbances

U rine turns yellow orange

S clera and skin orange

H emolytic anemia

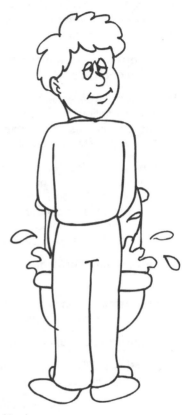

©2001 I CAN Publishing, Inc.

Mr. P. O. was not happy with his pain, but after taking Pyridium the pain from his UTI must be gone. Judging by the look on his face, Pyridium is obviously working. He can now pee out a "GUSH" without discomfort. Remember: **P**yridium turns urine **O**range!

URECHOLINE

Action: Stimulation of muscarine receptors of the GU tract, resulting in a relaxation of the trigone and sphincter muscles and contraction of the detrusor muscle.

Indications: Postpartum and postoperative nonobstructive urinary retention or urinary retention caused by neurogenic bladder.

Warnings: Hypersensitivity. Mechanical obstruction of the Gi or GU tract. Use cautiously in clients with a history of asthma; Ulcer disease; Cardiovascular disease; Epilepsy; Hyperthyroidism; OB, Lactation, Pediatrics: Safety not established.

Undesirable Effects: Headache, malaise; bronchospasm; Extreme muscarinic stimulation may result in sweating, tearing, urinary urgency, bradycardia and hypotension. *(Refer to next page for an easy way to remember these undesirable effects.)* Additional undesirable effects may include heart block, syncope/cardiac arrest. GI: abdominal discomfort, diarrhea, nausea, vomiting.

Other Specific Information: Sensitivity to cholinergic agents or effects.

Interventions: Administer by oral route either 1 hour prior to or 2 hours following meals. Evaluate Intake & Output.

Education: Teach client to report any of the undesirable effects.

Evaluation: Client will be relieved of urinary retention with no undesirable effects.

Drug: bethanechol (Duvoid, Urabeth, Urecholine)

URECHOLINE

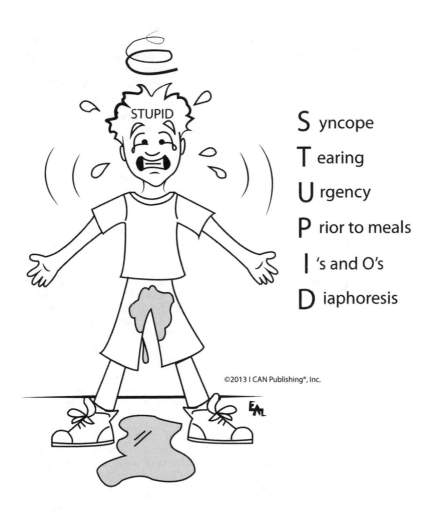

S yncope

T earing

U rgency

P rior to meals

I 's and O's

D iaphoresis

©2013 I CAN Publishing®, Inc.

MUSCARINIC ANTAGONISTS: DITROPAN

Action: Inhibits muscarinic receptors of the detrusor muscle of the bladder, which prevents contractions of the bladder and the urge to void.

Indications: Urinary symptoms that may be associated with neurogenic bladder including frequent urination, urgency, nocturia, urge incontinence. Clients with an overactive bladder with symptoms of urge incontinence, urgency, and frequency will benefit from these drugs.

Warnings: Hypersensitivity; uncontrolled angle-closure glaucoma; Intestinal obstruction or atony; Urinary retention. Use cautiously in hepatic/renal impairment; bladder outflow obstruction; ulcerative colitis; benign prostatic hypertrophy; cardiovascular disease; GI obstructive disorders; myasthenia gravis; pregnant, lactation; geriatrics poorly tolerated due to anticholinergic effects. Safety in children has not been established.

Undesirable Effects: Dizziness, drowsiness, confusion, insomnia; anticholinergic effects: urinary retention, blurred vision, dry mouth, constipation, nausea.

Other Specific Information: Tricyclic antidepressants, Anti-histamines, or phenothiazines used concurrently may result in muscarinic blockage. ↑ anticholinergic effects with other agents having anticholinergic properties such as amantadine, antidepressants, phenothiazines, disopyramide, and haloperidol. Additive CNS depression with other CNS depressants including alcohol, antihistamines, antidepressants, opioids, and sedative/hypnotics. Ketoconazole, itraconazole, erythromycin and clarithromycin may ↑ effects.

Interventions: Do not confuse Ditropan (Oxybutynin) with diazepam. Assess voiding pattern and output ratio, and assess abdomen for bladder distention prior to and periodically during therapy. Assess geriatric clients for anticholinergic effects (sedation and weakness). May be administered on an empty stomach or with meals or milk to prevent gastric irritation. Use extended-release formulations to minimize anticholinergic effects. Avoid chewing or crushing these extended–release tablets. Instruct that the shell of extended–release tablets will be eliminated whole in the stool. Apply patch on same two days each week to hip, abdomen, or buttock in an area that is clean, dry and without irritation. Rotate sites to minimize irritation.

Education: Instruct to increase dietary fiber, consume 2 to 3 L/day of fluid from beverage and food sources, sip fluids and avoid hazardous activities if vision is disturbed. Report symptoms of undesirable effects to provider of care. Review drugs to stay away from when taking muscarinic antagonists.

Evaluation: Client will experience decrease of urinary urgency and frequency, nocturia and urge incontinence.

Drugs: darifenacin (Enablex), oxybutynin (Ditropan)

DITROPAN (DI-TRO-PAN)

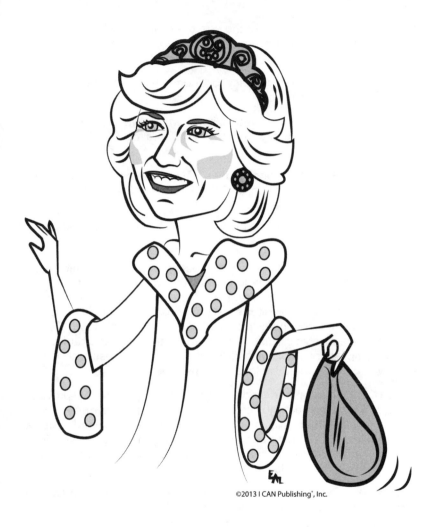

©2013 I CAN Publishing®, Inc.

"DI-TRO-PAN" - "DI" for Dianna. This med helped Dianna "TRO" (for throw) the bed "PAN" away, and she could finally sleep during the night without getting up and going to the bathroom all night. This is an image of Di throwing the bedpan out!

PROTEASE INHIBITORS

Action: Inhibits the binding of the enzyme protease, which is needed for the HIV protein to mature. These agents act only during viral replication. Antiretroviral.

Indications: HIV infection. May be combined with nucleoside or reverse transcriptase inhibitors.

Warnings: Use cautiously with clients who have liver impairment. Interactions include toxicity of drugs activated by CYP3A4 (a liver enzyme).

Undesirable Effects: Kidney stones; GI symptoms: abdominal pain, diarrhea, nausea and vomiting, and altered sense of taste. *Neurologic:* headache, insomnia, weakness.

Other Specific Information: Never give at the same time as didanosine (Videx).

Interventions: Assess for signs of infection or anemia. Monitor AST, ALT. Culture and sensivity before drug therapy and after treatment. Assess bowel pattern during treatment. Assess urine color, consistency, and ease in urinating. Monitor skin eruptions, rash, urticaria. Monitor CD4 cell count throughout treatment. Administer with food. Do not mix with juice or acidic fluids. Administer antiemetic, antidiarrheal as needed. Implement safety measures in case of weakness. Encourage sedatives and nonopoid analgesics as needed.

Education: Avoid other medications unless directed by provider of care. The drug does not cure, but does manage symptoms and does not prevent transmission of HIV to others. Recommend to use a nonhormonal form of birth control while taking the drug. If miss dose take as soon as remembered up to 1 hour before next dose; do not double dose. Take with food.

Evaluation: Client will have a therapeutic effect from the medication with no complications from undesirable effects.

Drugs: amprenavir (Agenerase); indinavir (Crixivan), nelfinavir (Viracept), ritonavir (Norvir), saquinavir (Invirase)

PECANS

P rotease enzyme is inhibited which is needed for HIV protein to mature. These agents act only during viral replication.

E ncourage sedatives and nonopioid analgesics as needed

C autiously use with liver impairment

A bdominal pain, nausea and vomiting
ltered sense of taste—undesirable effects
dminister antiemetic and antidiarrheal as needed

N eurological side effects: headache, insomnia, weakness

S tones, kidney—monitor

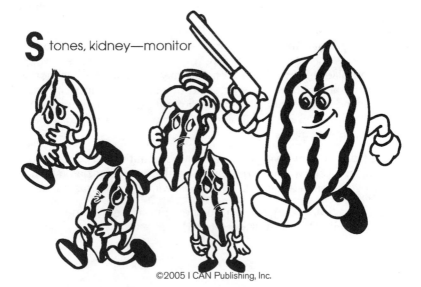

©2005 I CAN Publishing, Inc.

The chief PECAN is shooting to inhibit the binding of the enzyme protease. Note: This prevents maturity of the HIV protein.

NUCLEOSIDE INHIBITORS

Actions: Inhibits reverse transcriptase, that is needed to convert RNA into DNA in HIV infecion. HIV is a retrovirus, meaning that the genetic code is introduced opposite of a human gene (DNA to RNA).

Indications: HIV infections, both early onset and advanced stages. Lower transmission of HIV from mother to fetus.

Other Specific Information: Interactions can occur with other bone marrow depressants and certain antibiotics. Toxicity that occurs from the drugs may be difficult to distinguish from the symptoms of HIV infection.

Warnings: Hypersensitivity. Severe renal disease, impaired hepatic disease,

Undesirable Effects: Granulocytopenia and anemia; neurotoxicity: headache, insomnia, muscle pain, and nausea. Overdose: anemia, fatigue, leukopenia, severe nausea, thrombocytopenia, vomiting, seizures.

Interventions: Monitor CBC count. Perform a baseline neurologic assessment and check periodically thereafter. Monitor the effectiveness of the drug and the amount taken.

Education: Teach that drug is not a cure for AIDS but will control symptoms. Notify provider of care of sore throat, swollen lymph nodes, malaise, fever; other infections. Inform client that infection is still present and can be transmitted to others. Follow up visits must be continued since serious toxicity may occur; blood counts must be done q 2 weeks. Serious interactions may occur, so no OTC meds unless provider is aware.

Evaluation: Client will receive a therapeutic response from medication. Client will not experience any blood dyscrasias (anemia, granulocytopenia). Lab reports will remain with in the normal range.

Drugs: abacavir (Ziagen); lamivudine (Epivir), stavudine (Zerit), zalcitabine (HIVID), zidovudine (Retrovir)

REVERSE

R everse transcriptase is inhibited, which is needed to convert RNA into DNA in HIV infections. HIV is a retrovirus, meaning that the genetic code is introduced opposite of a human gene.

E valuate CBC

V ID or **VIR** are typically in the drug name (i.e., Retro**vir**, **Vid**ex, Epi**vir**, Hi**vid**)

E valuate neurological status

R eacts with bone marrow depressants and certain antibiotics

S ide effects—granulocytopenia and anemia, headache, insomnia, nausea

E valuate for overdose; some clients use as a suicide attempt (anemia, fatigue, leukopenia, thrombocytopenia, vomiting, seizures)

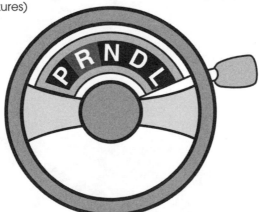

©2005 I CAN Publishing, Inc.

The steering wheel has been **reversed**. "REVERSE" will assist in recalling the most important facts about this category of drugs.

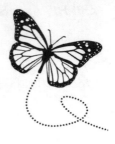

Caring is the essence of nursing—caring for, caring with, and caring about.

M. PATRICIA DONAHUE, PHD, RN

Antineoplastic Agents

UNDESIRABLE EFFECTS FROM ANTICANCER DRUGS

Bone marrow depression

Alopecia

Retching—nausea/vomiting

Fear and anxiety

Stomatitis

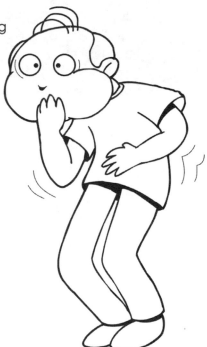

ANTINEOPLASTIC AGENTS

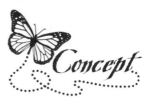

C B C, platelets—monitor

A ntiemetics before drug

N ephrotoxicity—undesirable effect

C ounseling regarding reproduction issues

E ncourage handwashing, avoid crowds

R ecommend a wig for alopecia

ALKYLATING AGENTS

Action: Causes cell death or mutation of malignant growths through inhibition of protein synthesis by interfering with DNA replication by alkylation of DNA. Action most evident in rapidly dividing cells.

Indications: Palliative treatment of chronic lymphocytic leukemia; malignant lymphomas; Hodgkin's disease; breast, lung and ovarian cancers.

Warnings: **HIGH ALERT DRUG** Hypersensitivity; bone marrow depression; active infections; recent immunization with live virus; renal or liver disease; concurrent radiation therapy; pregnancy, lactation.

Undesirable Effects: Tremors, muscular twitching, confusion; nausea, vomiting, hepatotoxicity; bone marrow depression; sterility; alopecia, urticaria; hemorrhagic cystitis; cancer, acute leukemia.

Other Specific Information: Individual drugs have specific interactions with meds. It is beyond the scope of this book to review.

Interventions: Monitor CBC with differential and platelets weekly. Monitor uric acid, liver and renal function tests before and throughout therapy. Hydrate client well before and after treatment. Premedicate with antietemics, ondansetron or granisetron are preferred. Have prn antiemetics available. Monitor IV site for irritation and phlebitis. Have epinephrine, corticosteroids, antihistamines and emergency equipment on hand for potential allergic reaction. Store drug in airtight container at room temperature.

Education: Consult with provider prior to receiving any vaccination. Instruct to report bleeding, signs of anemia, or infection to provider. Recommend a diet low in purines to alkalize urine. Review the importance of good oral hygiene with soft toothbrush. Do not use toothbrush when platelet count is < 50,000 cells/mm^3. Reduce nausea and vomiting by eating small meals and refer for dietary consultation. (Refer to "**CANCER**".)

Evaluation: Client will be free of cancer; blood counts will improve.

Drugs: busulfan (Busulfex, Myleran); carboplatin (Paraplatin); carmustine (BiCNU, Gliadel); chlorambucil (Leukeran); cisplatin (Platinol-AQ); cyclophosphamide (Cytoxan, Neosar); ifosfamide (Ifex); lomustine (CeeNU); mechlorethamine (Mustargen); melphalan (Alkeran); streptozocin (Zanosar); thiotepa (Thioplex)

NITROGEN MUSTARD

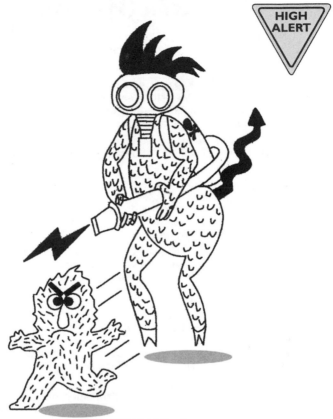

©2001 I CAN Publishing, Inc.

B one marrow depression (leukopenia, thrombocytopenia)

A norexia/alopecia

D istressful nausea and vomiting

Nitrogen Mustard, the alkylating agent, is destroying malignant neoplasm. Somewhat of a beast itself, it causes **"BAD"** undesirable effects.

185

TOPOISOMERASE INHIBITOR
TOPOTECAN (HYCAMTIN)

Action: Kills cancer cells by interrupting DNA synthesis by inhibiting the enzyme topoisomerase at the cell cycle phase S-specific.

Indications: Ovary and small cell lung tumors

Warnings: **HIGH ALERT DRUG** Contraindicated in hypersensitivity; Pregnancy or lactation; Pre-existing severe myelosuppression. Use with caution in impaired renal function (reduce dose if CCr < 40 ml/min); Platelet count < 25,000 cells / mm^3 (decrease dose); Childbearing potential.

Undesirable Effects: Headache, fatigue, weakness; dyspnea; abdominal pain, diarrhea, nausea, vomiting, anorexia; alopecia; anemia, leukopenia, neutropenia, thrombocytopenia.

Other Specific Information: Neutropenia is prolonged by concurrent use of filgrastim (do not use until day 6; 24 hr following completion of topotecan). Increase myelosuppression with other antineoplastics (especially cisplatin) or radiation therapy. May decrease antibody response to and increase risk of adverse reactions from live virus vaccines.

Interventions: Monitor for bleeding (bruising, bleeding gums)) or infection (temperature, sore throat). Instruct to avoid crowds and contact with infectious individuals. Monitor CBC. Administer antiemetic for nausea and vomiting such as ondansetron (Zofran) in combination with dexamethasone, granisetron (Kytril) or metoclopramide (Reglan) prior to initiating chemotherapy. Prior to administering agents, clarify all ambiguous orders; double check single, daily, and course-of-therapy dose limits; have second practitioner independently double–check original order, dose calculations, and infusion pump settings. If administered IV, solution should be prepared in a biologic cabinet. Wear gloves, gown, and mask while handling IV medication. Discard IV equipment in specially designated containers. Monitor labs.

Education: Advise client to perform excellent oral hygiene and avoid mouth wash with alcohol. Recommend that female clients use birth control during treatment. May be taken without regard to food. Capsules must be swallowed whole; do not open, crush, or chew. Do not replace dose if client vomits after taking dose. Do not take missed doses. If any capsules are leaking or broken, do not touch with bare hands. Dispose of capsules and wash hands with soap and water. Notify provider for signs of infection, bleeding, bruising. Review importance of being cautious with crowds or individuals with known infections. Instruct to use soft toothbrush and electric razor. No alcoholic beverages or products containing aspirin or NSAIDs. No OTC meds or any meds without consulting provider of care. Review with client that hair loss may occur 7 to 10 days after the beginning of treatment and will last for a maximum duration of 2 months after the last administration of the chemotherapeutic agent. Recommend that client selects a hairpiece prior to or at the occurrence of hair loss. No vaccinations without consulting provider.

Evaluation: Client will experience a decrease in size and spread of malignancy.

Drugs: topotecan (Hycamtin)

TOPOISOMERASE INHIBITORS
"TOPO-IS-OM-ERASE"

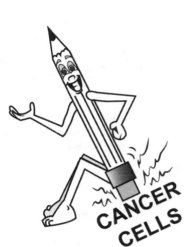

E nzyme topoisomerase is inhibited

R enal function, CBC, and bleeding
      should be monitored

A ntiemetic for nausea and vomiting
      (give Zofran)

S igns of infection should be
      monitored (sore throat, fever...)

E xtra care should be taken when
      handling medication (e.g., gloves,
      mask, gown...)

ANTIMETABOLITES

Action: Interferes with the building blocks of DNA synthesis, greatest activity is in the S phase of the cell cycle.

Indications: Myelocytic leukemia; acute lymphocytic leukemia; cancer of breast, cervix, colon, liver, ovary, pancreas, stomach, and rectum; combination treatment for non-Hodgkin's lymphoma in children.

Warnings: **HIGH ALERT DRUG** Allergy; myelosuppression; active infections; recent immunization with live virus; renal or hepatic disease; pregnancy, lactation.

Undesirable Effects: Anorexia, nausea, vomiting, diarrhea, oral and anal inflammation; bone marrow depression, thrombocytopenia, hemorrhage; alopecia, rash, fever; renal dysfunction.

Other Specific Information: ↓ effect of digoxin with cytarbine. ↑ toxicity of fluorouracil with leucovorin. May be fatal if methotrexate is taken with specific NSAIDs. Interactions may occur with live virus vaccines, bone marrow depressants, calcium, and cimetidine.

Interventions: Evaluate complete blood count, uric acid, kidney and liver chemistries before administration. Evaluate neurological status prior to and during therapy. Premedicate with antiemetics. Comfort measures if headache, inflammation, or other associated pain occurs with cytarabine syndrome. Safety measures if dizziness occurs. (Refer to "**METABOLITE**" on next page.)

Education: Client should report fever, sore throat, extreme fatigue, rash, ulcers, tarry stools, bleeding, or other unusual symptoms to provider. Do not use a toothbrush if platelet count is < 50,000/mm³. Reduce nausea and vomiting by eating small meals and refer for dietary consultation. (Refer to "**CANCER**" and "**METABOLITE**".)

Evaluation: Client's tumor will decrease in size and blood tests will remain in normal range.

Drugs: capecitabine (Xeloda); cytarabine (Ara-C, Cytosar-U, DepoCyt, Tarabine PFS); floxuridine (FUDR); fludarabine (Fludara); fluorouracil (Adrucil, Efudex, Fluoroplex, 5-FU); mercaptopurine (Purinethol); methotrexate (MTX); thioguanine (6-Thioguanine)

ANTIMETABOLITE

M onitor CBC and platelets weekly

E valuate renal function tests

T emperature assessment q 4–6 hrs.

A sepsis—strict

B leeding, anemia, infection, and nausea—report

O ral hygiene—brush with soft toothbrush

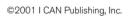

©2001 I CAN Publishing, Inc.

L ots of fluids (2–3 L/day)

I ntake and Output, nutritional intake—monitor

T he Protocols for handling and administering—follow

E mphasize protective isolation

ANTINEOPLASTIC AGENTS: ANTIBIOTICS

Action: Inhibits RNA synthesis and delays or inhibits mitosis. Interferes with DNA replication and messenger RNA production.

Indications: Most useful in treating slow growing tumors. Hodgkin's disease, testicular carcinoma, breast and bladder cancer.

Warnings: **HIGH ALERT DRUG** Hypersensitivites. Use cautiously with client who have cardiopulmonary disease, dose reduction may be necessary. Caution in client with depressed bone marrow function, active infections, recent immunization with live virus, impaired renal or hepatic function, history of cardiopulmonary disease or diminished cardiac function. Use with caution for those with antineoplastic or radiation therapy within 3–6 weeks. Dactinomycin is contraindicated for clients with viral infections. This drug should be used with caution for obese clients or those with gout.

Undesirable Effects: Most antitumor antibiotics are toxic to the heart and lungs.

Other Specific Information: Increased toxicity with other antineoplastics or radiation. Alopecia, stomatitis, nausea, and vomiting are the most commonly occurring nonorgan-specific undesirable effects. Daunorubicin and doxorubicin may cause dose-limiting myelosuppression.

Interventions: All are vesicants except bleomycin. Severe tissue damage if extravasation. Administer with precautions to avoid tissue damage. Avoid with live vaccines. Monitor the CBC. Evaluate the client's cardiac and pulmonary status prior to and during treatment.. Administer antiemetics before initiating therapy and provide with antiemetics for home use.

Education: When reconstituted, daunorubicin and doxorubicin have a bright, reddish-orange color, which causes the client's urine to turn a similar color. Dactinomycin is a radiation sensitizer and may cause a phenomenon called radiation recall. This condition means that tissue that was damaged by radiation may become reddened and inflamed in response to antineoplastic therapy. Provide comprehensive client education on management of the symptoms and when to seek medical support.

Evaluation: The client will experience a therapeutic effect from the drug. There will be a decreased tumor size and a decrease in the spread of the malignancy.

Drugs: bleomycin (Blenoxane), dactinomycin (Cosmegen), daunorubicin (DaunoXome), doxorubicin (Adriamycin PFS, Adriamycin RDF, Rubex), epirubicin (Ellence), idarubicin (Idamycin, Idamycin PFS), methotrexate (Folex, Folex PFS, methotrexate, Rheumatrex), mitomycin (Mitomycin, Mutamycin), mitoxantrone (Novantrone), plicamycin (Mithramycin, Mithracin)

CINEMANS

HIGH
ALERT

C olor of urine change.

I ncreased opportunistic infection

N ausea and vomiting

E xtravasation

M yelosuppression, mucositis

A lopecia

N ausea and vomiting

S terility

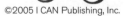

©2005 I CAN Publishing, Inc.

Mr. "CINemans" is mowing away at the slow growing weeds (cancer cells). Many of these agents end in "CIN"!

MITOTIC INHIBITORS

Action: Inhibits cell mitosis

Indications: Breast cancer, lymphomas, leukemia, Wilm's tumor, sarcomas

Warnings: **HIGH ALERT DRUG** Hypersensitivity; Paclitaxel (Taxol) is contraindicated for clients with a neutropenia count of less than 1500 cells/mm³. It is also used with caution in clients with cardiac dysrhythmias. Etoposide (VP-16) is contraindicated for clients with severe bone marrow depression, current or recent infection, and severe renal and hepatic dysfunction. Used with caution for clients with gout. Women during pregnancy; during lactation; and for children. Vincristine should be used cautiously in clients with infection, leukopenia, bone marrow suppression, chickenpox, current neurologic or neuromuscular hepatic dysfunction.

Undesirable Effects: Allergic interactions since all are plant derivatives. All of the vinca alkaloids are vesicants, which means that these drugs are capable of causing permanent tissue damage and necrosis when allowed to extravasate into tissues. VIncristine is fatal if given intrathecally.

Other Specific Information: When vinblastine is given concurrently with mitomycin, bronchospasms may occur. When paclitaxel and ketoconazole are given together, serious toxicities may occur.

Interventions: When giving vesicant drugs via a peripheral IV route, extreme caution must be taken to establish a reliable IV access that has not been subjected to a recent venipuncture. Vinca alkaloids (vesicant drugs) can cause leakage of drug into soft tissues around the venipuncture site (extravasation). Remember "V" for vesicant and use precautions with **V**elban, **V**incristine, **V**inblastine, **V**indesine. Establish a protocol for administration of antidotes and application of heat or cold before administering a vesicant drug. Administer antidotes to minimize the damage caused by extravasation. Verify that informed consent has been given before initiating treatment. Check the client's lab and diagnostic studies before beginning therapy with special attention being given to the CBC, platelet count, and liver function studies. Monitor for bone marrow depression and peripheral neuropathy.

Education: Instruct client about signs and symptoms of peripheral neuropathy, including paresthesias in the hands or feet, difficulty with fine-motor skills, and numbness. Other signs and symptoms include constipation, paralytic ileus, urinary retention, and jaw pain. Instruct client to report any of these complaints immediately to the health care provider. (Failure to report peripheral neuropathy immediately may result in irreversible neurological damage.)

Evaluation: Client's cancer will decrease and blood tests will remain in normal range.

Drugs: Etoposide (VP-16), Paclitaxel (Taxol), Vinblastine (Velban), Vincristine (Oncovin), vinorelbine (Navelbine)

MITOTIC INHIBITOR: ANTINEOPLASTIC AGENTS

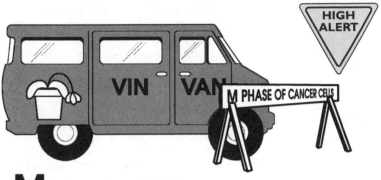

M ay cause hepatotoxicty

I nhibits cell mitosis

T ake precautions—vesicants (remember V's for vesicant: Vincristine, Vinblastine, Velban)

O ncovin (Vincristine)

T reat for breast cancer, lymphomas, leukemia, Wilm's Tumor

Rev **I** ew client's mobility and ADLs

C NS and neuro side effects such as peripheral neuropathy

©2005 I CAN Publishing, Inc.

The " VIN VAN" will help you remember that several of these agents start with "VIN". These agents block cell mitosis.

BIOLOGICAL RESPONSE MODIFIER (INTERFERON)

Action: Possess antiviral and antineoplastic effects, directly inhibit effects on DNA and protein synthesis, and increase cancer cell antigens on the cell surface. This enables the immune system to recognize the cancer cells more easily. These actions halt virus replication and prevent penetration into healthy cells. They enhance the activity of the other cells in the immune system and stop the division of the cancer cells.

Indications: Treatment of viral infections: rhinovirus, papillovirus, tetrovirus, hepatitis, chondyloma—a wart-like growth in the perineal area; transmitted sexually. Treatment of various cancers: Kaposi's sarcoma, mulitple myeloma, renal cell carcinoma, melanoma, bladder cancer, T-cell lymphoma. Treatments of some autoimmune diseases: multiple sclerosis.

Warnings: Allergies to egg protein or neomycin. If allergic, do not adminiter these agents. Hypersensitivity. Renal, cardiac, or hepatic disease.

Undesirable Effects: Flu-like symptoms: fever, chills, headache, malaise, myalgia, and fatigue. GI: nausea, vomiting, diarrhea, anorexia. CNS: dizzy, confusion, paranoia. CV: tachycardia, cyanosis, tachypnea. Hematologic neutropenia, thrombocytopenia. Renal: increased BUN and creatinine levels, proteinuria, and altered LFTs.

Other Specific Information: Interactions can occur with aminophylline therapy, and there are additive effects with other antiviral agents

Interventions: Determine if there are any egg allergies. If severe, do not start therapy. If reaction is mild, then give antihistamines and begin therapy. Monitor CBC, renal studies. Monitor vital signs. Assess for signs of bleeding and infections. Implement safety precautions if CNS effects occur. Use nonopoid analgesics prn for flulike symptoms.

Education: Discuss the importance for reporting any bleeding or signs of infection. Review safety precautions with client for both bleeding and infection. Provide client and/or family written directions regarding how to take medication safely.

Evaluation: Client will experience decreased serious infections, improvement in existing infections and inflammatory conditions.

Drugs: interferon-alfa (Roferon-A, Alferon N), interferon-beta (Betaseron), interfeon-gamma (Actimmune)

INTERFERON

F lu-like effect

E valuate for bleeding, ↑HR, ↑RR

V ertigo

E gg allergies

R eview CBC, BUN, creatinine

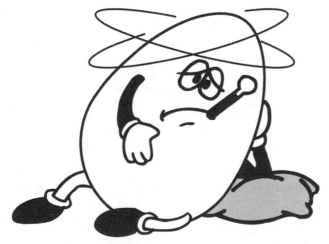

©2005 I CAN Publishing, Inc.

The sick Mr. Egg is reminding us not to administer these agents if client has any egg allergies. "FEVER" will help you remember some undesirable effects from these agents.

ANTI-ESTROGEN TAMOXIFEN

Action: Antineoplastic. Antiestrogen homone. Inhibits cell division by binding to cytoplasmic estrogen receptors; resembles normal cell complex but inhibits DNA synthesis and estrogen response of target tissue.

Indications: Advanced breast carcinoma not responsive to other therapy in estrogen-receptor-positive patients (usually post meno-pausal), prevention of breast cancer, following breast surgery/radiation in ductal carcinoma in situ.

Warnings: Hypersensitivity; Leukopenia, thrombocytopenia, cataracts.

Undesirable Effects: Thrombocytopenia, leukopenia, vaginal bleeding, DVT, PE, nausea, vomiting, anorexia, rash, alopecia, hot flashes, headache, light-headedness, depression. Visual acuity may be decreased and the loss is irreversible.

Other Specific Information: Increased chance of bleeding when taken with anticoagulants. Bromocriptine may increase tamoxifen levels.

Interventions: Assess CBC, differential, platelet count every week; hold drug if WBC < 3500 or platelet count is < 100,000; notify provider of care. Assess for bleeding q 8 hours: hematuria, guaiac, bruising, petechiae, mucosa or orifices. Assess for psychological effects to the alopecia. Assess for symptoms indicating severe allergic reactions: rash, pruritus, urticaria, purpuric skin lesions, itching, flushing. Administer antacid prior to the oral agent; administer after evening meal, before going to bed. Administer an antiemetic 30–60 min. before giving drug to prevent vomiting. Do not crush, break, or chew tablets.

Education: Review importance of a liquid diet, if necessary, including cola, jello; dry toast or crackers if client is having difficulties with nausea and vomiting. Advise client to increase fluid intake to 2–3 L/day to prevent dehydration. Discuss taking in a nutritious diet with iron and vitamin supplements as ordered. Store in a light-resistant container at room temperature. Review the undesirable effects with the client and family members and advise to report to provider of care. Apply sunscreen and protective clothes when out in the sun. Report any vaginal bleeding immediately. Routine eye exams. Premenopausal women must use mechanical birth control because ovulation may be induced. Advise that new hair growth may be different in color and texture.

Evaluation: The client will have a decrease in the tumor size or spread of malignancy.

Drugs: tamoxifen (Tamoxifen, Nolvadex, Tamofen, Tamoplex, Tamone)

"TAMI OX SUN"

T hrombocytopenia, leukopenia, visual acuity
decreased—warnings

dvanced breast cancer—indications
A ntacids prior to taking the oral agent
ssess CBC and hold if WBC< 3500 or platelet count < 100,000

M echanical birth control—for premenopausal women

I ncrease fluid intake to 2–3 per day
ron and vitamin supplements as ordered

R **O** utine eye exams

X out crushing, breaking, or
chewing tablets

S unscreen when in the sun
tore in a light-resistant container

U ndesirable effects—
DVT, PE, nausea and
vomiting

N utritious diet

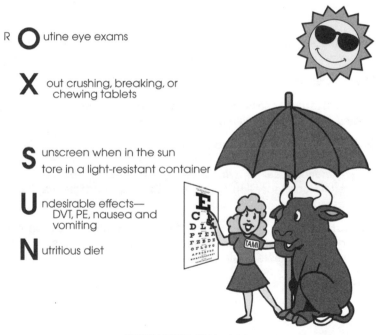

©2005 I CAN Publishing, Inc.

"TAMI" is evaluating the visual acuity of the "OX" since visual acuity
may be affected by the drugs. "TAMI" is protecting the "OX" from the
"SUN" due to photosensitivity. "TAMI OX SUN" will help you remember
the agent tamoxifen.

AROMATASE INHIBITOR
LETROZOLE (FEMARA)

Action: Inhibits the enzyme aromatase, which is partially responsible for conversion of precursors to estrogen. Decreases levels of circulating estrogen, which may halt progression of estrogen-sensitive breast cancer.

Indications: First-line treatment of post-menopausal women with hormone receptor positive or hormone receptor unknown metastatic or advanced breast cancer. Advanced breast cancer in postmenopausal clients with disease progression despite antiestrogen therapy.

Warnings: Hypersensitivity; Premenopausal women; pregnancy; Use cautiously in liver disease; Lactation or children (safety not established).

Undesirable Effects: Anxiety, depression, weakness; Nausea, abdominal pain, anorexia; musculoskeletal pain, arthralgia, fractures.

Other Specific Information: No significant drug-drug interactions.

Interventions: Assess for pain and other undesirable effect during therapy. May be taken with or without regard to food.

Education: Teach client to take as prescribed and directed. Inform of undesirable effects and to report to provider. Caution women who are perimenopausal or who recently became menopausal to use appropriate contraception throughout therapy; letrozole may result in fetal harm.

Evaluation: Client will experience the slowing of disease progression with advanced breast cancer. There will also be a decrease in the risk of recurrent / metastatic disease.

Drug: letrozole (Femara)

LETROZOLE (FEMARA)

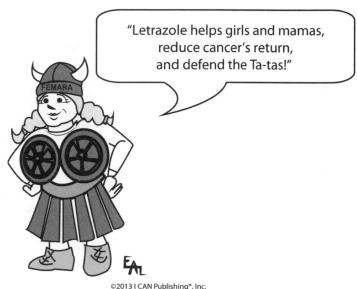

"Letrazole helps girls and mamas, reduce cancer's return, and defend the Ta-tas!"

©2013 I CAN Publishing®, Inc.

E strogen levels are ⬇ which may halt progression of estrogen-sensitive breast cancer

S afety not established in children and lactating mothers

T he A's are UE: anxiety, abdominal pain, anorexia, arthralgia

R eport the UE to provider of care

O mit pregnancy due to risks involved

This is Femara the warrior. She knows how to shield against breast cancer! She's no girly-girl, keeping **ESTRO**gen at bay!

IMMUNOSUPPRESSIVE AGENT (IMURAN)

Action: Produces immunosuppression by inhibiting purine synthesis in cells.

Indications: Renal tranplants to prevent graft refection, refractory rheumatoid arthritis, refractory ITP, glomerulonephritis, nephrotic syndrome, bone marrow transplant

Warnings: Hypersensitivity. Precautions with severe renal disease or hepatic disease. Elderly.

Undesirable Effects: GI: nausea, vomiting, stomatitis, pancreatitis, hepatotoxicity; HEMA: Leukopenia, thrombocytopenia, anemia, pancytopenia; INTEG: Rash, alopecia; MS: Arthralgia, muscle wasting; MISC: Serum sickness, Raynaud's symptoms.

Other Specific Information: Do not mix with other drugs. **(Imuran)** Leukopenia can result when taken with ACE inhibitors; cotrimoxazole, myelopoiesis. Decreased immune response when taken with vaccines. Decreased action of warfarin. Increased myelosuppression with cyclosporines and antineoplastics. Increased action of azathioprine when taken with allopurinol. Immunosuppression may result when taken with astragalus, echinacea, or melatonin.

Interventions: Assess for infection: increased temperature, WBC; sputum, urine. Assess for rheumatoid arthritis, pain, mobility, ROM; I&O, weight every day, report oliguria; Blood studies: Hgb, WBC, platelets during treatment monthly; if leukocytes are < 3000/mm³ or platelets < 100,000/mm³, drug should be discontinued. Monitor for hepatotoxicity such as dark urine, jaundice, itching, light-colored stools, increased LFTs; drug should be discontinued. Monitor LFTs: alk phosphatase, AST, ALT, bilirubin. Assess for arthritis: pain; location, ROM, swelling, before and during treatment. All medications po if possible, avoiding IM injections, since bleeding may occur. Administer po with meals to reduce GI upset. For IV route, prepare in biologic cabinet using gown, gloves, mask.

Education: Educate client to take as prescribed, do not miss any dose. If dose is missed on qd regimen, skip dose; if on multiple dosing/day, take as soon as remembered. Therapeutic response may take 3–4 mo. In rheumatoid arthritis; to continue with prescribed exercise, rest, other medication. Report rash, fever, diarrhea that is severe, chills, sore throat, fatigue, due to the fact that serious infections may occur. Instruct client to use contraceptive measures during treatment and for 12 wks after finishing treatment. Avoid vaccinations. Reduce risk of infection by avoiding crowds. Use soft-bristled toothbrush to prevent bleeding.

Evaluation: Absence of graft rejection; immunosuppression in autoimmune disorders.

Drugs: azathioprine (Imuran), tacrolimus (Prograf), cyclosporine (Sandimmune), mycophenolate (CellCept)

IMURAN

I muran, Prograf, Sandimmune, Cellcept—
lessen or prevent immune response

M onitor CBC and liver enzymes

U ses: organ transplantation and autoimmune diseases

R eport fever of 99° farenheit or higher, skin rash, joint pain,
swelling of lymph glands

A dvise to give oral forms with meals

N o liver vaccines

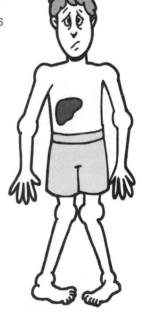

COLONY STIMULATING FACTORS

Action: Erythropoietin is one factor controlling rate of red cell production; drug developed by recombinant DNA technology. Stimulates production of red blood cells. Amino acid polypeptide.

Indications: Anemia resulting from reduced endogenous erythropoietin production, primarily end-stage renal disease; anemia due to AZT treatment in HIV clients; anemia due to chemotherapy.

Warnings: Hypersensitivity to mammalian cell-derived products, or human albumin, uncontrolled hypertension.

Undesirable Effects: Hypertensive encephalopathy, seizures; headache; joint pain

Other Specific Information: Need for increased anticoagulant during hemodialysis

Interventions: Assess renal studies; urinalysis, protein, blood, BUN, creatinine. Blood studies; ferritin, transferrin monthly. Evaluate for rising blood pressure as Hct rises; antihypertensives may be needed. Report drop in urine output less than 50 ml/hour. Administer only IV or Subcutaneously.

Education: Avoid driving or hazardous activity during beginning of treatment. Monitor Blood pressure. Take iron supplements, vitamin B12, folic acid as directed.

Evaluation: Client will have an increase in the reticulocyte count in 1–6 weeks, Hgb/Hct. Client will have an increased appetite and enhanced sense of well-being.

Drug: epoetin (EPO, Epogen, erythropoietin, Procrit); darbepoetin (Aranesp)

PROCRIT

P roduces erythropoietin

R ed blood cells ↑ (Epogen, Procrit, Aranesp)

O$_2$↑ ; decreases fatigue, weakness, SOB

C hemotherapy, cancer

R equires frequent HCTs for dosage adjustment

I V or SQ injection only

T hree times weekly

GRANULOCYTE COLONY-STIMULATING FACTOR

Action: Stimulates proliferation and differentiation of neutrophils.

Indications: To decrease infection in clients receiving antineoplastics that are myelosuppressive; to increase WBC in clients with drug-induced neutropenia; bone marrow transplantation. Investigational uses: Neutropenia in HIV infection.

Warnings: Hypersensitivity to proteins of E. coli. Pregnancy, lactation, cardiac conditions, children, myeloid malignancies.

Undesirable Effects: RESP: Respiratory distress syndrome; CNS: Fever; HEMA: Thrombocytopenia; INTEG: Alopecia, exacerbation of skin conditions; MS: Osteoporosis, skeletal pain; GI: Nausea, vomiting diarrhea, anorexia.

Other Specific Information: Do not use these agents concomitantly with antineoplastics.

Interventions: Assess blood studies: CBC, platelet count before treatment and twice weekly; neutrophil counts may be increased for 2 days after therapy. Assess B/P, respirations, pulse before and during therapy. Assess bone pain, give mild analgesics.

Education: Instruct client on the technique for self-administration: dose, side effects, disposal of containers and needles; provide written instructions.

Evaluation: Absence of infection.

Drugs: fil**grastim** (**Neu**pogen), pegfil**grastim** (**Neu**lasta)

NEUPOGEN

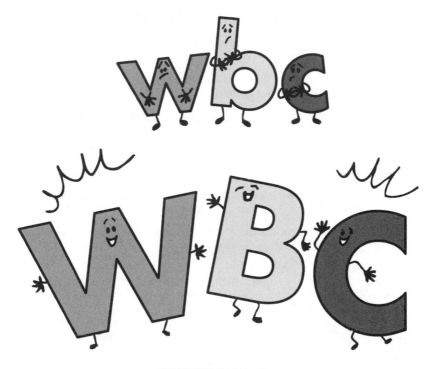

Neupogen is used to increase "new" white blood cells. The "NEU" will assist you in remembering this drug category.

GRANULOCYTE MACROPHAGE COLONY-STIMULATING FACTOR: SARGRAMOSTIM (LEUKINE)

Action: Acts on the bone marrow to increase the production of white blood cells (neutrophils, monocytes, macrophages, eosinophils).

Indications: Increases bone marrow function after bone marrow transplant. Used in treatment of failed bone marrow transplant.

Warnings: Contraindicated if clients are allergic to yeast products, or additives (mannitol, tromethamine, or sucrose); Products containing benzyl alcohol should not be used in newborns. Use cautiously in clients with heart disease, hypoxia, peripheral edema, or pleural or pericardial effusion. Use cautiously in clients with cancer of the bone marrow.

Undesirable Effects: Headache; fever; diarrhea, weakness, rash, malaise; arthralgia, bone pain, and myalgia; leukocytosis, thrombocytosis.

Other Specific Information: Lithium or corticosteroids may potentiate myeloproliferative effects of sargramostim (concurrent use should be undertaken cautiously).

Interventions: Monitor HR, BP, RR during and immediately after infusion. If dyspnea occurs, slow infusion rate by half. Reassess; med may need to be discontinued. Assess for peripheral edema daily throughout therapy. Monitor for first-dose reaction (flushing, hypotension, syncope, weakness). Assess for fever daily during therapy. Assess for arthralgias and myalgias, usually occur in lower extremities, which tend to occur when granulocyte counts are returning to normal. Treat discomforts with analgesics. Monitor renal and hepatic function before and biweekly throughout therapy in clients with renal or hepatic dysfunction. May cause ↑ BUN, creatinine, and hepatic enzymes. May cause ↓ serum albumin concentrations. Monitor for symptoms of undesirable effects and notify healthcare provider. Monitor CBC two times per week during treatment. Reduce dose or interrupt treatment for absolute neutrophil count > 20,000/mm^3, platelets > 500,000/mm^3. Sargramostim should not be agitated and should not be combined with other drugs. Administer by IV infusion.

Education: Instruct client to notify healthcare provider if dyspnea or palpitations occur.

Evaluation: Absence of infection. WBC and differential within normal ranges. Acceleration of bone marrow recovery.

Drugs: sargramostim (Leukine)

SARGRAMOSTIM

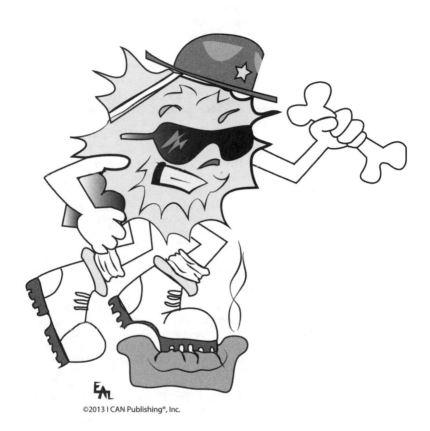

"Sarg."(Sergeant) RAM-O-STIM," is a WBC that is called to duty by the Granulocyte Macrophage Colony Stimulating Factor.

THROMBOPOIETIC GROWTH FACTORS
OPRELVEKIN (INTERLEUKIN-II, NEUMEGA)

Action: Increases the production of platelets.

Indications: Decreases thrombocytopenia and the need for platelet transfusions in clients receiving chemotherapy.

Warnings: Contraindicated in clients who have cancer of the bone marrow because they may stimulate tumor growth. Use cautiously in clients with heart failure and pleural effusion. Renal disease.

Undesirable Effects: Allergic reactions, possible anaphylaxis; fluid retention (peripheral edema, dyspnea on exertion); cardicac dysrhythmias (tachycardia, atrial fibrillation, atrial flutter); conjunctival injection, transient blurring of vision, papilledema; GI: anorexia, constipation, diarrhea, dyspepsia, nausea, oral moniliasis, vomiting; alopecia, ecchymoses, rash; chills, fever, infection, pain.

Other Specific Information: No significant drug-drug interactions, but do NOT combine with other medications. Diuretics can result in hypokalemia, which can be fatal.

Interventions: Assess for signs of fluid retention (dyspnea on exertion, peripheral edema) during therapy. Fluid retention is a common side effect that usually resolves within several days following discontinuation of oprelvekin. Monitor platelet count prior to and periodically during therapy, especially at expected nadir. Therapy is continued until postnadir platelet count is > 50,000/mm^3. Monitor CBC prior to and at regular intervals during therapy. Decrease in hemoglobin concentration, hematocrit, and RBC count may occur due to increased plasma volume (dilutional anemia); usually begins within 3-5 days of therapy and is reversible within a week of discontinuation of therapy. Monitor electrolyte concentrations in client receiving chronic diuretic therapy due to risk of developing hypokalemia which may be fatal. May cause an ↑ in plasma fibrinogen. Therapy should be started within 6-24 hours after completion of chemotherapy and continued for 10-21 days. Treatment should be discontinued at least 2 days prior to next planned chemotherapy cycle. Subcutaneous: Reconstitute with 1 ml of sterile water for injection without preservatives for a concentration of 5 mg/ml. Direct diluents to sides of vial and swirl gently. Solution is clear and colorless. Do not administer solutions that are discolored or contain particulate matter. Do not shake or agitate vigorously. Do not freeze or reuse vials. Administer within 3 hr of reconstitution as a single injection in abdomen, hip, thigh, or upper arm. Administer once daily by subcutaneous injection until platelet count reaches prescribed level.

Education: Teach client about proper technique for preparation and administration. Provide a puncture–resistant container for disposal of needles. Discuss the importance of reporting any transient blurred vision or dizziness. Caution to avoid driving or other activities requiring alertness until response to medication is assessed and determined. Advise healthcare provider if pregnancy is planned or suspected. Review undesirable effects.

Evaluation: Platelet count greater than or equal to 50,000/mm^3 in postnadir.

Drugs: oprelvekin (Interleukin –II, Neumega)

THROMBOPOIETIC GROWTH FACTORS

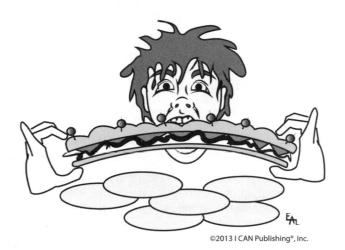

©2013 I CAN Publishing®, Inc.

S ubcutaneous injection once daily

U ndesirable effects: fluid retention, cardiac dysrhythmias, allergic reaction

B one cancer – oprelvekin is contraindicated

C onjunctival infection, transient blurring of vision, papilledema

U ndesirable effect of hypokalemia if receiving diuretic therapy (can be fatal)

T he CBC, platelet count, and electrolytes should be monitored

Here's an easy way to increase our plates (Platelets): Cut that sub! ("SUB-CUT")

HYDROXYUREA (HYDREA)

Action: Sickle cell anemia supplemental agent and antineoplastic agent. Increases production of fetal hemoglobin in sickle cell disease. Interferes in DNA synthesis, useful in treatment of many cancers.

Indications: Reduces frequency of vaso-occlusive pain crisis and need for blood transfusions in sickle cell anemia. Treatment of multiple carcinomas, including chronic myelocytic leukemia; ovarian cancer; and melanomas. Unlabeled uses: Used for treating HIV infections as a part of antiretroviral therapy.

Warnings: Carcinogenic agent that can cause infertility and birth defects. Caution with severe anemia-should be corrected before starting treatment. Caution in liver disease and renal impairment.

Undesirable Effects: Decreased WBCs and platelets, hepatotoxicity, secondary leukemia after treatment, GI effects (nausea, vomiting, diarrhea, poor appetite), dizziness, gangrene, hair loss, rashes, infertility, birth defects.

Other Specific Information: Some products contain tartrazine (FDC yellow dye #5) and should be avoided in clients with hypersensitivity.

Interventions: Monitor CBC, renal function, liver function, uric acid before and throughout therapy. Protect self from exposure to the medication, wearing gloves when handling. Adjust dose for renal insufficiency.

Education: Teach client to wear gloves when handling capsules and wash hands before and after contact. Advise on contraception for females of childbearing age-high risk of birth defects during use. Teach to notify provider of signs of infection or thrombocytopenia, including sore throat, fever, bruising, and bleeding. Recommend supplemental folic acid for sickle cell clients to prevent deficiency. For sickle cell disease, teach about lifestyle changes to improve quality of life and decrease complications-daily hydration, balanced nutrition, regular sleep pattern, and stress management.

Evaluation: Sickle cell clients will experience fewer pain crisis and require fewer blood transfusions within 18 months of starting medication. Clients with hematologic illnesses or carcinomas will go into remission.

Drug: hydroxyurea (Droxia, Hydrea, Mylocel)

HYDROXYUREA (HYDREA)

S ickle Cell Anemia supplemental agent

C ancer treatment; antineoplastic agent

A dvise to use contraception, as there is a high risk for birth defects

R enal and Liver function must be monitored

E ducate client on handling capsules; use gloves and handwashing before and after taking medication

D ecreases WBC's and platelets; danger of infection, bleeding and bruising

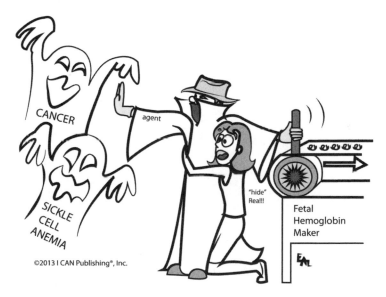

©2013 I CAN Publishing®, Inc.

This "agent" is going to "hide-Rea" (Hydrea), who is **SCARED** of having Sickle cell anemia or cancer. The agent is here to help by increasing the production of fetal hemoglobin and interfering with DNA synthesis. Note, the agent has on gloves to remind you to wear gloves when handling capsules.

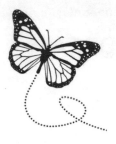

Courage is not the absence of fear, but rather the judgment that something else is more important than fear.

AMBROSE REDMOON

Anti-Inflammatory Agents

Editors' Note: *While we have made every effort to include the most up-to-date information regarding these agents, several of these medications were still under investigation for possible increased risk factors at the time of publication.*

—Loretta and Sylvia

NONSTEROIDAL ANTI-INFLAMMATORY DRUGS (NSAIDs)

Action: Inhibits prostaglandin synthesis; resulting in analgesic, anti-inflammatory, and antipyretic activities.

Indications: To reduce fever and inflammatory process. Musculoskeletal disorders (e.g., rheumatoid arthritis and osteoarthritis); analgesic for mild to moderate pain.

Warnings: Do NOT give if client is allergic to salicylates or NSAIDs, renal or hepatic disease, asthma, peptic ulcer, bleeding disorders, systemic lupus erythematosus (SLE). Caution with the elderly.

Undesirable Effects: Refer to next page.

Other Specific Information: ↑ the risk of bleeding with oral anticoagulants. ↑ effects of lithium. ↓ effect of loop diuretics; ↓ antihypertensive effects of beta blockers.

Interventions: Monitor CBC, renal and liver function tests. Observe client for bleeding. (Refer to education.)

Education: Instruct client to take with meals. Avoid alcohol and consult with provider about other meds. Advise not to take aspirin or acetaminophen when taking an NSAID. No driving or activities requiring motor response until certain there is no dizziness. Inform dentist and other providers of drug therapy. Discontinue these meds 5 to 7 days before any major procedure or surgery. Report if temperature does not subside, bleeding occurs, or inflammation does not decrease. Periodic eye exams for long-term therapy.

Evaluation: Client will have pain relief, decreased temperature, and improved mobility without undesirable effects from drugs.

Drugs: diclofenac (Voltaren); diflunisal (Dolobid); etodolac (Lodine); fenoprofen (Nalfon); flurbiprofen (Ansaid); ibuprofen (Advil, Medipren, Motrin, Nuprin); indomethacin (Indocin); ketoprofen (Orudis, Oruvail); ketorolac (Toradol); meclofenamate (Meclomen); meloxicam (Mobic); nabumetone (Relafen); naproxen (Aleve, Anaprox, Naprosyn); oxaprozin (Daypro); piroxicam (Feldene); sulindac (Clinoril); tolmetin (Tolectin)

NSAIDS

N o alcohol

S E: "BIRTH"—see below

A spirin sensitivity—do not give

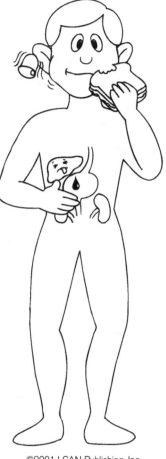

I nhibits prostaglandins

D o take with food

S top 5–7 days before surgery

©2001 I CAN Publishing, Inc.

Some side effects include **B**one marrow depression, **I**ncreased GI distress, **R**enal toxicity, **T**innitus and **H**epatotoxicity. Just think that NSAIDs can cause the "death" of inflammation, pain and fever, but the "birth" of undesirable effects.

NONSTEROIDAL ANTI-INFLAMMATORY DRUGS: COX$_2$ INHIBITORS

Action: Inhibition of prostaglandin synthesis, primarily through inhibition of cyclooxygenase-2 (COX$_2$). This results in anti-inflammatory, analgesic, and antipyretic activities.

Indications: Osteoarthritis, rheumatoid arthritis, acute pain in adults.

Warnings: Hypersensitivity; allergic-type reactions to sulfonamides; asthma; urticaria, or allergic-type reaction after taking aspirin or other NSAIDs. GI ulceration, bleeding, or perforation; renal/hepatic; disease; anemia; fluid retention, hypertension, or heart failure; pregnancy/lactation. Bextra can cause Steven-Johnson type reaction.

Undesirable Effects: Refer to next page.

Other Specific Information: Ace Inhibitors and furosemide given concurrently with these drugs may have ↓ effects. Aspirin may result in ↑ rate of GI ulceration. Fluconazole may ↑ celebrex levels. Lithium levels may ↑ when given with celebrex. Warfarin may have ↑ risk of bleeding with celebrex predominantly in the elderly.

Interventions: Monitor CBC, liver/renal function tests, and for signs and symptoms of GI bleeding.

Education: Instruct to take with food or meals. Educate client regarding the importance of reporting any signs of GI bleeding or ulceration, skin rash, weight gain or edema, tinnitus, headache, blurred vision, fever, or chills to the health care provider. If visual or CNS disturbances occur, discuss safety measures. Review comfort measures to decrease pain and inflammation (i.e., positioning, warmth, rest, etc.). (Refer to "**NSAIDs**".)

Evaluation: Client will have pain relief, decreased temperature, or improved mobility without undesirable effects.

Drugs: celecoxib (Celebrex); valdecoxib (Bextra)

COX$_2$ INHIBITORS

N o alcohol

S E: "BIRTH"—see below

A spirin sensitivity—do not give

I nhibits COX$_2$ enzyme

D o take with food

S top 5–7 days before surgery

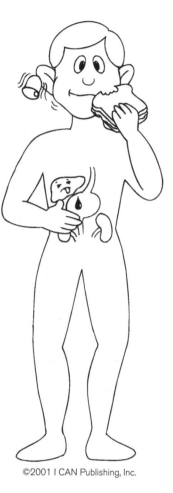

©2001 I CAN Publishing, Inc.

Some side effects include **B**one marrow depression, **I**ncreased GI distress, **R**enal toxicity, **T**innitus and **H**epatotoxicity. Just think that NSAIDs can cause the "death" of inflammation, pain and fever, but the "birth" of undesirable effects.

MOBIC

Action: Decreases pain and inflammation associated with osteoarthritis. (Nonsteroidal anit-inflammatory drug)

Indications: Relief of signs and symptoms of osteoarthritis and rheumatoid arthritis(including juvenile rheumatoid arthritis).

Warnings: Contraindicated in clients that may have severe renal impairment or peri-operative pain from coronary artery bypass graft. Needs to be cautious in clients that have cardiovascular disease or risk factors for cardiovascular disease. Clients that may have coagulation disorders.

Undesirable Effects: GI bleeding, Nausea, vomiting, abdominal pain, and gas; Steven-Johnson Syndrome, bleeding may be prolonged. May cause anemia. Pruritus.

Other Specific Information: Mobic may alter the effects of Lithium. May interfere with ace inhibitors and Lasix resulting in hypertension.

Interventions: Evaluate BUN, serum creatinine, CBC, and liver function periodically.

Education: Educate/Inform client to take medication with a full glass of water and remain in an upright position for at least 15 minutes after administration. Avoid use of alcohol, aspirin, acetaminophen or other OTC medications while taking this medication.

Evaluation: Relief of pain and improved joint mobility.

Drugs: meloxicam (Mobic)

MOBIC "MOBY DICK"

M obility of joints is improved

O T C medications should be avoided

B leeding may be prolonged

I nform to take with full glass of water

C B C, creatinine and LFT, monitor

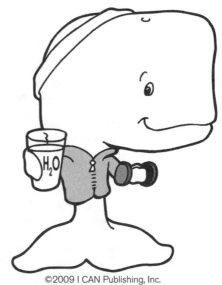

©2009 I CAN Publishing, Inc.

Moby Dick the whale remembers to take his Mobic with a full glass of water and sits upright for 15 minutes afterwards.

ACETAMINOPHEN

Action: Inhibits the synthesis of prostaglandins that may operate as mediators of pain and fever, primarily in the CNS.

Indications: Mild pain. Fever.

Warnings: Contraindicated if there was a previous hypersensitivity. Products containing alcohol, aspartame, saccharin, sugar, or tartrazine should be avoided if client has hypersensitivity to these compounds. Caution in hepatic/renal disease, alcohol abuse, and/or clients who are malnourished.

Undesirable Effects: Hepatic failure or hepatotoxicity if overdose occurs. Renal failure if use high doses or chronic use. Neutropenia, leukopenia, pancytopenia; rash, urticaria.

Other Specific Information: Doses of greater than 2 g/day may increase risk of bleeding with warfarin. (PT should be assessed on a routine basis and INR should not exceed 4). Other hepatotoxic substances if given with acetaminophen may result in hepatotoxicity such as concurrent use of substances containing alcohol. Concurrent use of isoniazid, rifampin, rifabutin, phenytoin, barbiturates, and cabamazepine may result in acetaminophen-induced liver damage and decrease the effects of acetaminophen. NSAIDs taken along with acetaminophen may increase the risk of adverse renal effects. Propranolol may decrease the metabolism and may increase effects.

Interventions: Assess health status and alcohol usage prior to administering acetaminophen. Administer with a glass of water. May be taken with food or on an empty stomach. Assess amount, type and frequency of OTC drugs. Prolonged use increases risk of undesirable renal effects. Do not exceed the recommended dose. Assess characteristics of pain 30-60 min. prior to and after administration. Assess temperature and note presence of associated signs such as diaphoresis, tachycardia, and malaise. Evaluate renal, hepatic, and hematologic function. Increase in the serum bilirubin, LDH, AST, ALT and prothrombin time may indicate hepatotoxicity. If overdose occurs, acetylcysteine (Mucomyst) is the antidote.

Education: Review the importance of taking exactly as prescribed. Advise not to exceed 4 G / day. Avoid alcohol (3 or more glasses per day increase risk of liver damage). Instruct to observe for signs of bleeding. Inform parents regarding importance of checking concentrations of liquid preparations. Errors may result in liver damage. Discuss with clients with diabetes that acetaminophen may alter results of blood glucose monitoring. Notify provider of care if discomfort or temperature is not relieved by routine dose or if T > 103 degrees F or lasts longer than 3 days.

Evaluation: Client will experience a relief of mild pain and / or a reduction in the fever.

Drugs: acetaminophen (Abenol, Acephen, Aceta, Aminofen, Apacet, APAP, Apo-Acetaminophen, Aspirin Free Anacin, Aspirin Free Pain Relief, Children's Pain Reliever, Dapacin, Feverall, Extra Strength Dynafed E.X., Extra Strength Dynafed (Billups, P.J.), Genapap, Genebs, Halenol, Infant's Pain Reliever, Liquiprin, Mapap, Maranox, Meda, Neopap, Novo-Gesic, Oraphen-PD, Panadol, paracetamol, Redutemp, Ridenol, Silapap, Tapanol, Tempra, Tylenol, Uni-Ace)

ACETAMINOPHEN

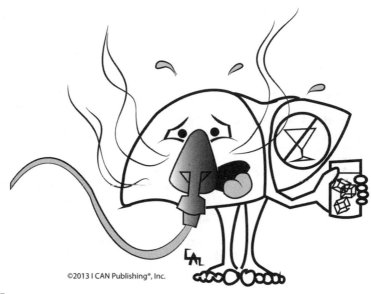

©2013 I CAN Publishing®, Inc.

L ook for diaphoresis, tachycardia and malaise

I ntake of one glass of water is recommended

V ia nebulizer, administer Mucomyst - the antidote for O.D.

E rrors in dosing may result in liver damage

R enal disease, alcohol abuse and hepatic disease - use cautiously

ANTIGOUT: ALLOPURINOL (ZYLOPRIM)

Action: Reduces production of uric acid by inhibiting xanthine oxidase.

Indications: Gout, recurrent calcium oxalate stones, secondary hyperuricemia which may occur during treatment of leukemia and tumors.

Warnings: Hypersensitivity, renal disease, hepatic disorder.

Undesirable Effects: Anorexia, nausea, vomiting, diarrhea, stomatitis; dizziness, headache; rash, pruritus; metallic taste; retinopathy; bone marrow depression.

Other Specific Information: Alcohol and antacids ↓ effectiveness. Amoxicillin or ampicillin may ↑ incidence of skin rash. Thiazide diuretics ↑ the risk of reactions and ↓ effect. ↑ effect of warfarin, phenytoin, theophylline, anticancer drugs, and ACE inhibitors.

Interventions: Monitor renal and liver functions (i.e., BUN, serum creatinine, ALP, AST, and ALT), serum uric acid levels, and CBC prior to initiating therapy, and periodically during therapy. (Refer to Education.)

Education: Increase fluids. May take 1 or more weeks for full therapeutic response. Administer drug following meals; encourage fluid intake (3000 ml/day); monitor intake and output (urinary output should be at least 2000 ml/day). Low purine food intake. Advise to avoid alcohol, caffeine, and large doses of vitamin C. Contact provider if any undesirable effects occur. Recommend a yearly eye examination since visual changes may occur from prolonged use of allopurinol. Driving or activities requiring alertness should be avoided until the response to the medication has been determined.

Evaluation: Client will experience a decrease in joint tenderness, swelling, redness, and fewer acute gout attacks.

Drug: allopurinol (Zyloprim)

GOUT

G ulp 10–12 glasses (8 oz.) of fluid daily
I distress–undesirable effect

O utput and input–monitor closely

U ric acid production decreased
se no alcohol

T ake after meals

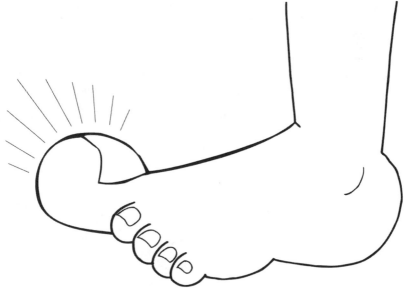

©2001 I CAN Publishing, Inc.

COLCHICINE

Action: Decreases leukocyte motility, phagocytosis, lactic acid production, resulting in decreased urate crystal deposits, inflammatory process.

Indications: Antigout during an initial or acute exacerbation. This may arrest the progression of neurological disability in multiple sclerosis.

Warnings: Severe gastrointestinal, renal, hepatic, or cardiac disorders; blood dyscrasias.

Undesirable Effects: Oliguria, anemias, hypersensitivity, nausea, vomiting, anorexia, diarrhea, cramps.

Other Specific Information: NSAIDs may increase risk of GI distress and anemias. Decrease action of B12.

Interventions: Monitor intake and output. Monitor CBC every 3 months. Evaluate for signs of toxicity including: weakness, abdominal pain, and nausea and vomiting, diarrhea. Discontinue if client experiences weakness, abdominal pain, nausea, vomiting, diarrhea.

Education: Recommend taking with food. Only taken PO or slow IVP (2–5 minutes); never mix with D_5W. Avoid any OTC preparation containing alcohol. Report pain, rash, sore throat, bleeding, and/or weakness to the provider of care.

Evaluation: The client will have a decrease stone formation exemplified on x-ray and decrease in the pain in the kidney and/or joints.

Drugs: colchicine; febuxostat (Uloric)

COLCHICINE

A lcohol is out

C uts down on effects of B 12
supplements

U ndesirable effects—oliguria, anemia,
nausea, vomiting, anorexia, diarrhea

T ake with food

E xacerbation—gout

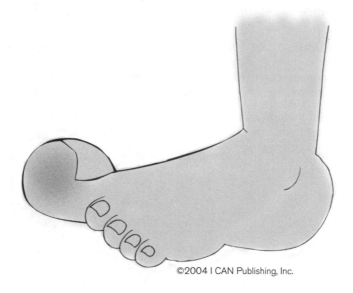

ULORIC

Action: Xanthine oxidase inhibitor that reduces the production of uric acid in the body.

Indications: High blood concentrations of uric acid.

Warnings: Contraindicated in hypersensitivity; pregnant; being treated with azathioprine (Azasan, Imuran), mercaptopurine (Purinethol), or theophylline (Elixophyllin, TheoCap, Theochron, Uniphyl). Use cautiously with kidney disease, liver disease, diabetes, heart disease, cancer, Lesch-Nyhan syndrome, a history of heart attack or stroke, or if client has ever received an organ transplant.

Undesirable Effects: *Less serious:* Uloric undesirable effects may include: nausea; joint pain, swelling, or stiffness; mild skin rash; or dizziness. *Late and serious undesirable effects include*: hives; difficulty breathing; swelling of the face, lips, tongue, or throat; chest pain or heavy feeling, pain spreading to the arm or shoulder, nausea, sweating, general ill feeling; sudden numbness or weakness, especially on one side of the body; sudden headache, confusion, problems with vision, speech, or balance; or nausea, stomach pain, low fever, loss of appetite, dark urine, clay-colored stools, jaundice (yellowing of the skin or eyes).

Other Specific Information: Theophylline (Elixophyllin, TheoCap, Theochron, Uniphyl) may result in a drug interaction.

Interventions: Client may have an increase in gout symptom flares when first starting to take Uloric. For best results, have client keep taking the medication as directed. Provider may prescribe other gout medications to use during the first 6 months of treatment with Uloric.

Education: Instruct client to store Uloric at room temperature away from moisture and heat. Instruct how to safely take Uloric.

Evaluation: Client will experience less pain and a reduction of uric acid in the body.

Drugs: febuxostat (Uloric)

ULORIC

Too much uric acid?
Don't just store it!
Sweep-clean your blood,
And use Uloric!

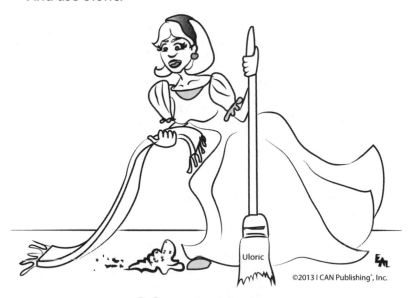

©2013 I CAN Publishing®, Inc.

M ercaptopurine

A zathioprine

T heophylline

Don't forget to check the "M.A.T.!" (Contraindicated
with these drugs!)

DEMARDS II–
MAJOR BIOLOGIC DMARDS

Action: Binds to tumor necrosis factor (TNF) and makes it inactive. TNF is a mediator of inflammatory response.

Indications: Decrease progression, signs and symptoms of rheumatoid arthritis, juvenile arthritis, ankylosing spondylitis, psoriatic arthritis, or plaque psoriasis when response has been inadequate to other disease-modifying agents.

Warnings: Hypersensitivity. Sepsis; Untreated Infections; Wegener's granulomatosis (receiving immunosuppressive agents); Concurrent cyclophosphamide or ankainra. Use cautiously in pre-existing or recent demyelinating disorders (multiple sclerosis, myelitis, optic neuritis); History of tuberculosis (increased risk of reactivation); Underlying chronic diseases which may predispose to infections (advanced or poorly controlled diabetes); Latex allergy (needle cover of diluents syringe contains latex); Geriatrics may experience increase risk of infections. Children with significant exposure to varicella virus.

Undesirable Effects: Headaches, dizziness, weakness; rhinitis, pharyngitis; upper respiratory tract infection, cough; Injection site reactions; Infections, Increase risk of maglignancies.

Other Specific Information: Use with anakinra ↑ risk of serious infections. Use of cyclophosphamide may ↑ risk of malignancies. May ↓ the antibody response to live-vaccine and ↑ risk of adverse reactions.

Interventions: Assess range of motion, characteristics of swelling, and pain in affected joints prior to and periodically throughout therapy. Assess injection sites for reaction (pain, itching, erythema, swelling). Reactions are typically mild to moderate and last 3-5 days following injection. Discontinue therapy in clients who develop a serious infection or sepsis. Needle cover of the pre-filled syringe contains latex and should not be handled by individuals with latex allergies. Solution in pre-filled syringe may be allowed to reach room temperature (15-30 min); do not remove needle cap during this time. May be injected into abdomen, thight, or upper arm. Rotate sites. Do not administer within 1 inch of an old site or into area that is tender, red, hard, or bruised. Do not mix with other solutions or dilute with other diluents.

Education: Instruct client on technique for self-administration. Review importance of not receiving live vaccines during therapy. Advise parents that children should not receive meds until immunizations complete. Clients with consistent exposure to varicella virus (chickenpox) should DC therapy temporarily and consider administering varicella immune globulin. Advise clients that analgesics, methotrexate, NSAIDs, corticosteroids, and salicylates may be continued during therapy.

Evaluation: Client will experience a ↓ in the symptoms of rheumatoid arthritis.

Drugs: Abatacept (Orencia), Adalimumab (Humira), Etanercept (Enbrel), Infliximab (Remicade), Rituximab (Rituxan)

DMARDS

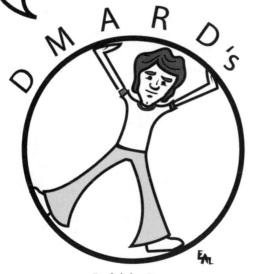

"Darn Medicine Alters Resistance Dude!"

latex allergy

for arthritis

immune system; high risk for Infections and URI's

to infection is reduced

Danger if exposed to varicella or live vaccines

Bubble Boy

Keep him in the DMARD's bubble because he is immunocompromised on this medicine!

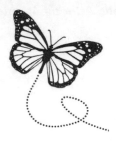

Do not go where the path may lead, go instead where there is no path and leave a trail.

RALPH WALDO EMERSON

The elevator to success is out of order. You'll have to use the stairs … one step at a time.

JOE GIRARD

Gastrointestinal Agents

ANTACIDS

Action: Neutralizes gastric acid; decreases pepsin activity.

Indications: Hyperacidity, peptic ulcer, reflux esophagitis.

Warnings: Hypersensitivity to aluminum products, hypophosphatemia, renal failure, obstructive bowel disease, CHF or HTN (Na Citrate). In renal failure, avoid products containing magnesium.

Undesirable Effects: Constipation (Aluminum), diarrhea (Magnesium). Hypercalcemia (in calcium-based antacids); hypermagnesemia (magnesium-calcium containing antacids); hypophosphatemia (long term, aluminum-containing antacids); systemic alkalosis, sodium overload, and rebound acid production (sodium preparation). Renal calculi; all may accumulate in clients with renal failure.

Other Specific Information: Bind, inactivate and/or decrease the absorption of many drugs (too numerous to include total list in this book). Of significant importance is the ↓ in absorption of antibiotics, digoxin, isoniazid, phenothiazine, phenytoin, quinidine.

Interventions: Monitor urinary pH, calcium, electrolytes, and phosphate levels. Record amount and consistency of stools. Clients on low - sodium diets should evaluate sodium content of antacids. (Refer to education)

Education: Instruct to shake suspension well before taking, follow with water. Take 1-3 hours after meals. Do not take within 1-2 hours of other medications. Do not take within 1-2 hours of eating fiber-rich foods. Do not combine with other antacids, calcium supplements (if using calcium-based antacid), or large amounts of caffeine or alcohol. Take calcium carbonate with large amounts of water or orange juice. Advise client to avoid foods or liquids that can cause gastric irritation.

Evaluation: Client will experience relief of heartburn or be absent of pain with no undesirable effects.

Drugs: *Aluminum-based agents:* ALternaGel; Amphogel. *Magnesium-based agents:* Milk of Magnesia. *Aluminum and Magnesium:* Gaviscon; Maalox; Mylanta; Riopan, Riopan Plus. *Calcium-based agents:* Citracal;Titrilac; Tums. *Sodium-based agents:* Sodium Citrate (Bicitra)

AUNT ACID'S FAMILY

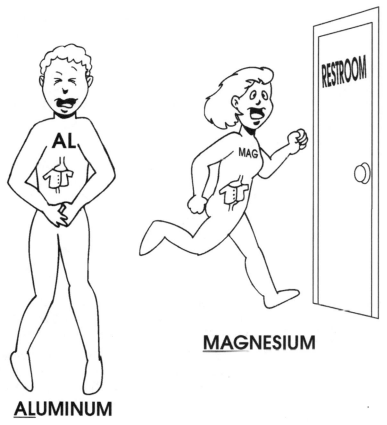

MAGNESIUM

ALUMINUM

©2001 I CAN Publishing, Inc.

Mag and Al have a history of an ulcer. While the ant-acids, may help in coating their stomachs, they may also experience undesirable effects. **Al's** problem is constipation. **Mag** has a problem with diarrhea.

ANTI-ULCER MEDICATIONS: H₂ HISTAMINE ANTAGONISTS

Action: Reduces gastric acid secretions; prevents histamine-induced acid release by competing with histamine for H2 receptors in the stomach.

Indications: Hypersecretion of stomach acids, gastroesophageal reflux, short-term treatment of duodenal ulcers, long-term prophylaxis of duodenal ulcer, prevention of upper GI bleed in critically ill clients.

Warnings: Hypersensitivity; caution with administering cimetidine in clients > 50 years old with renal or liver failure.

Undesirable Effects: Confusion, headache; nausea, diarrhea or consipation; depression; rash; blurred vision. Hepatic/renal toxicity—more profound with cimetidine. Blood dyscrasias are rarely seen.

Other Specific Information: Cimetidine ↑ serum concentrations of many drugs by inhibiting liver P450 enzymes: oral anticoagulants, theophylline, lidocaine, phenytoin, benzodiazipines, nephedipine, propranolol, procainamide. ↓ absorption of ketoconazole. ↓ absorption with antacids.

Interventions: Monitor GI discomfort. Periodic evaluation of blood counts, gastric acid secretion tests, and renal and hepatic function tests. Be alert that the elderly need a decrease in the drug dosage.

Education: Avoid antacids for 1 hour before taking drug. Advise to take with meals. Take Zantac, Pepcid, or Axid at 6pm for better suppression of nocturnal acid secretion. To assist in ↓ acid reflux, advise client to elevate the head of the bed with 6 inch blocks during sleep; wear loose clothing; no meal intake 2 hours prior to hs; eliminate caffeine, alcohol, harsh spices, chocolate, peppermint from diet; stop smoking; no ASA or NSAIDS. Notify provider of blood in emesis or stool or an increase in the abdominal pain.

Evaluation: Peptic ulcer disease eradicated in 4–8 weeks. GERD eradicated in 6–12 weeks. Client will be free of discomfort with no undesirable effects from the medication.

Drugs: *(These drugs end in "dine".)* cimeti**dine** (Tagamet); famoti**dine** (Pepcid); nizati**dine** (Axid); raniti**dine** (Zantac)

NO WINE, JUST DINE

D on't take with antacids

I nform provider of bleeding

N o smoking, alcolhol or NSAIDs

E levate head of bed

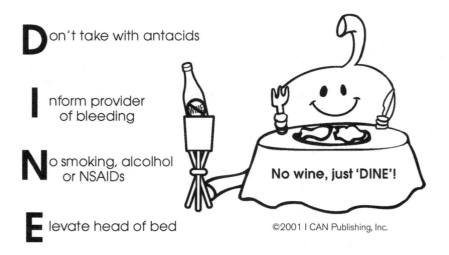

No wine, just 'DINE'!

©2001 I CAN Publishing, Inc.

CIMETI**DINE**
FAMOTI**DINE**
NIZATI**DINE**
RANITI**DINE**

CHOLINERGIC BLOCKERS (ANTICHOLINERGICS)

Action: Blocks cholinergic receptor sites so response to acetylcholine is decreased.

Indications: Bradycardia and heart block; gastrointestinal disorders related to increased motility and secretion (peptic ulcers, diverticulitis, ulcerative colitis); urinary spasms; Parkinson's disease (may also be used to treat extrapyramidal symptoms associated with administration of Thorazine); dilates pupils of the eye. Preoperatively to decrease secretions and vagal stimulation.

Warnings: Glaucoma, myasthenia gravis, obstructive GI disorders, prostatic hypertrophy, children less than 3 years of age; elderly.

Undesirable Effects: Dilated pupils, distended bladder, dry mucous membranes, constipation, increased heart rate.

Other Specific Information: ↑ anticholinergic effect with anti-depressants, MAOIs, and phenothiazines.

Interventions: Monitor VS, report ↑ HR; monitor for constipation, oliguria. Atropine could result in CNS stimulation (confusion, excitement), or drowsiness.

Education: Instruct to take 30 minutes before meals; eat foods high in fiber and drink plenty of fluids. Avoid OTC antihistamines. Instruct client not to drive a motor vehicle or participate in activities requiring alertness. Advise to use hard candy, ice chips, etc. for dry mouth. Recommend artificial tears.

Evaluation: The client will experience symptomatic relief with no undesirable effects.

Drugs: atropine (Isopto Atropine); benztropine mesylate (Cogentin); dicyclomine (Bentyl); glycopyrrolate (Robinul); procyclidine (Kemadrin); propantheline (Pro-Banthine); scopolamine (Isopto Hyoscine, Transderm-Scop); trihexyphenidyl (Artane)

ANTICHOLINERGICS

Can't pee
Can't see
Can't spit
Can't sh*t

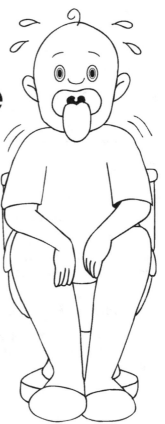

PROTON PUMP INHIBITOR

Action: Suppresses the final step in gastric acid production by forming a covalent bond to two sites of the (H^+, K^+)-ATPase enzyme system at the surface of the gastric parietal cell. This results in an increase in the gastric pH, reducing gastric acid production.

Indications: Short-term treatment of erosive esophagitis associated with gastroesophageal reflux disease (GERD). Omeprazole–Long-term treatment of active duodenal ulcer. Maintenance of erosive esophagitis. Treatment of H. Pylori (with amoxicillin), active benign gastric ulcers. Prevacid and Protonix are available in IV. May see off-label use for stress ulcer prophylaxis and GI bleed. Prevacid IV must be administered with a filter. Both may be given as a continuous infusion.

Warnings: Hypersensitivity; pregnancy/lactation; safety and efficacy of pantoprazole for maintenance therapy beyond 16 weeks have not been established.

Undesirable Effects: Headache, dizziness, diarrhea, abdominal discomfort, flatulence.

Other Specific Information: May ↑ concentration of oral anticoagulants, diazepam, phenytoin when administered with omeprazole. No clinically relevant interactions with pantoprazole.

Interventions: Monitor for GI symptoms or headache.

Education: Take omeprazole before meals; pantoprazole once or twice a day. Instruct client to report headache to the provider of care. Emphasize the importance of only remaining on the pantoprazole for a maximum of 16 weeks. Omeprazole may need to be taken for up to 8 wks. Regular medical follow-ups are important for evaluation.

Evaluation: Client should experience relief of gastrointestinal symptoms.

Drugs: ome**prazole** (Prilosec); panto**prazole** (Protonix), lanso**prazole** (Prevacid), rabe**prazole** (Aciphex), esome**prazole** (Nexium)

PROTON PUMP INHIBITOR

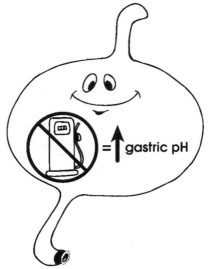

©2001 I CAN Publishing, Inc.

P rilosec—only p. o.

U E: headache, G I disturbances

M aximum of 16 weeks for Protonix

P rotonix—can be given IV
revacid

PEPSIN INHIBITOR: CARAFATE

Action: Forms a protective covering on the ulcer surface, protecting ulcer from acid, bile salts, and pepsin; also inhibits pepsin activity in gastric juices.

Indications: Short-term treatment of duodenal ulcers (up to 8 weeks); NSAID or aspirin induced GI symptoms; prevention of stress ulcers in critically ill clients.

Warnings: Hypersensitivity, renal failure, pregnancy, lactation.

Undesirable Effects: Dizziness, nausea, constipation.

Other Specific Information: ↓ effectiveness of ciprofloxacin, norfloxacin, penicillamine, phenytoin. Altered absorption with antacids. Risk of aluminum toxicity with aluminum-containing antacids.

Interventions: Monitor the characteristics of the abdominal pain, renal function, fluid and electrolytes, and gastric pH (> 5 is desired).

Education: Instruct to administer drug on an empty stomach. Administer antacids 30 minutes before or after sucralfate. Allow 1 to 2 hours between sucralfate and other medications; sucralfate binds with certain drugs, reducing the effect of the drugs. Instruct to take drug as ordered. It usually takes 4–8 weeks for optimal ulcer healing. Recommend fluid, fiber, and exercise to decrease constipation. Recommend no smoking and no foods and liquids that can cause gastric distress. Report pain or vomiting of blood.

Evaluation: Client will be free of pain and will experience no undesirable effects of med.

Drug: sucralfate (Carafate)

CARA

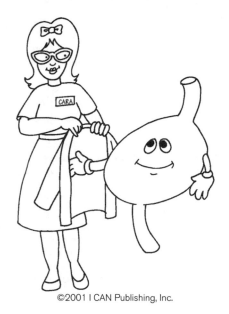

©2001 I CAN Publishing, Inc.

C onstipation—undesirable effect

A dminister on an empty stomach

R isk of aluminum toxicity with aluminum antacids

A dminister antacids 30 min. before or after med.

Cara is holding the coat that goes on the stomach. Carafate will form a protective coating on the ulcer surface. It protects against pepsin and acid.

PROSTAGLANDIN E ANALOG

Action: Acts as an endogenous prostaglandin in the GI tract to decrease acid secretion, to increase the secretion of bicarbonate and protective mucus, and to produce vasodilation to maintain submucosal blood flow. This will prevent gastric ulcers.

Indications: Long-term use of NSAIDs to prevent gastric ulcers. Prostaglandin E Analog is also used for duodenal ulcers. (Unlabeled use)

Warnings: Pregnancy. Use extreme caution when used for cervical ripening (unlabeled use) may cause uterine rupture; risk factors are late trimester pregnancy, previous cesarean section or uterine surgery or ≥ 5 previous pregnancies.

Undesirable Effects: Abdominal pain and diarrhea. Women may experience spotting along with dysmenorrhea. May result in a miscarriage.

Other Specific Information: Increased risk of diarrhea with magnesium-containing antacids.

Interventions: Assess client routinely for epigastric or abdominal pain and for occult blood in the stool, emesis, or gastric aspirate. Misoprostol is usually begun on 2nd or 3rd day of menstrual period following a negative pregnancy test. **Do not confuse Cytotec (misoprostol) with Cytoxan (cyclophosphamide).** Misoprostol therapy should be initiated at the onset of treatment with NSAIDs. Administer at bedtime and with meals to decrease severity of diarrhea. Antacids may be administered prior to or after misoprostol for relief of pain. Avoid those containing magnesium due to increased risk with diarrhea with misoprostol.

Education: Instruct clients to notify provider of symptoms of diarrhea and abdominal pain. May need to reduce dosage. Instruct to notify provider if spotting and dysmenorrheal occur. Medication may be needed to be discontinued. Teach to take misoprotol with meals and at bedtime. Avoid alcohol and foods that may increase GI irritation.

Evaluation: Clients, who are receiving chronic NSAID therapy, will not experience a gastric ulcer.

Drug: misoprostol (Cytotec)

PROSTAGLANDIN E ANALOG (CYTOTEC)

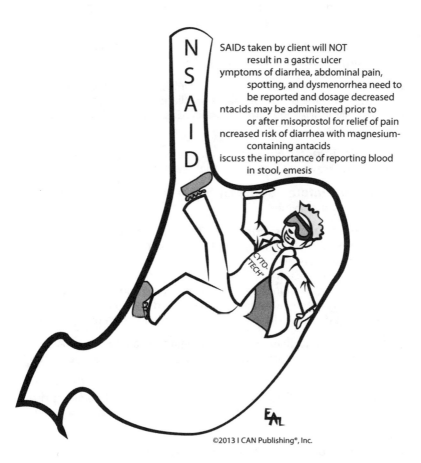

N SAIDs taken by client will NOT
result in a gastric ulcer
S ymptoms of diarrhea, abdominal pain,
spotting, and dysmenorrhea need to
be reported and dosage decreased
A ntacids may be administered prior to
or after misoprostol for relief of pain
I ncreased risk of diarrhea with magnesium-
containing antacids
D iscuss the importance of reporting blood
in stool, emesis

This Cyto - "technician" is blocking the stomach from the irritation caused by NSAIDs.

Anti-Emetic: Zofran

Action: Blocks the effects of serotonin at 5-HT$_3$ - receptor sites (selective antagonist) located in vagal nerve terminals and the chemoreceptor trigger zone in the CNS.

Indications: Prevention of nausea and vomiting associated with chemotherapy or radiation therapy.

Warnings: Hypersensitivity; orally disintegrating tablets contain aspartame and should not be used in clients with phenylketonuria. Use cautiously in liver impairment (daily dose not to exceed 8 mg); abdominal surgery.

Undesirable Effects: Headache, dizziness; constipation, diarrhea, increased liver enzymes; extrapyramidal reactions.

Other Specific Information: May be affected by drugs altering the activity of the liver enzymes.

Interventions: Do not confuse Zofran (ondansetron) with Zosyn (piperacillin/tazobactam). Assess for nausea, vomiting, abdominal distention, and bowel sounds before administering and during treatment. Assess client for extrapyramidal effects (facial grimacing, rigidity, Involuntyary movements, shuffling walk, trembling of hands) during therapy. Monitor AST/ALT and serum bilirubin during treatment. First dose is adminstered prior to chemotherapy.

Education: Instruct client to take ondansetron as directed. Advise client to noitfy HCP immediately if involuntary movement of eyes, face, or limbs occurs.

Evaluation: The client will not experience nausea and vomiting due to radiation, initial and repeat courses of chemotherapy, and/or during the postoperative period.

Drug: ondansetron (Zofran), granisetron (Kytril)

ANTI-EM

A ction: blocks the effects of serotonin at
5-HT$_3$-receptor sites (selective antagonist)

N ausea/vomiting from
chemotherapy or
radiation (prevents)

T ake before chemotherapy

I nteractions with drugs
that affect AST/ALT

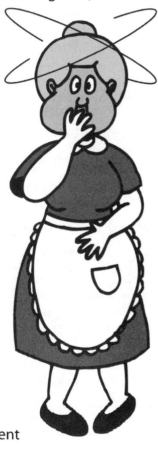

E xtrapyramidal effects:
undesirable effect and
must REPORT!

M onitor AST/ALT during treatment

LAXATIVES: STIMULANT/EMOLLIENT

Action: *Stimulant:* Increases peristalsis by direct effect on colonic smooth musculature. Laxative effect is a result of the promotion of fluid and ion accumulation in the colon. *Emollient:* Softens stools by increasing the water and fat penetration in the intestines.

Indications: Constipation, Evacuation of colon for bowel examination, rectal, and/or elective colon surgery. Stool softener; facilitates passage of stools. Prevention of constipation in cardiac/post surgical procedures.

Warnings: Hypersensitivity, fecal impactions, intestinal/biliary obstruction, nausea and vomiting, acute hepatitis, appendicitis, and/or acute surgical abdomen.

Undesirable Effects: Nausea, anorexia, cramping, and/or diarrhea.

Other Specific Information: *Stimulant:* Gastric irritation if taken with antacids, H2-blockers, and gastric proton pump inhibitors, and milk. *Emollient:* If taken with mineral oil, may result in toxicity.

Interventions: Monitor intake and output, bowel sounds, and serum electrolytes, and/or abdominal pain and cramping.

Education: *Emollients:* May take up to 3 days to soften stools. Take tablets whole. Do not take for long term therapy. *Both:* Report cramping, weakness, dizziness, and an increase in being thirsty. Inform provider if constipation is unrelieved or symptoms of electrolyte imbalance occur: muscle cramps, pain, weakness, dizziness, excessive thirst. Teach family and client that normal bowel movements do not always occur daily.

Evaluation: Client will have regular bowel movements with no constipation or straining.

Drug: *Stimulant:* bisacodyl (Carter's Little Pills, Dulcolax, Dacodyl, Feen-a-mint, Fleet Laxative, Therelax). *Emollient:* docusate calcium (Surfax, DC Softgels); docusate sodium (Colace, Ex-Lax, Modane, Silace)

COLACE

Cause of constipation (fluids, bulks, decrease exercise)

Dulc**O**lax—most common drug producing bowel stimulation

F**L**uid—increase intake

T**A**ste bitter; give in milk or juice to mask

Cardiac/surgical procedures—to minimize straining

Electrolytes

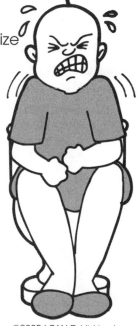

©2005 I CAN Publishing, Inc.

BULK-FORMING: METAMUCIL

Action: Bulk-forming laxative by drawing water.

Indications: Chronic constipation.

Warnings: Hypersensitivity, abdominal discomfort, fecal impaction, intestinal obstruction.

Undesirable Effects: Anorexia, cramps, nausea, vomiting, diarrhea, intestinal obstruction if not taken with adequate water.

Other Specific Information: ↓ absorption of aspirin, oral anticoagulant, digoxin, nitrofurantoin.

Interventions: Monitor VS, I & O, signs of fluid and electrolyte imbalance, and bowel sounds. Assess cause of constipation.

Education: Instruct to mix the drug in 8-10 oz. of water, stir, and drink immediately. Do not swallow in dry form. Follow drug with 1 extra glass of water. Instruct client to drink a minimum of eight 8 oz. glasses of water per day and to increase foods high in fiber. Review the nonpharmacologic methods for decreasing constipation. Review the importance of not becoming a habitual user of laxatives.

Evaluation: Client will have regular bowel movements with no constipation.

Drug: psyllium (Metamucil)

SILLY PSYLLIUM

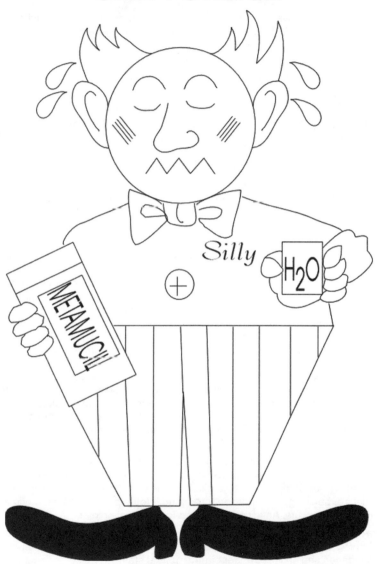

Silly got his name by taking psyllium (Metamucil) with a jigger of water instead of a BIG glass of water. Now he's sweating because this bulk-forming laxative that expands has bulked his bow tie instead of his stool.

LAXATIVES: LACTULOSE

Action: Increases water content and softens the stool. Lowers the pH of the colon, which inhibits the diffusion of ammonia from the colon into the blood, resulting in a reduction in the blood ammonia levels.

Indications: Chronic constipation in adults and geriatric clients. Adjunct in the management of portal-system (hepatic) encephalopathy (PSE). Decreased blood ammonia levels with improved mental status in PSE.

Warnings: Contraindicated in clients on low-galactose diets. Use cautiously in clients with Diabetes Mellitus; excessive or prolonged use (may lead to dependence); OB, Lactation, Pediatric clients (safety has not been determined.

Undesirable Effects: Belching, cramps, distention, flatulence, diarrhea; hyperglycemia (diabetic clients).

Other Specific Information: Should not use with other laxatives in the treatment of hepatic encephalopathy (unable to evaluate optimal dose of lactulose). Anti-infectives may diminish effectiveness in treatment of hepatic encephalopathy.

Interventions: Assess client for abdominal distention, presence of bowel sounds, and normal bowel function. Assess color, consistency, and amount of stool produced. For PSE: Assess orientation and/or level of consciousness prior to and periodically during course of therapy. Will decrease blood ammonia concentrations by 25-50%. May cause increased blood glucose levels in diabetic clients. Monitor serum electrolytes periodically. May cause diarrhea with can result in hypokalemia and hypernatremia. When used in hepatic encephalopathy, dosage should be adjusted until client averages 2-3 soft bowel movements per day. During the initial therapy, 30-45 ml may be administered hourly to induce rapid laxation. Darkening of solution does not alter potency. PO: Mix with fruit juice, water, milk, or carbonated citrus beverage to enhance flavor. Administer with a full glass (240 ml) of water or juice. May be administered on an empty stomach for more rapid results. Dissolve single dose packets in 4 oz of water. Solution should be colorless to slightly pale yellow. Rect: To administer enema, use rectal balloon catheter. Mix 300 ml of water or 0.9% NaCl. Enema should be retained for 30-60 min.

Education: Encourage clients to adapt other forms of bowel regulation such as increasing fluid intake, increasing bulk and fiber in diet, and increasing ambulation and activity. Caution clients that this medication may result in flatulence, belching, or abdominal cramping. Notify provider if this continues or if diarrhea occurs. Anticipate the need for low-protein diet.

Evaluation: Client will experience the passage of a soft, formed stool, usually within 24-48 hours. Client will experience the clearing of confusion, apathy, and irritation and an improvement in the mental status in PSE.

Drugs: lactulose (Cephulac, Cholac, Chronulac, Constilac, Constulose, Duphalac, Enulose, Evalose, Heptalac, Kristalose, Lactulax, Lactulose PSE, Portalac)

LACTULOSE (LAXATIVE)

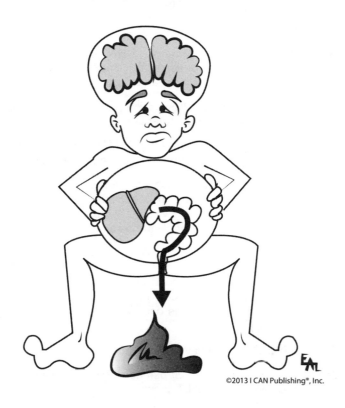

©2013 I CAN Publishing®, Inc.

P SE and constipation are indications

O rientation (LOC) should be monitored

O utput (stool) and electrolytes should be monitored

ANTIDIARRHEAL: LOMOTIL

Action: Inhibits gastric motility.

Indications: Acute diarrhea.

Warnings: Child < 2; pregnancy; elderly; antibiotic associated colitis or ulcerative colitis; hepatic/renal disease; glaucoma; electrolyte imbalance. Do not use if client has C. diff.

Undesirable Effects: Drowsiness, dizziness, constipation, dry mouth, blurred vision, urinary retention.

Other Specific Information: Alcohol, MAO inhibitors, antihistamines, narcotics, and sedative-hypnotics may interact with drugs.

Interventions: During the history, determine cause of diarrhea. Monitor stools for frequency and consistency, bowel sounds, I & O, vital signs, and electrolytes. Evaluate hydration especially in the very young and very old. Report if client has a narcotic drug history.

Education: Encourage clear liquids. Avoid OTC drugs and alcohol. Avoid activities requiring alertness, motor activities, until response to drug is evaluated. Notify provider for diarrhea that persists longer than 2 days, high fever, blood in stool, or acute abdominal pain. Advise client that these drugs can be habit forming, so only take the prescribed dose.

Evaluation: Client will have no diarrhea.

Drugs: *(C-V Controlled Substance)* diphenoxylate with atropine (Logen, Lomanate, Lomotil, Lonox)

ANTIDIARRHEALS

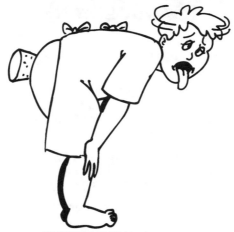

©1999 I CAN Publishing, Inc.

D rowsiness, dizziness, dry mouth, dehydration

I nhibits gastric mobility

A lcohol is OUT!

R eport if there is a narcotic drug history

R esponse of drug determined prior to driving

H abit-forming; only take prescribed dose

E lectrolytes—monitor with severe diarrhea; encourage clear liquids

A ssess frequency of bowel movements; bowel sounds

ANTIDIARRHEAL: OCTREOTIDE (SANDOSTATIN)

Action: Suppresses secretion of serotonin and gastroenterohepatic peptides. Increases absorption of fluid and electrolytes from the GI tract and increases transit time.

Indications: Severe diarrhea and flushing episodes in clients with GI endocrine tumors, including metastatic carcinoid tumors and vasoactive intestinal peptide tumors. Unlabeled use: Management of diarrhea in clients with AIDS or with fistulas.

Warnings: Contraindicated in hypersensitivity. Use cautiously in Gallbladder disease; Renal impairment; Hyperglycemia or hypoglycemia; Fat malabsorption may be aggravated; Pregnancy or lactation.

Undesirable Effects: Dizziness, drowsiness, fatigue, headache, weakness; visual disturbances; orthostatic hypotension, palpitations; abdominal pain, cholelithiasis, diarrhea, nausea, vomiting; hyperglycemia, hypoglycemia. May cause a slight $\uparrow$ in the liver enzymes. May cause a $\downarrow$ in the serum thyroxine (T_4) levels.

Other Specific Information: May alter insulin or oral hypoglycemic requirements. May $\downarrow$ blood levels of cyclosporine.

Interventions: Assess frequency and characteristics of stools and bowel movements during therapy. Assess HR and BP prior to initiating therapy. Evaluate client's fluid and electrolyte balance and skin turgor for dehydration/hypovolemia. Assess client for hypoglycemia if diabetic. May require a decrease in insulin and sulfonylureas and treatment with diazoxide. Review for gallbladder disease; assess for pain and assess ultrasound examinations of gallbladder and bile ducts prior to and during prolonged therapy. Do not use solution that contains particulate matter or that is discolored. Ampules should be refrigerated but may be stored at room temperature for the time they will be used. Discard any solution that is not used.

Education: Instruct client that this medication may result in dizziness, drowsiness, or visual disturbances. Avoid driving or other activities that require alertness until cognitive response to drug has been determined. Review the importance of changing positions slowly to decrease risk of orthostatic hypotension. Review correct technique for administering at home. Review importance to take as prescribed. Do not double up on doses.

Evaluation: Client will experience a decrease in severity of diarrhea and improvement of electrolyte imbalances.

Drugs: octreotide (Sandostatin)

OCTREOTIDE/SANDOSTATIN (ANTIDIARRHEAL)

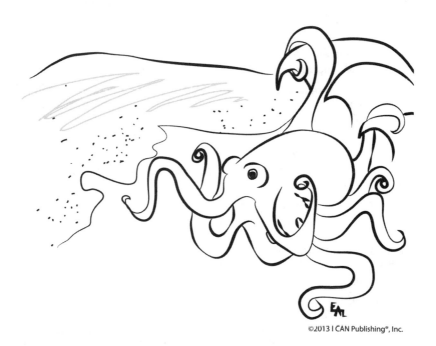

"Octreo-Tide"

Octreo-octopus is doing the unthinkable! She's holding back the tide of diarrhea! The Sand-o-statin will absorb the moisture (fluids and electrolytes) from the GI tract to decrease diarrhea!

PROKINETIC AGENT
METOCLOPRAMIDE (REGLAN)

Action: Controls nausea and vomiting by blocking dopamine and serotonin receptors in the chemoreceptor trigger zone (CTZ) of the central nervous system. Stimulates motility of the upper GI tract and accelerates gastric emptying.

Indications: Prevention of chemotherapy induced emesis. Treatment of postsurgical and diabetic gastric stasis. Facilitation of small bowel intubation. Management of GERD and gastroparesis.

Warnings: Contraindicated in clients with GI perforation, GI bleeding, bowel obstruction, and hemorrhage. History of seizure disorder. Pheochromocytoma; Parkinson's disease. Use cautiously in children and older adults due to risk for extrapyramidal side effects (EPS).

Undesirable Effects: Drowsiness, extrapyramidal symptoms, tardive dyskinesia; diarrhea, restlessness; neuroleptic malignant syndrome; dry mouth, hypotension.

Other Specific Information: Additive CNS depression may occur if taken concurrently with other CNS depressants, including alcohol, antidepressants, opioid analgesics and sedative/hypnotics. May decrease the absorption of other orally administered drugs as a result of effect on GI motility. Anticholinergics and opioids may decrease the effects of metoclopramide.

Interventions: Monitor clients for CNS depression, EPS, and neuroleptic malignant syndrome. Assess hepatic function test results. May cause an increase in the serum prolactin and aldosterone concentrations. Monitor the client's bowel function and for signs of dehydration. Medication may be given IV or orally.

Education: Instruct client that drug may cause drowsiness. Caution to avoid driving or other activities requiring alertness until medication response has been established. Recommend to avoid concurrent use of alcohol, other CNS depressants, and medications with anticholinergic effects while taking this medication. Discuss the importance of reporting any involuntary movement of eyes, limbs, or undesirable effects to provider of care.

Evaluation: Client will experience no nausea and vomiting, a decrease in the symptoms of gastric stasis, and decrease in the symptoms of esophageal reflux.

Drugs: metoclopramide (Reglan)

METOCLOPRAMIDE (REGLAN)

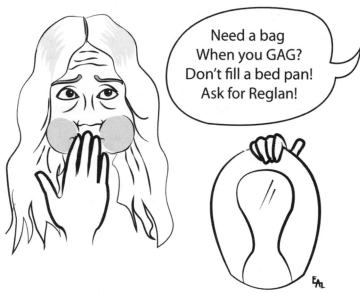

Need a bag
When you GAG?
Don't fill a bed pan!
Ask for Reglan!

N ausea and vomiting are controlled

A ccelerates gastric emptying

U ndesirable Effects: Tardive Dyskinesia, drowsiness

S tay away from anticholinergics and opioids; no alcohol or CNS depressants

E ducate about no driving until mental alertness determined

A ssess for CNS depression and EPS

ALOSETRON (LOTRONEX)

Action: Selective blockade of 5-HT$_3$ receptors, which innervate the viscera and result in increased firmness in stool. This will decrease the urgency and frequency of defecation.

Indications: Female clients with irritable bowel syndrome with diarrhea that has lasted more than 6 months and has been resistant to conventional treatment.

Warnings: Chronic constipation, history of bowel obstruction, Crohn's disease, ulcerative colitis, impaired intestinal circulation or thrombophlebitis.

Undesirable Effects: Constipation which may cause GI complications such as impaction, perforation, bowel obstruction, or ischemic colitis.

Other Specific Information: Medications that induce cytochrome P450 enzymes such as phenobarbital may decrease levels of alosetron.

Interventions: Clients must sign a treatment agreement and meet specific criteria to be treated with this medication. Dosage may start as once a day, and then may be increased to BID.

Education: Review the importance of observing for rectal bleeding, bloody diarrhea, or abdominal pain and report to provider of care. Medication should be discontinued. Discuss with client that symptoms should subside within 1 to 4 weeks, but will return 1 week after medication is discontinued.

Evaluation: Client should experience relief of diarrhea and a decrease in urgency.

Drugs: alosetron (Lotronex)

ALO-SET-RON

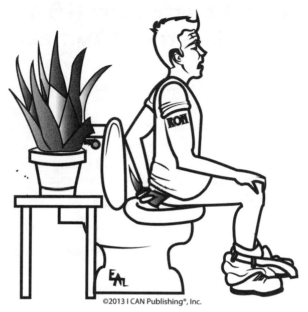

©2013 I CAN Publishing®, Inc.

L asting more than 6 months with diarrhea from IBS, nothing else helping; makes one a candidate for this drug.

O nce a day to start medication, then increase to BID.

O bserve for rectal bleeding, bloody diarrhea, or abdominal pain, and report to care provider.

S tool firmness as a result of the selective blockade of 5-HT3 receptors (which innervate the viscera).

E nzymes induced by medications (P450/ phenobarbital) may decrease levels of Alosetron.

IRRITABLE BOWEL SYNDROME WITH CONSTIPATION (IB-C): LUBIPROSTONE (AMITIZA)

Action: Increases fluid secretion in the intestine to promote intestinal motility.

Indications: Irritable bowel syndrome with constipation; chronic constipation.

Warnings: Contraindicated if a client has a history of bowel obstruction, Crohn's disease, ulcerative colitis, or diverticulitis

Undesirable Effects: Nausea and diarrhea

Other Specific Information: No significant interactions

Interventions: Monitor frequency of stools. Notify provider if severe diarrhea occurs.

Education: Instruct client to take medication with food. Oral dose should be taken BID.

Evaluation: Client should be relieved of constipation.

Drugs: lubiprostone (Amitiza)

LUBI-PRO-STONE (AMITIZA)

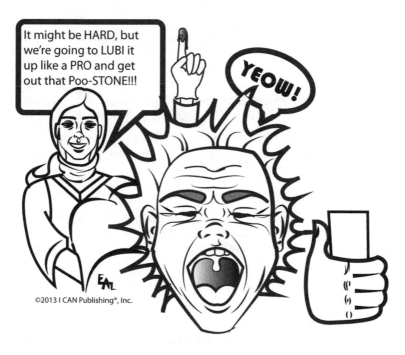

It might be HARD, but we're going to LUBI it up like a PRO and get out that Poo-STONE!!!

YEOW!

©2013 I CAN Publishing®, Inc.

H istory of bowel obstruction:
DO NOT GIVE DRUG!

A ction: Increases fluid secretion in the
intestine - promotes intestinal motility.

R eview: The importance of taking medication
with food.

D iarrhea may be an undesirable effect; report
to provider of care.

5-AMINOSALICYLATES
SULFASALAZINE (AZULFIDINE)

Action: Decreases inflammation by inhibiting prostaglandin synthesis.

Indications: Inflammatory bowel disease: Crohn's disease, ulcerative colitis

Warnings: Contraindicated if sensitive to sulfonamides, salicylates, and/or thiazide diuretics. Use with caution in clients with kidney, liver disease or blood dyscrasias.

Undesirable Effects: Agranulocytosis, hemolytic and macrocytic anemia.

Other Specific Information: No significant interactions.

Interventions: Administer in 4 divided dosages in a 24 hour period. Monitor client's complete blood count. *(The 5 part train: The Engine and 4 Doses on next page will assist you in remembering this information.)*

Education: Advise client to report sore throat and to have CBC monitored.

Evaluation: Client will demonstrate evidence of decreased bowel inflammation and bowel function will return to normal.

Drug: sulfasalazine (Azulfidine)

5-AMINOSALICYLATES
SULFASALAZINE (AZULFIDINE)

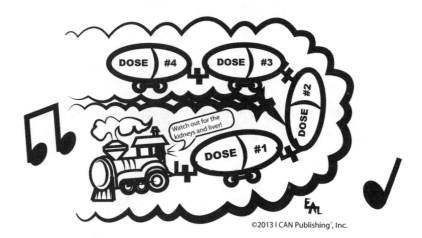

©2013 I CAN Publishing®, Inc.

(To the tune of "Down by the Station")
"Decreases inflammation; inhibits prostiglandins...
Check the CBC; as you go...
Give in 4 doses; watch the cleansing organs...
Chug-chug, choo-choo! Now he can go!"

(To the tune of "Little Red Caboose")
"Sulfa-sala-zine! Sulfa-sala-zine!
Sulfa-sala-zine behind the train!
Sore-throat coming back, back, back, back...
Anemia on the track, track, track, track...
Sulfa-sala-zine behind the train!"

5- Aminosalicylates (5 part train; the engine and 4 doses). Sulfasalazine (Asulfidine) give in 4 divided doses. It moves down the G.I. track decreasing inflammation...

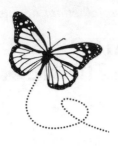

There is no medicine like hope, no incentive so great, no tonic so powerful as the hope of a better tomorrow.

UNKNOWN

Endocrine
Agents

CORTICOSTEROIDS

Action: Synthesized by adrenal cortex. Exhibits antiinflammatory properties; suppresses the normal immune response. Increases carbohydrate, fat, and protein metabolism.

Indications: Antiinflammatory; immunosuppressant; dermatological disorders; replacement in adrenal cortical insufficiency.

Warnings: Hypersensitivity; PUD; tuberculosis, fungal infections or any suspected infection; HIV; blood clotting disorders; renal hepatic impairment; cardiac disease, congestive heart failure, hypertension; diabetes mellitus; geriatric client, and postmenopausal women.

Undesirable Effects: Undesirable effects rarely seen with short-term high dose or replacement therapy. "**CUSHING**" will help you in recalling effects that may occur with long-term use. Cushing-like symptoms (moon-face, excess fat deposits at trunk, wasting of arms and legs—refer to Cushy Carl on next page). To assist you in remembering that the sodium ↑, potassium ↓, glucose ↑, and calcium levels ↓, refer to next page.

Other specific information: ↑ risk of hypokalemia with diuretics, amphotericin B, ticarcillin. ↓ effects of antidiabetics, vaccines, potassium supplements. May ↑ digoxin toxicity (due to hypokalemia).

Interventions: Monitor VS, BP, weight, blood glucose, electrolytes, EKG, and TB skin test results.

Education: Instruct to administer oral drugs with food or milk early in the morning; withdraw medication slowly. Follow-up visits and lab tests are essential. Avoid infection. Taper off gradually under medical supervision. Report visual disturbance or severe GI distress, sudden weight gain, swelling, sore throat, fever, or signs of infection. Wounds may heal slowly. Avoid crowds and known infection. Do not receive vaccination. Don't take aspirin or any medication without consulting provider. Discuss a diet low in sodium, high in vitamin D, protein and potsassium. Inform provider of therapy. Don't overuse. For topical applications, apply after shower. Do not cover. Avoid sun light on treated area. Recommend wearing a medical alert tag.

Evaluation: The client will experience an improvement in the underlying condition for which the corticosteroids were given and will have no undesirable effects.

Drugs: *(Many of these end in "one")* **Topical:** alclometas**one** (Acolvate); amcinonide (Cyclocort); betamethas**one** (Celest**one**, Dipros**one**, Uticort, Valis**one**–O, IV, IL, IA); clobetasol (Temovate); cortis**one** (Cort**one**–O); desoride (Tridesil**one**); desoximetas**one** (Topicort); dexamethas**one** (Decadron–O, IM, IV, OP, IN, IH); fluocinol**one** (Synalar, Synemol); flurandrenolide (Cordran); fluticas**one** (Cutivate, Flonase–IN); halcinonide (Halog); halobetasol (Ultravate); hydrocortis**one** (Cort-Dome, Cortef, Hydrocort**one**, Solu-Cortef–O, IM, IV, SubQ, R); mometas**one** (Elocon); prednicarbate (Dermatop); **Inhalation, intranasal:** beclomethas**one** (Beclovent, Vanceril, Beconase, Vancenase); budesonide (Rhinocort–IN only); flunisolide (Aerobid, Nasalide); triamcinol**one** (Azmacort, Kenalog, Nasacort–O); **Oral:** fludrocortis**one** (Florinef); methylprednisol**one** (Medrol, Solu-Medrol–IM, IV); prednisol**one** (Delta-Cortef, Hydeltra, Hydeltrasol –IM, IV, IL, IA); prednis**one** (Deltas**one**, Meticorten, Oras**one**). **Ophthalmic:** fluoromethol**one** (FML); rimexol**one** (Vexol).

Key: Intraarticular = IA, Inhalation = IH, Intralesional = IL, Intramuscular = IM, Intranasal = IN, Intravenous = IV, Oral = O, Ophthalmic = OP, Rectal = R, Subcutaneous = SubQ

CUSHY CARL

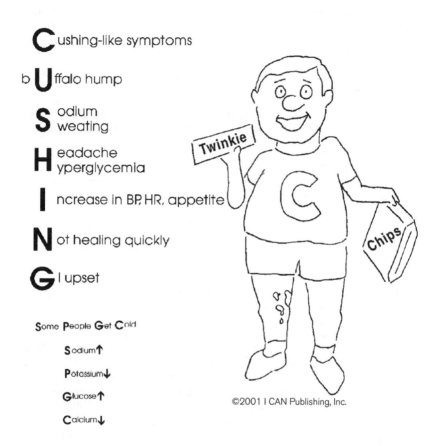

C ushing-like symptoms

b **U** ffalo hump

S odium
     weating

H eadache
     yperglycemia

I ncrease in BP, HR, appetite

N ot healing quickly

G I upset

Some People Get Cold

S odium ↑

P otassium ↓

G lucose ↑

C alcium ↓

©2001 I CAN Publishing, Inc.

Cushy Carl has taken cortisone for a long time and illustrates some of the undesirable effects with his moon face, buffalo hump, and delay in wound healing (sore on leg). Twinkies and chips are a no-no! **"Some People Get Cold"** is a way to help you remember some lab changes that can occur with **"Cushy Carl"**. The labs would be opposite for Addison's Disease.

THYROID PREPARATIONS

Action: Increases the metabolic rate, oxygen consumption, and body growth.

Indications: Hypothyroidism, myxedema, cretinism.

Warnings: Thyrotoxicosis, MI, cardiovascular disease, hypertension, renal disease. Caution in the elderly client.

Undesirable Effects: Vomiting, diarrhea, weight loss; tachycardia, palpitations, angina; nervousness, tremors, irritability, insomnia; menstrual irregularities, sweating, heat intolerance.

Other Specific Information: ↓ effects of antidiabetic agents and digtialis preparation. ↑ effects of oral anticoagulants, sympathomimetics, and antidepressants. ↓ absorption with cholestyramine, colestipol.

Interventions: Monitor serum T_3, T_4, and TSH levels. Obtain baseline vital signs and weight to compare with future assessments. If converting levothyroxine po to IV while in hospital, the IV dose should be 1/2 the oral dose!

Education: Advise client that within 3–4 days there should be improvement and the maximum effect is usually in 4–6 weeks. Teach to take a single daily dose on an empty stomach before breakfast. Do not discontinue without consulting provider. Review the importance of lifelong replacement (even when symptoms improve). Keep scheduled appointments to have periodic blood tests and medical evaluation. Instruct to report signs and symptoms of hypothyroidism (T, P, and BP are usually decreased) and hyperthyroidism (tachycardia and palpitations usually occur). Instruct how to take pulse and to hold medication if > 100. Do not change brands since they are not bioequivalent. Instruct client to have a medic alert tag, card, or bracelet in case of emergency.

Evaluation: The client will be involved in the activities of daily living without becoming tired. Adequate thyroid hormone levels will be attained.

Drugs: levothyroxine T_4 (Eltroxin, Levothroid, Levoxyl, Synthroid)

MORBID MATILDA

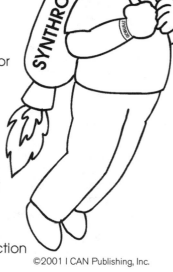

T SH, T_3, T_4—monitor

H ypo/hyperthyroidism—monitor

R eview how to take a pulse

O bserve clinical improvement
in 3—4 days

I ncrease metabolic rate—action

©2001 I CAN Publishing, Inc.

D o NOT change brands of drug

Synthroid gives Morbid Matilda a boost so she will be less tired.

ANTITHYROID

Action: Inhibits the synthesis of thyroid hormones.

Indications: Hyperthyroidism.

Warnings: Hypersensitivity, lactation.

Undesirable effects: Paresthesia, neuritis, drowsiness, vertigo, nausea, vomiting, agranulocytosis, granulocytopenia, thrombocytopenia, bleeding, skin rash.

Other Specific Information: Altered effects of oral anticoagulants. $\uparrow$ concentration of digoxin. ^{131}I may be $\downarrow$.

Interventions: Regular blood tests to monitor bone marrow depression and bleeding tendencies. Assess for signs and symptoms of a thyroid crisis (thyroid storm). Monitor vital signs (with hyperthyroidism, tachycardia and palpitations usually occur).

Education: Instruct to take the drug with meals; take 3 equal doses at 8-hour intervals around the clock; do not abruptly stop. Foods containing iodine may be restricted such as salt, shellfish, and OTC cough medicines. Report fever, sore throat, unusual bleeding or bruising, headache or general malaise. Advise client that signs and symptoms of hyperthyroidism should be alleviated in 1-3 weeks. Review signs and symptoms of hypothyroidism since it can occur as a result of treatment. Inform medical staff that client is taking this drug due to increase risk of bleeding.

Evaluation: Client will have a decrease in signs of hyperthyroidism with no undesirable effects.

Drugs: methimazole (Tapazole), propylthiouracil (PTU)

GO GETTER GERTRUDE

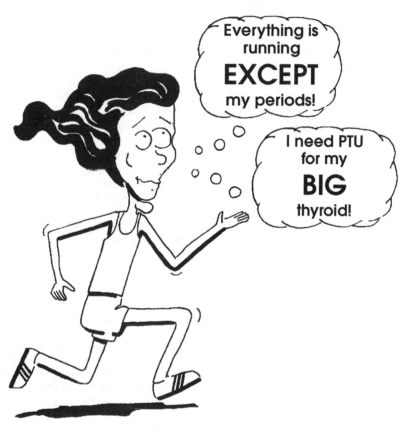

©2001 I CAN Publishing, Inc.

Gertrude Graves needs some PTU for her **"BIG"** thyroid. These antithyroid drugs can cause some problems with bleeding and infection. Taking them with food will decrease GI distress.

LUGOL'S SOLUTION

Action: Thyroid-nonradioactive iodine creates high levels of iodide resulting in a reduction of the iodine uptake by the thyroid gland. This will inhibit thyroid hormone production, and block the release of the thyroid hormones into the blood stream.

Indications: Used for the development of euthyroid state and reduction of thyroid gland size prior to thyroid surgery and/or emergency treatment of thyrotoxicosis.

Warnings: Contraindicated in pregnancy. Hypersensitivity; hyperkalemia; pulmonary edema; impaired renal function. Use with caution if client has tuberculosis; bronchitis; cardiovascular disease.

Undesirable Effects: Metallic taste, diarrhea, nausea, vomiting, stomatitis, sore teeth and gums, gastric distress that may result in GI bleeding, and small bowel lesions. Confusion; hypothyroidism; hypersensitivity.

Other Specific Information: Lithium may ↑ hypothyroidism. ↑ antithyroid effect of methimazole and propylthiouracil. ↑ hyperkalemia may result from combined use with potassium-sparing diuretics, ACE inhibitors, angiotensin II receptor antagonists or potassium supplements. Concurrent intake of foods high in iodine (e.g., iodized salt, seafood) increases risk for iodism.

Interventions: Assess for signs and symptoms of iodism (metallic taste, stomatitis, skin lesions, cold symptoms, severe GI upset) and report. Monitor symptoms of hyperthyroidism (tachycardia, palpitations, nervousness, insomnia, diaphoresis, heat intolerance, tremors, weight loss) and report. Monitor for hypersensitivity (rash, pruritus, laryngeal edema, wheezing), DC drug, and report. Assist client to drink through a straw to prevent tooth discoloration. Mix solutions in a full glass of fruit juice, water, broth, formula, or milk. Administer medication with or after meals to reduce gastrointestinal distress. Solution is normally clear and colorless. Darkening upon standing does not affect potency of drug. Solutions that are brownish yellow should be discarded. Crystals may form, especially if refrigerated, but redissolve upon warming and shaking. **Do not confuse iodine with Lodine (etodolac).** Monitor thyroid function before and periodically during therapy. Monitor serum potassium levels periodically during therapy.

Education: Teach client to report symptoms of iodism promptly to healthcare provider. Teach client signs and symptoms of hyperthyroidism to report. Instruct to take as ordered. Missing a dose may precipitate hyperthyroidism. Do not double doses. Take missed dose as soon as possible, but not just prior to next dose. Instruct client to report suspected pregnancy to provider prior to initiating therapy. Advise to avoid foods high in iodine (seafood, iodized salt, cabbage, kale, turnips) or potassium. Review the importance of increasing fluid intake, unless contraindicated due to medical condition. Advise to consult healthcare provider before using OTC or herbal cold remedies.

Evaluation: Resolution of the signs and symptoms of the thyroid crisis. ↓ in size of gland before surgery.

Drug: strong iodine solution (Lugol's Solution)

STRONG IODINE SOLUTION

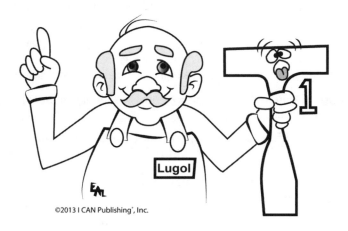

©2013 I CAN Publishing®, Inc.

"If your thyroid is going crazy,
Lugol's solution will help you baby!
If your mouth tastes like metal,
And your tummy is sore,
You must call your healthcare provider
Before taking more!
This may indicate a problem with iodism,
So also stay away from foods
with potassium and iodine in them!"

    Lugol's "solution" is a thyroid-nonradioactive iodine that creates high levels of iodide resulting in a reduction of the iodine uptake by the thyroid gland. This will block the release of the thyroid hormones into the blood stream.

RADIOACTIVE IODINE (^{131}I)

Action: Absorbed by the thyroid and destroys some of the thyroid producing cells. At high doses, thyroid-radioactive iodine destroys thyroid cells.

Indications: High doses: Hyperthyroidism, Thyroid cancer; Low doses: Thyroid function studies (visualization for the uptake of the iodine by the thyroid gland) is useful in diagnosing thyroid disorders.

Warnings: Contraindicated in pregnancy, clients of childbearing age/ intent, and lactation.

Undesirable Effects: Hypothyroidism—depression, edema, brady-cardia, weight gain, intolerance to cold; Bone marrow depression—anemia, leukopenia, thrombocytopenia; Radiation sickness—intense nausea, vomiting, hematemesis, epistaxis.

Other Specific Information: Use of other antithyroid meds reduces uptake of radioactive iodine. If client is taking any of these other meds, discontinue for a week prior to therapy.

Interventions: Encourage to increase fluid intake, usually 2 to 3 L/ day. Limit contact with clients to 30 min/day/person. Encourage to void frequently to avoid irradiation of gonads.

Education: Advise client to discontinue other anti-thyroid meds for a week prior to therapy. Review the importance of disposing of body wastes per protocol. Instruct the client regarding the importance of not coughing and expectorating (source of radioactive iodine).

Evaluation: Client will have a diagnosis confirmed.

Drugs: Radioactive iodine (^{131}I)

RADIOACTIVE IODINE (^{131}I)

G iven for Hyperthyroidism and Thyroid cancer

O ffspring may be harmed by treatment-
Do not give if pregnant or breastfeeding

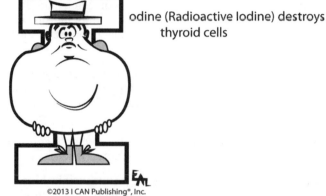

odine (Radioactive Iodine) destroys
thyroid cells

©2013 I CAN Publishing®, Inc.

T hyroid function studies are an indication for taking
this med (to visualize iodine uptake)

E ncourage client to increase fluid intake and to void
frequently; eliminate coughing and expectorating

R adiation sickness may occur- intense
nausea, vomiting, hematemesis, and epistaxis

GROWTH HORMONE
ANTERIOR PITUITARY HORMONES:
SOMATROPIN

Action: Stimulates overall growth and the production of protein, and decreases use of glucose.

Indications: Growth hormone deficiencies in children due to chronic renal insufficiency. Growth failure in children due to deficiency of growth hormone. Short stature associated with Turner's syndrome.

Warnings: Contraindicated if hypersensitive to growth hormone or who are severely obese or have severe respiratory impairment (sleep apnea). Acute critical illness (therapy should not be initiated) or respiratory failure. Use cautiously in clients with diabetes mellitus due to risk of hyperglycemia. Treatment should be discontinued prior to epiphyseal closure.

Undesirable Effects: Edema of the hands and feet. Hyperglycemia—assess for polydipsia, polyphagia, polyuria. Hypothyroidism—assess for depression, bradycardia, weight gain, anorexia, cold intolerance, dry skin. Monitor thyroid function and assess for signs of hypothyroidism.

Other Specific Information: Glucocorticosteroids when taken with somatropin can counteract growth-promoting effects.

Interventions: Monitor the client's baseline height and weight. Monitor the trends for growth patterns during medication administration, usually monthly. Reconstitute medication per protocol, rotating gently, and do not shake prior to administration. Monitor thyroid function prior to and during therapy. Monitor serum glucose during therapy. Rotate injection sites with each injection.

Education: Instruct client and parents on correct procedure for reconstituting medication, site selection, technique for IM or subcut injection, disposal of needles and syringes. Review schedule for administration. Report persistent pain or edema at injection site. Emphasize importance for regular follow-up with endocrinologist to ensure appropriate growth rate, to evaluate lab work, and to determine bone age by x-ray exam.

Evaluation: Client increases in height and attainment of adult height in growth failure secondary to pituitary growth hormone deficiency.

Drugs: somatropin (Genotropin, Nutropin)

GROWTH HORMONES
ANTERIOR PITUITARY HORMONES

G rowth hormone deficiencies in children (indication)

R ate of growth sould be monitored (ht, wt, trends...)

O besity and respiratory impairment are contraindications

W atch for hyperglycemia and hypothyroidism

I nstruction for administration (reconstitution, site, schedule...)

N utropin

G enotropin

©2013 I CAN Publishing®, Inc.

POSTERIOR PITUITARY HORMONES

Action: Alters permeability of the renal collecting ducts, allowing reabsorption of water. In high doses acts as a nonadrenergic peripheral vasoconstrictor.

Indications: Central diabetes insipidus due to deficient antidiuretic hormone.

Warnings: **HIGH ALERT DRUG** Chronic renal failure with increased BUN; Hypersensitivty to beef or pork proteins. Use cautiously in perioperative polyuria (increased sensitivity to vasopressin); comatose clients; seizures; migraine headaches; asthma; heart failure; cardiovascular disease; renal impairment; pregnancy, geriatric, and children.

Undesirable Effects: Dizziness, "pounding" sensation in head. Angina, chest pain (from vasoconstriction); abdominal cramps, belching, diarrhea, flatulence, heartburn, nausea, vomiting; paleness, allergic reactions, fever, water intoxication (higher doses). If DDAVP is administered intranasal, then assess for rhinitis, nasal congestion.

Other Specific Information: Antidiuretic effect may be decreased by concurrent use of alcohol, lithium, heparin, or norepinephrine. Antidiuretic effect may be increased by concurrent use of carbamazepine, clofibrate, tricyclic antidepressants, or fludrocortisone.

Interventions: Assess BP, HR, CVP, I & O, specific gravity, daily weight and lab studies (potassium, sodium, BUN, creatinine), and ECG periodically throughout therapy. Review the importance of reporting chest pain, tightness, and diaphoresis. Assess urine osmolality and urine volume frequently to evaluate effects of medication. Assess client for symptoms of dehydration (excessive thirst, dry skin, and mucous membranes, tachycardia, poor skin turgor). Assess for signs and symptoms of water intoxication including confusion, drowsiness, headache, weight gain, seizures, coma, and difficulty urinating. Treatment of overdose includes water restriction and temporary discontinuation of vasopressin until polyuria occurs. If symptoms are severe, administration of mannitol, hypertonic dextrose, urea, and / or furosemide may be used. **Do not confuse Pitressin (vasopressin) with Pitocin (oxytocin).** If administering IV, monitor site carefully due to extravasation which can result in gangrene. If DDAVP is administered intranasal then instruct on intranasal administration.

Education: Instruct client to take medication as directed. Review importance of not using more than prescribed amount. Advise to drink 1-2 glasses of water with med to decrease effects of blanching of skin, abdominal cramps, nausea. Discuss with client that these effects are not serious and usually disappear in a few minutes. Review the importance of not taking in any alcohol while taking vasopressin. Recommend carrying identification at all times describing disease process and medication regimen. Advise client to notify provider of care about chest pain, tightness, or diaphoresis.

Evaluation: Decrease in urine output associated with diabetes insipidus to normal levels of urine output.

Drugs: vasopressin (Pitressin Synthetic), desmopressin (DDAVP, Stimate)

VAS-O-PRESSIN
(ANTIDIURETIC HORMONE)

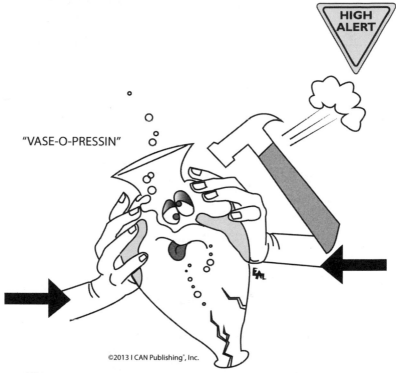

"VASE-O-PRESSIN"

©2013 I CAN Publishing®, Inc.

C ardiac Monitoring - B/P, HR, EKG

R ecommend carrying an identification about med regimen

A ssess urine osmolality and urine volume frequently, I & O, weight, edema

C entral diabetes insipidus - Indication

K now signs of water intoxication (confusion, dizziness, drowsiness, "pounding" headache)

S obriety is best - avoid alcolol

HYPOGLYCEMIA

T remors, tachycardia

I rritability, insomnia

R estless

E xcessive hunger

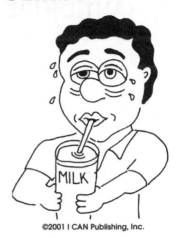

©2001 I CAN Publishing, Inc.

D iaphoresis, drowsiness, difficulty in concentration

HYPERGLYCEMIA

F lushed skin and fruit-like breath odor

L istless/lethargic

U nusual thirst, urine output increased

S kin dry

H yperventilate (rapid breathing)

E levated respirations and increased nausea
and vomiting

D rowsiness, decrease in appetite (nausea/vomiting)

©2013 I CAN Publishing®, Inc.

DIABETES

D iet, weight loss, exercise

I dentification—medical alert bracelet
V only Regular Insulin/Lispro (Humalog)

A void alcohol and other meds
lert (High)—oral hypoglycemics and insulin

B lood sugar and urine sugar, Hb A1c

E d. about antidiabetic agents

T ranscribe orders—"units" not "u"
herapy decreases signs, not a cure
wo nurses verify dosage administration

E d.—foot care, no smoking, stressors

S igns and symptoms of hyper/hypoglycemia—
show to do self-monitoring
kin care

ANTIDIABETIC: METFORMIN

Action: Decreases hepatic glucose production and intestinal absorption of glucose; increases peripheral insulin uptake and utilization.

Indications: Non-insulin dependent diabetes.

Warnings: Hypersensitivity; renal/hepatic disease; metabolic acidosis. Clients undergoing radiological studies involving parenteral administration of iodinated contrast materials should be temporarily stopped. Use caution when giving to elderly or malnourished client.

Undesirable Effects: Anorexia, abdominal gas or pain, headache, nausea, vomiting, possible metallic taste; hypoglycemia. *Toxic:* Lactic acidosis.

Other Specific Information: Calcium channel blockers, alcohol, digoxin, vancomycin, furosemide, may ↑ metformin concentration. ↑ risk of hypoglycemia with celery, coriander, dandelion root, garlic, ginseng. Concurrent use of iodine media contrast ordered for many diagnostic tests/procedures, may result in acute renal failure when administered with metformin.

Interventions: Monitor CBC, blood and urine for glucose and ketones, and HbA1c. Monitor renal function prior to therapy and at least annually to determine normal renal function. Discontinue if the client enters a hypoxic state.

Education: Instruct to take with meals and encourage adequate hydration. Instruct client to discontinue drug and notify provider immediately if experiences unexplained hypoxemia, dehydration, or signs of lactic acidosis (unexplained hyperventilation, muscle aches, fatigue, and lethargy). Inform client to Notify provider for problems with diarrhea and vomiting. (Refer to "**DIABETES**".)

Evaluation: The client's HbA1c and serum glucose level will remain within the normal limit, and client will experience no undesirable effects.

Drug: metformin (Glucophage)

METFORMIN

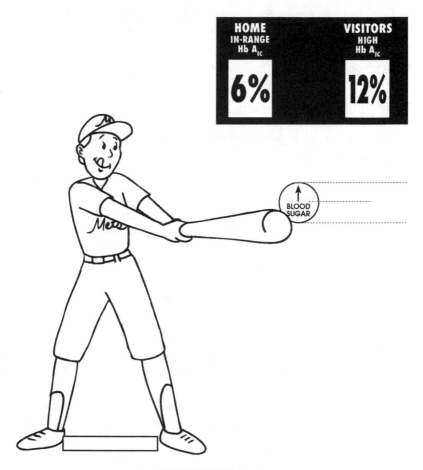

HOME
IN-RANGE
Hb A$_{1c}$

6%

VISITORS
HIGH
Hb A$_{1c}$

12%

BLOOD
SUGAR

©2001 I CAN Publishing, Inc.

Metformin "The Mets" (glucophage) bats against high blood sugar. He scores the winning home run by decreasing hepatic glucose production and intestinal absorption of glucose, while improving insulin sensitivity. Prior to playing in the big league, he must have a sports physical to check his renal function. A major complication with this medicine is lactic acidosis.

ANTIDIABETIC DRUGS: SULFONYLUREAS

Action: Not fully known. Stimulates insulin release from the pancreatic beta cells and reduces glucose output by the liver. Increases peripheral sensitivity to insulin.

Indications: Non-insulin dependent diabetes Type 2 (maturity-onset diabetes).

Warning: Allergies to sulfonylureas; Type 1 insulin dependent diabetes except in conjunction with insulin; diabetes complicated by ketoacidosis; renal/ hepatic disease; cardiac or thyroid disease.

Undesirable Effects: Nausea, vomiting, diarrhea, rash, pruritis, headache, hypoglycemia.

Other Specific Information: ↑ hypoglycemic effect with aspirin, alcohol, anticoagulants, anticonvulsants, sulfonamides, oral contraceptives, MAOIs, and some NSAIDs. ↓ hypoglycemic effect with cortisone, thiazide diuretics, calcium channel blockers, estrogen, phenytoin, thyroid drugs. ↑ risk of hypoglycemia with celery, coriander, dandelion root, garlic, ginseng.

Interventions: Monitor vital signs, BUN, serum creatinine, liver function tests, blood and urine glucose, and HbA1c. Chlorpropamide is not a desirable choice for the elderly client due to long duration of action. The second-generation agents may be safer for this group of clients with respect to drug interactions. Monitor elderly for hypersensitivity. Drug may accumulate in client with renal insufficiency. (Refer to "**DIABETES**".)

Education: Instruct client to take with food. Review with client that insulin might be necessary instead of an oral antidiabetic medication during a serious infection, stressful time, or surgery. Discuss the importance of eating meals on schedule since missing a meal can result in hypoglycemia. (Refer to "**DIABETES**".)

Evaluation: The client's HbA1c and serum glucose level will be within the normal range, and the client will be able to safely manage the oral antidiabetic agents.

Drugs: *first generation:* acetohexamide (Dymelor); chlorpropamide (Diabinese); tolazamide (Tolinase); tolbutamide (Orinase); *second generation:* glimepiride (Amaryl); glipizide (Glucotrol, Glucotrol XL); glyburide (Diabeta, Glynase PresTab, Micronase)

SULFONYLUREAS

G limepiride lipizide   are better for   **G** randmother

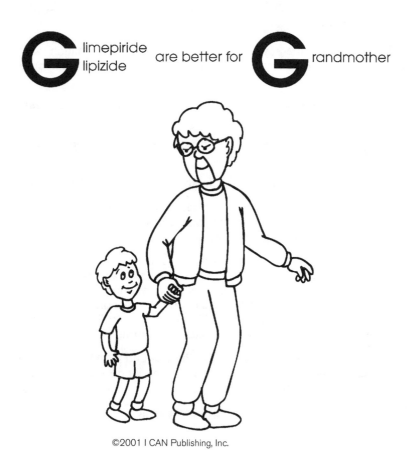

©2001 I CAN Publishing, Inc.

Chlorpropamide is not good for Grandmother (geriatic client) due to its long duration of action. Grandmother has a shorter span to live than her grandchild, so she needs the agent with the shorter duration of action.

INSULIN SENSITIZER: AVANDIA

Action: Stimulates insulin receptor sites to lower serum glucose and improve the action of insulin.

Indication: Monotherapy for Type II diabetes; combination with metformin when diet, exercise, and either agent alone are not effective with Type II diabetes.

Warnings: Hepatic disease, Class III-IV cardiac disease, premenopausal anovulatory women.

Undesirable effects: Headache, hypoglycemia, elevations in liver enzymes, anemia.

Other Specific Information: ↓ effectiveness of oral contraceptives.

Interventions: Monitor liver function tests, serum and urine glucose, and CBC. If client switches from troglitazone, do not start rosiglitazone for 7 days after stopping the troglitazone.

Education: Advise client to take with meals. If dose is missed, it may be taken at the next meal. Do not double dose the next day, if dose is missed for an entire day. Provide educational offerings regarding the disease, dietary control, exercise, avoidance of infection, hygiene, and signs and symptoms of hypo/hyperglycemia. Review the importance of using a barrier contraceptive if taking oral contraceptives.

Evaluation: Client's serum and urine glucose and HbA1c will remain within the normal range, and client will experience no undesirable effects from the medication.

Drug: rosiglitazone (Avandia), pioglitazone (Actos)

AVANDIA

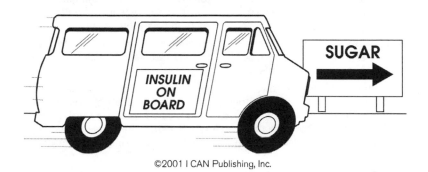

©2001 I CAN Publishing, Inc.

S igns of anemia. ↑ liver enzymes: UE

U se barrier contraceptives

G lucose urine and serum—monitor

A dminister with meals

R osiglitazone (Avandia)

This van is improving the action of insulin, which helps in the management of diabetes. "**SUGAR**" will assist you with the key points.

ALPHA-GLUCOSIDASE INHIBITORS

Action: Lowers blood glucose by inhibiting the enzyme alpha-glucosidase in the GI tract. Slows carbohydrate absorption and digestion. Lowers blood glucose in diabetic clients, especially postprandial hyperglycemia.

Indications: Management of non-insulin dependent diabetes in conjunction with dietary therapy and exercise life style changes. May be used with insulin or other hypoglycemic agents.

Warnings: Hypersensitivity; Diabetic ketoacidosis; Cirrhosis; Serum creatinine > 2 mg/dL; Inflammatory bowel disease or other chronic intestinal conditions resulting in impaired absorption or predisposition to obstruction; OB, Lactation, and/or Pediatrics- safety not established. Use cautiously in presence of a fever, infection, trauma, stress (may result in hyperglycemia, mandating alternative therapy).

Undesirable Effects: Intestinal effects (abdominal distention and cramping, hyperactive bowel sounds, diarrhea, excessive gas); risk for anemia due to the decrease of iron absorption; hepatoxicity with long-term use.

Other Specific Information: Concurrent use with sulfonylureas or insulin increase the risk for hypoglycemia. Concurrent use of metformin causes additive gastrointestinal effects and risk for hypoglycemia.

Interventions: Assess for drug-drug interactions. Assess for signs and symptoms of hypoglycemia when taking with other oral hypoglycemic agents. Monitor serum glucose and glycosylated hemoglobin periodically during therapy to evaluate effectiveness. Monitor AST and ALT every 3 mo for the first year and then periodically. Discontinue if liver function tests increase. Symptoms of flatulence, diarrhea, and abdominal discomfort are indicative of overdose and are transient. If client experiences stress, fever, trauma, infection or surgery, insulin may need to be added to regimen. Does not cause hypoglycemia when taken while fasting, but may increase hypoglycemic effect of other hypoglycemic agents. Administer with first bite of each meal 3 times per day.

Education: Instruct client to take med at same time each day. If a dose is missed and the meal is complete without taking the dose, skip missed dose and take next dose with the next meal. Do not double doses. Explain that these meds control hyperglycemia, but do not cure. Review signs and symptoms of hypoglycemia and hyperglycemia. Review importance of following prescribed diet, medication, and exercise regimen to prevent hypoglycemic or hyperglycemic episodes. Review proper testing of serum glucose and urine ketones. Notify healthcare provider if significant changes occur. Consult healthcare provider before treatment with other meds or surgery. Advise client to carry a form of oral glucose and identification describing disease process and medication regimen at all time. Review importance of follow-up examinations.

Evaluation: Control of blood glucose levels without the signs of hypoglycemia or hyperglycemia.

Drugs: acarbose (Precose), miglitol (Glyset)

ALPHA-GLUCOSIDASE INHIBITORS

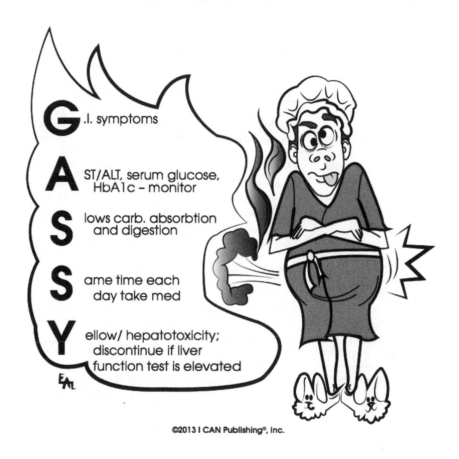

G.I. symptoms

AST/ALT, serum glucose, HbA1c – monitor

Slows carb. absorbtion and digestion

Same time each day take med

Yellow/ hepatotoxicity; discontinue if liver function test is elevated

"It's A G.I. antidiabetic agent, and it may make you very GASSY!!!"

AMYLIN MIMETICS

Action: Acts as a synthetic analogue of amylin, an endogenous pancreatic hormone that helps to control postprandial hyperglycemia; effects include slowed gastric emptying, suppression of glucagon secretion and regulation of food intake.

Indications: Improved control of postprandial hyperglycemia with clients with type 1 or type 2 diabetes. Noted: for concurrent use with insulin or an oral hypoglycemic agent, usually metformin or a sulfonylurea.

Warnings: **HIGH ALERT DRUG** Hypersensitivity; inability to identify hypoglycemia; gastroparesis or need for medications to stimulate gastric motility; Poor compliance with current insulin regimen or self-monitoring; HbA1c > 9%; recurrent severe hypoglycemia within the last 6 mo, requiring treatment; Pediatrics. Contraindicated for clients who have renal failure or are receiving dialysis. Use cautiously in clients who have thyroid disease, osteoporosis, or alcoholism.

Undesirable Effects: Dizziness, fatigue, headache; cough; nausea, abdominal pain, anorexia, vomiting; hypoglycemia; local allergy; arthralgia; systemic allergic reactions.

Other Specific Information: Insulin increases risk for hypoglycemia, usually requiring a 50% decrease of rapid or short-acting insulin. Concurrent use of pramlintide with medications that slow gastric emptying such as opioids, or medications that delay food absorption, such as atropine and other anticholinergics. Acarbose and miglitol may also further slow gastric emptying. May delay oral medication absorption with concurrently administered drugs; if prompt absorption desired, administer 1 hr prior or 2 hrs after pramlintide.

Interventions: Pramlintide and insulin should be administered as separate injections; do not mix. Avoid use in clients unable to self-monitor blood glucose levels. Administer oral medications 1 or 2 hrs after injection of parmlintide. Administer subcut prior to meals, using the thigh or abdomen. Assess HbA1c, recent blood glucose monitoring data, history of insulin-induced hypoglycemia, current insulin regimen, and body weight prior to initiation of therapy. Assess for signs and symptoms of hypoglycemia. Pramlintide alone does not cause hypoglycemia; may increase risk when administered with insulin. Monitor serum glucose frequently. *High Alert:* Dose errors are a potential problem with administration of pramlintide. It is available in a concentration of 0.6 mg/ml, dosing is in mcg, and insulin syringe for administration is in units. Carefully review dosing and conversion table prior to administration.

Education: Instruct clients to keep unopened vials in the refrigerator and not to freeze. Opened vials may be kept cool or at room temperature but should be discarded after 28 days. Keep vials out of direct sunlight. Instruct clients not to mix medication with insulin in the same syringe. Do not administer solutions that are cloudy. (Refer to **"DIABETES."**)

Evaluation: Client will experience a reduction in postprandial glucose concentration.

Drug: Pramlintide (Symlin)

AMYLIN MIMETICS (PRAMLINTIDE)

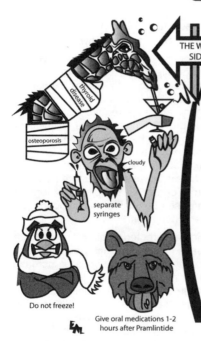

"Don't walk on the wild side when using Pram-lin-tide!"

THE WILD SIDE

thyroid disease

osteoporosis

cloudy

separate syringes

Do not freeze!

Give oral medications 1-2 hours after Pramlintide

D osing must be CAREFUL

O steoporosis, thyroid disease, or alcoholism; use with caution

S olution is cloudy - Do NOT use!

I nsulin and Pramlintide must be in separate syringes

N ot to freeze unopened vials

G ive oral medication 1-2 hours after injection of Pramlintide

INCRETIN MIMETICS

Action: Mimics the effects of naturally occurring glucagon-like peptide-1, and thereby promotes release of insulin which decreases secretion of glucagon, and delays gastric emptying. Fasting and postprandial blood glucose levels are lowered.

Indications: Supplemental glucose control for clients with type 2 diabetes. May be used in conjunction with an oral hypoglycemic agent, usually metformin or a sulfonylurea.

Warnings: Contraindicated with clients with renal failure, ulcerative colitis, Crohn's disease. Use cautiously in older adult clients and clients with renal impairment or thyroid disease.

Undesirable Effects: GI effects (nausea, vomiting and diarrhea). Pancreatitis (severe and intolerable abdominal pain).

Other Specific Information: Oral medication absorption is delayed, especially oral contraceptives and antibiotics. Sulfonylurea ↑ hypoglycemia.

Interventions: Assess for signs and symptoms of hypoglycemia("**TIRED**"); monitor serum glucose and HbA1c periodically during therapy to evaluate effectiveness. Some meds may need to be taken 1 hr before exenatide. Clients stabilized on diabetic regimen, but who are in an accident and exposed to stress, fever, infection, surgery, etc. may require insulin to be added to regimen. This med is supplied in prefilled injector pens. Administer in thigh, abdomen, or upper arm at any time within the 60-min. period before the morning and evening meals. Do not administer after a meal. Solution should not be administered if cloudy. Refrigerate; discard 30 days after 1st use, even if some drug remains in pen. Do not freeze. Do not store pen with needle attached. Medication may leak from pen or air bubbles may form in the cartridge. Drug is available in 10 mcg/dose (2.4 ml pen) for 60 doses (30 days of twice daily dosing) or 5 mcg/dose (1.2 ml pen).

Education: Instruct client to take exenatide as directed within 60 min. before a meal. Do not take after a meal. If a dose is missed, skip the dose and take the next dose at the prescribed time. Do not take an extra dose or increase the amount of the next dose to make up for missed dose. Review technique of administration, timing of dose and concurrent oral medications, storage of medication disposal of used needles. Discuss the importance of only inserting prior to initiation of therapy and with each prescription refill. Advise client that with New Pen Setup this should be done only with each new pen, not with each dose. Review the importance of purchasing pen needles separately, since they are not included with setup. Review that therapy is not a cure, but helps control hyperglycemia. (Review "**DIABETES**.")

Evaluation: Preprandial glucose levels of 90 to 130 mg/dL and postprandial levels of less than 180 mg/dL. HgbA1c less than 7%.

Drug: exenatide (Byetta)

EXENATIDE (BYETTA)

P.

Pen set up is only done with each new pen, not each dose.

E.

Evaluate for nausea, vomiting and diarrhea.

N.

Not = X ("eXenatide")

X...with oral contraceptives
X...to be used after 30 days
X...after meals
X...to be stored with needle attached

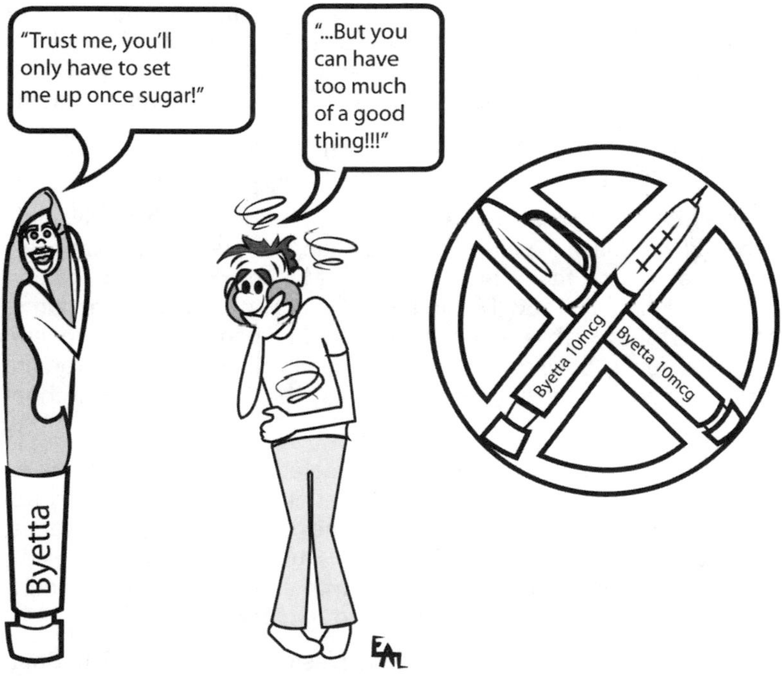

"Trust me, you'll only have to set me up once sugar!"

"...But you can have too much of a good thing!!!"

Byetta

Byetta 10mcg

Byetta 10mcg

GLIPTINS: SITAGLIPTIN (JANUVIA)

Action: Inhibits the enzyme dipeptidyl peptidase–4 (DPP-4), that slows the inactivation of incretin hormones, resulting in increased levels of active incretin hormones. These hormones are released by the intestine throughout the day, and are involved in regulation of glucose homeostasis. Increased/prolonged incretin levels, increase insulin release and decrease glucagon levels.

Indications: Use with diet and exercise to improve glycemic control in clients with type 2 diabetes mellitus. May be used as monotherapy or combination therapy with metformin and a thiazolidinedione and/or a sulfonylurea (glimepiride).

Warnings: Type 1 diabetes mellitus; diabetic ketoacidosis; hypersensitivity. Use cautiously in clients with renal impairment. (dose reduction required for CCr < 50 ml/min); Geriatrics: Consider age-related decrease in renal function when determining dose.

Undesirable Effects: Headache; nausea and diarrhea; upper respiratory tract infection; nasopharyngitis; hypersensitivity reactions including anaphylaxis, angioedema, and exfoliative skin conditions (Stevens-Johnson syndrome), rash, urticaria. Generally well tolerated.

Other Specific Information: May slightly increase serum digoxin levels; monitoring recommended. There are no significant interactions.

Interventions: Assess for signs and symptoms of hypoglycemic reactions (abdominal pain, sweating, hunger; weakness; dizziness, headache, tremor; tachycardia, anxiety). Monitor HbA1c prior to and routinely during therapy. Monitor renal function prior to and during therapy. Clients stabilized on a diabetic regimen who are exposed to stress, fever, physical trauma, infection, or surgery may require administration of insulin. Sitagliptin may be administered without regard to food.

Education: Instruct to take med as directed. Take missed doses as soon as remembered, unless it is almost time for next dose; do not double doses. Explain that sitagliptin helps control hyperglycemia, but does not cure diabetes. Therapy is usually ongoing and long term. Remind client not to share med with another client with similar symptoms due to risk involved. (Refer to "**DIABETES**.")

Evaluation: Improved HbA1c, fasting plasma glucose and 2-hr post-prandial glucose levels.

Drug: sitagliptin (Januvia)

GLIPTINS: SITAGLIPTIN (JANUVIA)

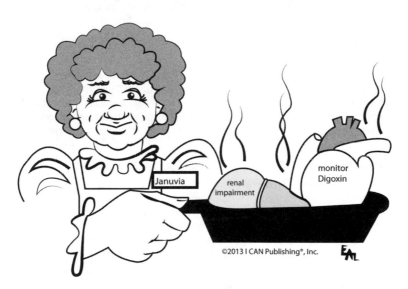

Januvia

renal impairment

monitor Digoxin

©2013 I CAN Publishing®, Inc.

F ood is not necessary when taking this drug

R enal impairment; use cautiously

I Increased levels of active incretin hormones, increase insulin release

E Evaluate HbA1c and symptoms of hypo/hyperglycemia

D igoxin serum levels may be increased; monitoring recommended

This is Januvia Sitagliptin... Sometimes it's hard for her to regulate her diabetes because she loves her food FRIED!

Meglitinides Repaglinide (Prandin)

Action: Insulin release from the pancreatic beta cells by closing potassium channels, which results in the opening of calcium channels in beta cells. This is followed by release of insulin.

Indications: Type 2 diabetes mellitus, with diet and exercise; may be used with metformin, rosiglitazone, or pioglitazone.

Warnings: Hypersensitivity; lactation; diabetic ketoacidosis; Insulin-dependent diabetes. Use cautiously in impaired liver function (longer dosing intervals may be necessary); severe renal impairment (dosage reduction recommended); Geriatrics (Consider age-related decrease in renal/hepatic/cardiovascular function); pregnancy and pediatrics: safety not established.

Undesirable Effects: Angina, chest pain; hypoglycemia

Other Specific Information: Concurrent use of gemfibrozil may lead to an increased risk for hypoglycemia by inhibiting the repaglinide metabolism. Effects may be decreased by corticosteroids, phenothiazines, thyroid preparations, estrogens, hormonal contraceptives, phenytoin, nicotinic acid, sympathomimetics, isoniazid, and calcium channel blockers. Glucosamine may worsen blood glucose control.

Interventions: Assess for signs and symptoms of hypoglycemia. It is more difficult to assess hypoglycemia in geriatric clients and in clients taking beta blockers. Monitor serum glucose and glycosylated hemoglobin per protocol. Administer up to 30 min. before meals (3 times/day). Clients who skip a meal or add an extra meal should skip or add a dose, as necessary for that meal. Encourage clients to consistently exercise and follow dietary guidelines. Advise clients to maintain a log of glucose levels and to note patterns that impact glucose levels (such as increase in dietary intake and infection). Refer to dietician and/ or diabetic nurse educator.

Education: Instruct client regarding signs and symptoms of hypo and hyperglycemia. Report to provider of care if there is a recurrent problem. Instruct to eat within 30 min of taking a dose of the medication. Instruct to self-administer a snack of 15 g of carbohydrate (4 oz orange juice, 2 oz grape juice, 8 oz milk, glucose tablets per manufacturer's suggestion to equal 15 g). Encourage clients to consistently exercise and to follow appropriate dietary guidelines. If severe hypoglycemia occurs, IV glucose may be needed. (Refer to "**DIABETES**.")

Evaluation: Control of blood glucose levels without the appearance of hypoglycemic or hyperglycemic episodes.

Drugs: repaglinide (Gluconorm, Prandin)

REPAGLINIDE
(GLUCONORM, PRANDIN)

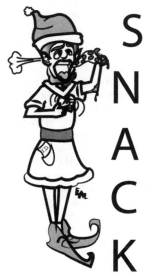

S nack on 15 grams of carbs after meals

N ote what impacts ⬆ glucose
such as food, infection and stress

A ngina, chest pain, hypoglycemia
undesirable effects

C oncurrent use of gemfibrozil (Lopid)
may ⬆ the risk of hypoglycemia

K eep identification with client at all times
describing disease and treatment

Repaglinide Song
(to the tune of,"Oh, Christmas Tree")

"Re-pag-lin-ide, Re-pag-lin-ide,
My 15 carbs are for you!
Re-pag-lin-ide, Re-pag-lin-ide,
Chest pain, low sugar from you!

A diet change may harm me most,
infection, stress, hurts my glucose...

Re-pag-lin-ide, Re-pag-lin-ide,
I.D. is always with me!"

Holidays are the best time to SNACK!

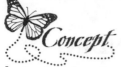

Concept: INSULIN

Instruct on how to administer insulin: Instruct clients to administer SC insulin in one general area to have consistent rates of absorption. Absorption rates from subcutaneous tissue increase from thigh to upper arm to abdomen. Select an appropriate needle length to ensure insulin is injected into subcutaneous tissue. Store vials in refrigerator. Vials may also be kept at room temperature for up to 28 days. Do not use if cloudy, discolored, or unusually viscous. Cartridges and pens should be stored at room temperature and used within 28 days. Unopened vials may be stored in the refrigerator until expiration date. Vials of premixed insulins may be stored for up to 3 months. Instruct client on proper technique for administration. Include type of insulin, equipment (syringe, cartridge pens, external puml, alcohol swabs), storage, and proper place to discard syringes. Review the importance of not changing brands of insulin or syringes, selection and rotation of injection sites, and compliance with therapy. Demonstrate technique for mixing insulins by drawing up aspart, insulin glulisine, or insulin lispro first. Roll intermediate-acting insulin vial between palms to mix, rather than shaking (may result in inaccurate dose). Review that medication is to control hyperglycemia, but does not cure diabetes. Review importance of systematically rotating injection sites and to allow 1 inch between injection sites. Insulin premixed in syringes may be kept for 1 to 2 weeks under refrigeration. Keep syringes in a vertical position, with needles pointing up. Store the vial that is in use at room temperature, avoiding proximity to sunlight and intense heat. Discard after 1 month. Never use mixed insulins in a pump or IV infusion.

Nutritional guidelines and exercise: Emphasize the importance of compliance with nutritional guidelines and regular exercise as prescribed.

Signs and symptoms of hyperglycemia and hypoglycemia: Hyperglycemia – "**FLUSHED**" and Hypoglycemia "**TIRED**"

Use source of sugar: (candy, glucose gel) If hypoglycemia occurs, advise client to take a glass of orange juice, 2-3 tsp of sugar, honey, or corn syrup dissolved in water, and notify health care provider. For conscious clients, administer a snack of 15 g of carbohydrate (4 oz orange juice, 2 oz grape juice, 8 oz milk, glucose tablets per manufacturer's suggestion to equal 15 g). If client is not fully conscious, do not risk aspiration. Administer glucose parenterally such as IV glucose, or SC/IM glucagon.

Look at office visits and reinforce the importance of going on a regular basis. During the first few weeks of therapy, the office visits must be regular.

Identification: Review the importance of wearing an alert bracelet, etc. for identification that describes their disease and treatment regimen at all times.

Note how to test serum glucose and ketones and no meds without consulting provider of care. These tests should be closely monitored during periods of stress or illness and health care professional notified of significant changes. Review the importance of notifying health care professional prior to using alcohol or other OTC, or herbal products concurrently with insulin.

PROTOTYPE MEDICATION (INSULIN)

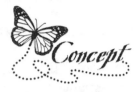
Concept

CLASSIFI-CATION	GENERIC (TRADE NAME)	ONSET	PEAK	DURATION
Rapid-Acting	Lispro insulin (Humalog)	< 15 min.	0.5–1 1/2 hr.	3–4 hr.
Short-Acting	Regular insulin (Humulin R)	30 to 60 min.	2–3 hr.	5–7 hr.
Intermediate-Acting	NPH insulin (Humulin N)	1–2 hr.	4–12 hr.	18–24 hr.
Long-Acting	Insulin glargine (Lantus)	1–1 1/2 hr.	None	20–24 hr.
70% NPH and 30% Regular	Humulin 70/30	30 min.	2–4 hr	14–24 hr.
75% insulin lispro protamine and 25% insulin lispro	Humalog 75/25	15–30 min.	30 min.–2 1/2 hr.	16–20 hr.

Hypoglycemia
(sung to the tune of

"Row, Row, Row Your Boat")

Hot and dry
Your sugar's high.
Your insulin is what you need.

Cold and clammy
You need some candy,
And milk will help indeed.

INSULIN

Action: Reduces blood sugar level by increasing glucose transport across muscle and fat cell. Promotes conversion of glucose to glycogen. Moves potassium into cells (along with glucose).

Indications: Diabetes Mellitus; diabetic ketoacidosis; to lower blood sugar.

Warnings: **HIGH ALERT DRUG** Pregnancy/lactation.

Undesirable Effects: Hypoglycemia (refer to **"TIRED"**) Tremors, tachycardia, Irritability, Restless, Excessive hunger, Diaphoresis, depression. Rebound hyperglycemia (Somogyi effect); redness, irritation or swelling at injection site; flushing; urticaria; lipodystrophy.

Other Specific Information: ↑ hypoglycemic effect with aspirin, oral anticoagulant, alcohol, beta blockers, oral hypoglycemics, MAOIs, tricyclic antidepressants, tetracycline. ↓ hypoglycemic effect with thiazides, glucocorticoids, oral contraceptives, thyroid drugs, smoking. ↑ risk of hypoglycemia with celery, coriander, dandelion root, garlic, ginseng.

Interventions: Monitor vital signs, blood and urine glucose levels, and HbA1c. Insulin can be used to manage diabetes in the pregnant woman; however, client must be monitored closely. Dosage is always expressed in USP units. Use syringes calibrated for the particular concentration of insulin administered. Humalog is the fastest acting insulin, acting within 15 minutes; may be given I.V. (Refer to **"INSULIN"** on page 298.)

Education: Whenever NPH or Lente is mixed with regular insulin in the same syringe, give it immediately to avoid loss of potency. (Refer to image for mixing insulin.) Avoid insulin that changes color or becomes clumped or granular in appearance. Dosage may vary with activities, diet, or stress. Chart and rotate injection sites. Store in refrigerator. (Refer to **"DIABETES"**.)

Evaluation: Blood sugar and HbA1c will be within normal limits, and client will manage insulin safely.

Drugs: *Rapid-Acting:* Lispro Insulin (Humalog); Insulin aspart (NovoLog); Insulin glulisine (Apidra); *Short-Acting:* Regular Insulin (Humulin R, Novolin R); *Intermediate-Acting:* NPH insulin (Humulin N); Insulin detemir (Levemir); *Long-Acting:* Insulin glargine (Lantus); *Premixed Insulins*: 70% NPH and 30% Regular (Humulin 70/30)-mixture of intermediate acting and short-acting insulin; 75% insulin lispro protamine and 25% insulin lispro (Humalog 75/25) - mixture of intermediate acting and rapid-acting insulin

INSULIN

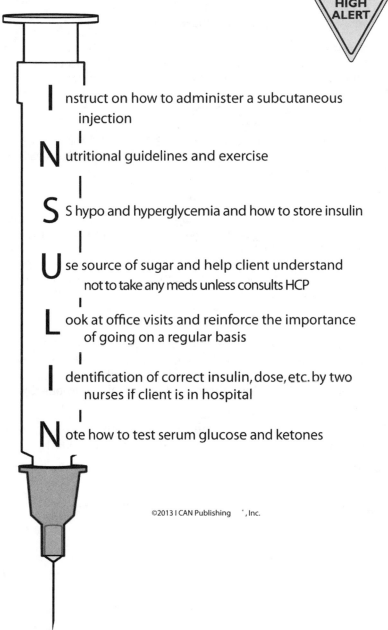

HIGH ALERT

I nstruct on how to administer a subcutaneous injection

N utritional guidelines and exercise

S hypo and hyperglycemia and how to store insulin

U se source of sugar and help client understand not to take any meds unless consults HCP

L ook at office visits and reinforce the importance of going on a regular basis

I dentification of correct insulin, dose, etc. by two nurses if client is in hospital

N ote how to test serum glucose and ketones

INSULIN LISPRO (HUMALOG)

Action: Antidiabetic (pancreatic hormone)

Indications: Rapid-acting insulin used to treat elevated glucose levels in type 1 and type 2 diabetes (usually in addition to intermediate and long-acting insulins, or, with type 2 diabetes, oral hypoglycemic agents).

Warnings: **HIGH ALERT DRUG** Allergy or hypersensitivity.

Undesirable Effects: Urticaria, HYPOGLYCEMIA, rebound hyperglycemia (Somogyi effect), lipodystrophy, itching, redness, swelling, allergic reactions including ANAPHYLAXIS.

Other Specific Information: Refer to Insulin.

Interventions: *Adults:* 5–10 units up to 15 min. before meals. Use only U-100 insulin syringes to draw up insulin lispro dose. Do not accept insulin orders that contain the abbreviation "U" for units. It has been misread as a zero, which resulted in serious, ten-fold over dose. Clarify any order that contains this abbreviation. Assess client for signs and symptoms of hypoglycemia. (For onset, peak, and duration times refer to chart on page 299.)

Education: Instruct client when mixing insulins to draw insulin lispro into syringe first to avoid contamination of insulin lispro vial. Instruct client and family about signs and symptoms of hyper and hypoglcemia. Instruct client regarding importance of eating meal after receiving medication. Do not wait for an extended period of time to eat. Client may get hypoglycemic.

Staff Education: Do not confuse Humalog with Humulin. (Refer to "**DIABETES**" on page 281 and "**INSULIN**" on page 298.)

Evalution: Client's blood sugar will remain within the therapeutic range.

Drugs: Insulin Aspart (Novolog), Insulin Lispro (Humalog)

LISPRO

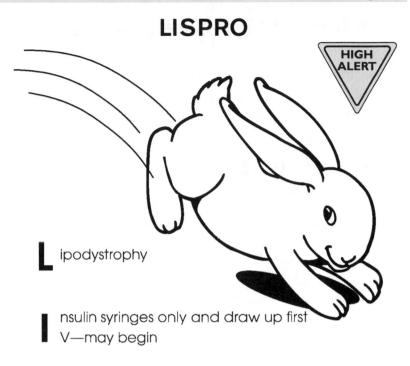

HIGH ALERT

L ipodystrophy

I nsulin syringes only and draw up first
V—may begin

S taff education—don't confuse Humalog
with Humalin

P refilled syringes stable for one week

R apid action, have food nearby

O bserve for hypoglycemic reactions

©2005 I CAN Publishing, Inc.

Hoppy Humalog is quick! He rapidly decreases glucose levels.

Insulin Glargine (Lantus)

Action: Pancreatic hormone. Antidiabetic agent.

Indications: Type 1 and 2 diabetes. Long-acting insulin with a constant concentration over 24 hours and with no pronounced peak. Provides a continuous level of insulin similar to the steady secretion of insulin provided by the normal pancreas.

Warnings: **HIGH ALERT DRUG** Allergy or hypersensitivity.

Undesirable Effects: Urticaria, HYPOGLYCEMIA, rebound hyperglycemia (Somogyi effect), lipodystrophy, itching, redness, swelling, allergic reactions including ANAPHYLAXIS.

Other Specific Information: Lantus insulin cannot be mixed with other insulins; action may be affected in an unpredictable manner.

Interventions: Assess client for signs of hypoglycemia (cool, clammy skin, difficulty concentrating, drowsiness; excessive hunger; headache; irritability; nausea; rapid pulse; shakiness) and hyperglycemia (hot, flushed skin; fruity breath; polyuria; loss of appetite; tiredness; thirsty) throughout therapy.

Education: Usually begin with 10 units at bedtime and titrate according to glucose levels. Use only insulin syringes to draw up dose. Rotate injection sites. Never mix with any insulin and do not administer IV.

Staff Education: Do not accept insulin orders that contain the abbreviation "U" for "units." It can be misread as a zero and has resulted in serious, tenfold overdoses. Clarify any order that contains this abbreviation. Do not confuse Lantus insulin with Lente insulin.

Evaluation: Client's blood glucose levels will remain within normal range.

Drugs: Insulin Glargine (Lantus)

LANTUS

L evel relatively constant

A lert for name confusion with lente

N ever mix with anything

T ake once a day

U ndesirable effects

S tore in cool place

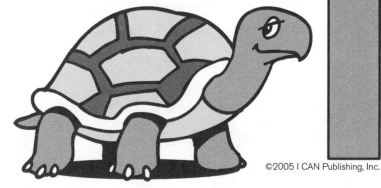

©2005 I CAN Publishing, Inc.

Lazy Lantus is in no hurry to peak. In fact, he is constant for one day or 24 hours.

MIXING INSULIN

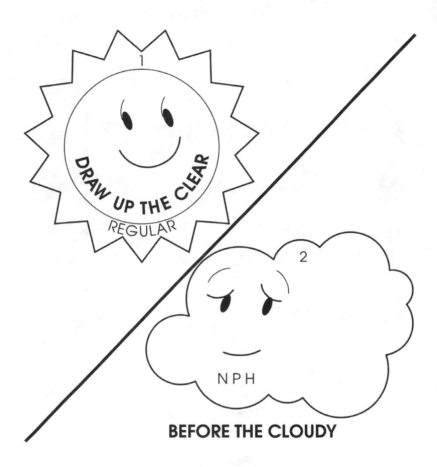

BEFORE THE CLOUDY

To prevent contaminating a short-acting insulin **"R**egular" with an intermediate insulin **"N**PH", draw the clear before the cloudy. Another way to remember is to think **RN** (**R**egistered **N**urse).

THE CONTESTANTS

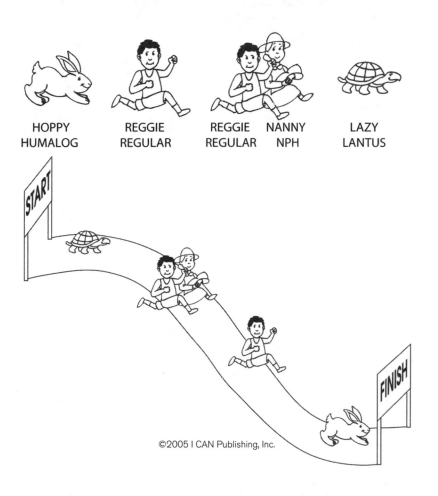

HOPPY
HUMALOG

REGGIE
REGULAR

REGGIE
REGULAR

NANNY
NPH

LAZY
LANTUS

©2005 I CAN Publishing, Inc.

Insulins vary in their onset, peak and duration.

HYPERGLYCEMIC AGENT

Action: Increases blood glucose levels by increasing the breakdown of glycogen into glucose. This results in a decrease in the glycogen synthesis which facilitates the synthesis of glucose.

Indications: Emergency care for a client who presents with hypoglycemic reaction resulting in an insulin overdose who may not have IV glucose available or who are not able to take oral glucose. Decrease in GI motility for clients who are undergoing radiological procedures of the stomach and intestines.

Warnings: **HIGH ALERT DRUG** Hypersensitivity; Pheochromocytoma; Some products contain glycerin and phenol-avoid use in clients with hypersensitivities to these ingredients. Ineffectifve if hypoglycemia is a result from inadequate glycogen stores such as what happens with starvation. Pregnancy Risk B. Use cautiously in clients who have cardiovascular disease.

Undesirable Effects: GI: N/V; hypotension; hypersensitivity; ↓ K$^+$.

Other Specific Information: Large doses may enhance effect of warfarin. Counteracts response to insulin or oral hypoglycemic agents. Phenytoin inhibits the stimulant effect of glucagon on insulin release. Hyperglycemic effect is increased and prolonged by epinephrine. Clients on concurrent beta blockers may experience an increase in heart rate and blood pressure.

Interventions: Assess for signs of hypoglycemia "TIRED". Assess neurologic status throughout therapy. Protect from injury caused by falling, aspiration, or seizures. Feed client supplemental carbohydrates orally to replenish liver glycogen and prevent secondary hypoglycemia as soon as possible after awakening. Assess nutritional status. Clients who lack liver glycogen stores (starvation, chronic hypoglycemia, adrenal insufficiency) will require glucose instead of glucagon. Assess for nausea and vomiting following administration of dose. Protect clients with depressed LOC from aspiration by repositioning on side; ensure a suction unit is available. Administer glucagon SC, IM, or IV following reconstitution parameters. As soon as client is able to swallow and is awake, administer food. Maintain a source of glucose and glucagon kit at all time. Monitor serum glucose and serum potassium.

Education: Review signs and symptoms of hypoglycemia and hyperglycemia and how to manage prior to getting into trouble with an alteration in the LOC. Review the importance of keeping a source of glucose and glucagon kit close by at all times and teach how to use kit. Health care provider must be contacted immediately after each dose for orders regarding further therapy or adjustment of insulin dose or diet. Advise family that client should receive oral glucose when alertness returns. Instruct client to be positioned on side due to risk of vomiting from glucagon. Instruct client to check expiration date monthly and to replace outdated medication immediately. Review hypoglycemic medication regimen, diet, and exercise program. Clients with diabetes mellitus should carry a source of sugar (such as a packet of sugar or candy) and identification describing disease process and treatment regimen at all times.

Evaluation: Elevation in serum glucose to be greater than 50 mg/dL.

Drug: glucagon (GlucaGen)

GLUCAGON (GLUCAGEN)

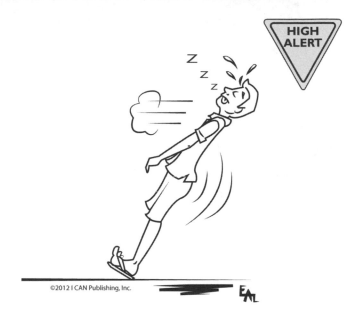

©2012 I CAN Publishing, Inc.

S ymptoms of hypoglycemia - Emergency care!

Y ummy candy/snack should be available

N ausea and vomiting may occur

C aution in clients with cardiovascular disease

O verdose of insulin requires Glucagon administration via IM, IV, or SQ

P rotect client with ⬇ LOC from aspiration

E mergency kit education is important

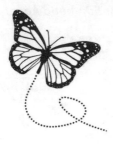

Vision without action is merely a dream. Action without vision merely passes the time. Vision and action can change the world.

JOEL BARKER

Central Nervous System Agents

MESCLIZINE

Action: CNS depressant, central anticholinergic and antihistaminic properties. It also decreases excitability of the middle ear labyrinth and depresses conduction in the middle ear.

Indications: Prevention and/or management of motion sickness, nausea, vomiting, and vertigo.

Warnings: Use cautiously in clients with prostatic hyperplasia, Closed-angle glaucoma and children.

Undesirable Effects: Drowsiness, fatigue, dry mouth, blurred vision.

Other Specific Information: CNS depressants including alcohol or other antihistamines, opioid analgesics, and sedative/hypnotics may result in additive CNS depression. Drugs possessing anticholinergic properties such as antihistamines, antidepressants, atropine, haloperidol, phenothiazines, quinidine and disopyramide.

Interventions: Assess for level of sedation after administered. Assess for nausea and vomiting before and 60 min. after administration. Assess for vertigo periodically in clients receiving mesclizine for labyrinthitis. May cause a false-negative result in skin tests using allergen extracts. Drug will need to be discontinued 72 hours before testing. Adminsiter oral doses with water, food, or milk.

Education: Advise client that medication may cause drowsiness, dry mouth, if used for motion sickness. Advise client to take at least 1 hour before any exposure to conditions that may cause motion sickness Client may need to use frequent mouth rinses, good oral hygiene, and sugarless gum or candy for dry mouth. Caution to avoid driving or other activities requiring mental alertness until response from medication has been determined. Discuss the importance of not taking alcohol and other CNS depressants with this medication.

Evaluation: Client will have relief of symptoms in motion sickness.

Drugs: meclizine (Antivert, Antrizine, Dramamine II, Bonine, D-vert, Medivert, Meclicot, Ru-Vert-M, Meni-D)

MESCLIZINE

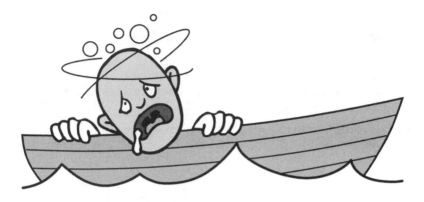

©2005 I CAN Publishing, Inc.

Bart is ready to throw up from his vertigo! Being in a boat does not help because now he has motion sickness.

NONBARBITURATES
SEDATIVE-HYPNOTICS

Action: CNS depression. Induces quiet, deep sleep.

Indications: Short-term treatment of insomnia.

Warnings: Hypersensitive to non-benzodiazepines. Sleep apnea. Anemia, hepatic, renal impairment, cardiac disease, gastritis, suicidal individuals, drug abuse, elderly, psychosis, seizure disorder, pregnancy, lactation, children <18 yr.

Undesirable Effects: Amnesia, daytime drowsiness, dizziness, "drugged" feeling, diarrhea, nausea, vomiting, hypersensitivity reactions, physical dependence, psychological dependence, tolerance.

Other Specific Information: Increased action of both drugs: alcohol, CNS depressants. Increased CNS depression with chamomile, kava, skullcap, valerian.

Interventions: Protect client from injury—raise bedside rails or assist with ambulation. Comply with federal narcotic laws regarding schedule IV drugs. Gastric irritations decrease by diluting dose. Baseline vital signs. Provide environment conducive to sleep. Assess sleep pattern of client. Evaluate elderly/children for paradoxical reaction. Assess blood studies, AST, ALT, bilirubin if liver damage has occurred. Assess mental status, signs of blood dyscrasias, and type of sleep problems.

Education: Take with a full glass of water or juice. Swallow whole, don't chew. Avoid alcohol and other CNS depressants. May cause dependence. Avoid abrupt discontinuation after prolonged use. Review alternative measures to improve sleep (reading, exercise several hours before hs, warm bath, warm milk, TV, self-hypnosis, etc). Clients > 65 years old, usual dose 5mg.

Evaluation: Client will be able to sleep at night, decreased amount of early morning awakening if taking drug for insomnia.

Drugs: Chloral Hydrate, zolpidem (Ambien)

AMY IS NOT AN "AM BIEN"

A nxiolytic and hypnotic effects

M orning drowsiness or hangover (modulates GABA receptors to cause suppression of neurons)

B eware of drug/drug toxic effects with Rifampin (blurred vision common side effect, so avoid tasks requiring driving)

I nsomnia treatment

E ffects REM sleep pattern by suppressing it

N on-barbituate (not for long term use)

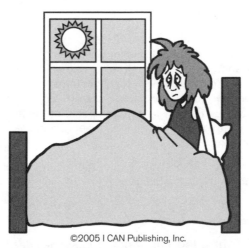

©2005 I CAN Publishing, Inc.

After Amy has taken her "AMBIEN" she goes in a deep sleep and is not ready to get up in the AM. Amy is not an "AM BIEN" (BEING).

NARCOTIC ANALGESICS

Action: Combines with opiate receptors in CNS. Reduces stimuli from sensory nerve endings; pain threshold is increased.

Indications: Moderate to severe pain, preoperative medication, and obstetrical analgesia. Methadone is used as part of heroin detoxification; hydrocodone and codeine have an antitussive effect.

Warnings: **HIGH ALERT DRUG** Alcoholism, respiratory, renal or hepatic disease, increased intracranial pressure, severe heart disease. Don't use Demerol in elderly clients or those with renal dysfunction.

Undesirable effects: "Droopy Deuteronomy" will help review the 6 D's.

Other Specific Information: Alcohol and/or CNS depressants may ↑ undesirable effects of CNS and/or respiratory depression. MAOIs may result in a fatal reaction. Note: IV doses are less than IM doses.

Interventions: Maintain records (most are class II drugs). Monitor urine output, bowel sounds, VS, and pain for type location, intensity, and duration. Dilute and administer IV solution slowly to prevent CNS depression and possible cardiac arrest. Do not mix with barbiturates. Hold medication if respirations < 12/min. with the adult or < 20/min. with the child. Have Narcan available.

Education: No alcohol or CNS depressants. Recommend nonpharmacological interventions for decreasing pain. No ambulating without assistance; no driving. Instruct to take before pain is too severe. Dependence on drug is not likely for short-term medical needs. Do not abruptly withdraw medication. Teach client with a patient-controlled analgesia (PCA) pump how to safely administer the medicine. Instruct about deep breathing and coughing, especially in clients with altered pulmonary function.

Staff Education: Do not confuse with oxycontin, oxycodone, MS Contin, morphine regular release.

Evaluation: The client's pain will be relieved without any undesirable effects from the medication.

Drugs (C-II controlled substance): Codeine; dezocine (Dalgan); fentanyl (Sublimaze); hydrocodone (Hycodan); hydromorphone (Dilaudid); levomethadyl (ORLAAM); levorphanol (Levo-Dromoran); meperidine (Demerol); methadone (Dolophine); morphine (Roxanol, MS Contin); oxycodone (Roxicodone); oxymorphone (Numorphan); propoxyphene (Darvon); remifentanil (Ultiva); sufentanil (Sufenta)

DROOPY DEUTERONOMY

HIGH ALERT

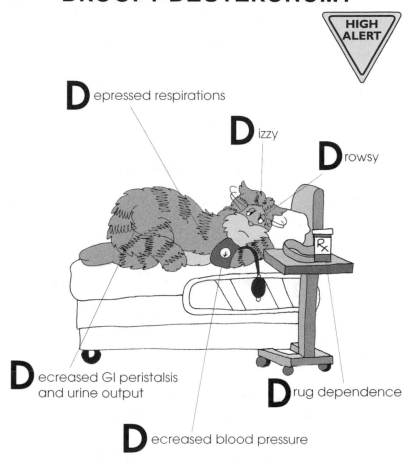

Depressed respirations

Dizzy

Drowsy

Decreased GI peristalsis and urine output

Drug dependence

Decreased blood pressure

©2001 I CAN Publishing, Inc.

"Droopy Deuteronomy" is drooping in his hospital bed from too much morphine. These drugs can make him throw up so he needs his emesis basin.

NARCOTIC ANTAGONISTS

Action: Reverses the effects of opioid agonist (narcotic analgesic) by competing for the receptor sites.

Indications: Reverses narcotic induced respiratory depression. Naloxone–drug for reversing respiratory depression.

Warnings: Hypersensitivity. Respiratory depression, narcotic addiction, cardiac disease, acute hepatitis or liver failure.

Undesirable effects: Negligible effects with no narcotics in body. The 5 P's demonstrated by **"PERKY PERKOLATOR"** will assist you in remembering these effects when the med is in the body. Pulse, pressure (blood), perspiration, pain, and puke (nausea and vomiting) are increased.

Other Specific Information: Verapamil can precipitate withdrawal in a client addicted to narcotic analgesics.

Interventions: Monitor client carefully as Naloxone "wears off" and opioid is still present; client may go back into a respiratory arrest. Nalmefene is longer acting than Naloxone, but client should still be observed until there is no risk of recurrent respiratory depression. Be aware of pain intensity when narcotic action is reversed. Have antagonist agent available. Have resuscitative equipment available immediately.

Education: Review the action of the drug with the client and family.

Evaluation: Client's respiratory rate and vital signs will remain within normal range.

Drugs: nalmefene (Revex); naloxone (Narcan); naltrexone (ReVia)

PERKY PERKOLATOR

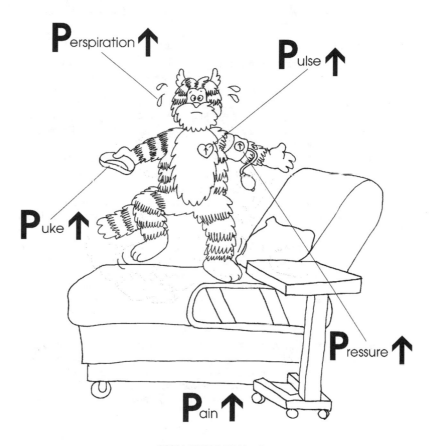

"Perky Perkolator" is experiencing some of the undesirable effects from these drugs (the 5 P's).

ANALGESIC (CENTRALLY ACTING): TRAMADOL

Action: Binds to mu-opioid receptors. Inhibits reuptake of serotonin and norepinephrine in the CNS.

Indications: Moderate to moderately severe pain.

Warnings: Contraindicate in hypersensitivity; Cross-sensitivity with opioids may occur. Intoxicated with alcohol, sedative/hypnotics, centrally acting analgesics, opioid analgesics, or psychotropic agents; A physical dependence on opioid analgesics; Pregnant or lactation. Use cautiously in geriatrics; clients at risk for seizures; Renal impairment; Hepatic impairment; Client receiving MAO inhibitors or CNS depressants; Increased intracranial pressure or head trauma; Acute abdomen; A history of opioid dependence or have recently received large doses of opioids. Children < 16 (safety not yet determined).

Undesirable Effects: Seizures, dizziness, headache, somnolence, anxiety, CNS stimulation, confusion, coordination disturbance; constipation, nausea, abdominal pain, anorexia, diarrhea, dry mouth, dyspepsia; physical dependent. May increase serum creatinine, elevated liver enzymes, decreased hemoglobin and proteinuria.

Other Specific Information: Increased risk of CNS depression when taken with other CNS depressants, including alcohol, antihistamines, sedative/hypnotics, opioid analgesics, anesthetics, or psychotropic agents. ↑ risk of seizures with high doses of penicillins, cephalosporins, phenothiazines, opioid analgesics, or antidepressants. Carbamazepine ↑ metabolism and ↓ effectiveness of tramadol (increased doses may be required). Kava kava, valerian, or chamomile can ↑ CNS depression.

Interventions: Do not confuse tramadol with Toradol (ketorolac). Assess characteristics of pain. Baseline vital signs. Assess bowel function. Assess previous analgesic history. Tramadol is not recommended for clients dependent on opioids or who have received opioids for more than 1 week since this may result in withdrawal symptoms. If tolerance develops, change to an opioid agonist. Monitor for seizures. Risk is increased with higher doses and in clients taking antidepressants (SSRIs, tricyclics, or MAO inhibitors), opioid analgesics or other drugs that alter the seizure threshold.

Education: Teach to administer as prescribed. Tramadol may be administered without regard to meals. Extended-release tablets should be swallowed whole; do not crush, break, or chew. Instruct client on how and when to ask for pain medication. Caution not to drive until cognitive response has been determined, since this drug may result in drowsiness and dizziness. Review the importance of changing positions slowly to decrease orthostatic hypotension. Caution client to avoid use of alcohol or other CNS depressants with this medication. Review importance of T, C, and DB every 2 hr to prevent atelectasis.

Evaluation: Client will experience a decrease in the severity of pain without a significant alteration in the level of consciousness or respiratory status.

Drugs: tramadol (Ralivia, Ultram, Ultram ER)

TRAMADOL (UL "TRAM")

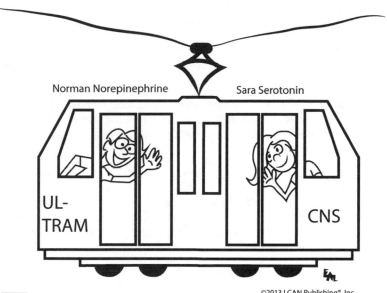

Norman Norepinephrine   Sara Serotonin

UL-
TRAM   CNS

©2013 I CAN Publishing®, Inc.

T reatment for moderate to severe pain

R euptake of serotonin and norepinephrine
      are inhibited; renal and hepatic
      impairment may occur

A ssess characteristics of pain; bowel function

M onitor serum creatinine; liver enzymes;
      hemoglobin

Norman Norepinephrine and Sara Serotonin will not
get taken up again on the TRAM (reuptake is inhibited).

SKELETAL MUSCLE RELAXERS
(SMRs)

Action: Act with the central nervous system, not directly on the muscles except for Dantrium that acts directly upon the muscle cells by interfering with the movement of Calcium ions which relaxes the muscle. May provide temporary relief of pain. These are considered a controlled substance.

Indications: To relax muscles, ease pain, and reduce spasm and stiffness. Used to treat injury or other acute or chronic conditions affecting muscles, such as fibromyalgia, arthritis chronic pain, multiple sclerosis, or spinal injury.

Warnings: Cyclobenzaprine (Flexeril), when combined with other medications that increase serotonin can cause a sometimes fatal side-effect–"Serotonin Syndrome". Muscle relaxers can be addictive. When mixed with some types of medications the efficacy of muscle relaxers are increased, making the drug dangerous. In women, muscle relaxers can interact with estrogen supplements.

Undesirable Effects: Drowsiness, dizziness, fatigue, muscle weakness, nausea, diarrhea, difficulty swallowing, dry mouth, blurred vision, headache, fever, impaired thinking, functioning and decision making.

Other Specific Information: Valium, a depressant, should not be used long term and can worsen depression associated with chronic pain. Flexeril can impair mental and physical function, and may lead to urinary retention in males with enlarged prostates. Avoid use if taking tricyclic antidepressants (e.g., Elavil), SSRI's, MAO inhibitors (e.g., Parnate), other drugs that effect the heart rhythm.

Interventions: Monitor liver function tests, falls precautions.

Education: Review potential side effects with client and instruct to report to the healthcare provider. Instruct client not to drive or operate machinery because of drowsiness, avoid alcohol and other antidepressants while taking muscle relaxants.

Evaluation: Improve quality of life, no pain, or decreased pain.

Drugs: carisoprodol (Soma), cyclobenzaprine (Flexeril, Flexmid, Amrix), diazepam (Valium), dantrolene (Dantrium), metaxalone (Skelaxin), methocarbamol (Robaxin), tizanidine (Zanaflex), orphenadrine (Norflex)

CARISOPRODOL (SOMA)
CYCLOBENZAPRINE (FLEXERIL)
DIAZEPAM (VALIUM)

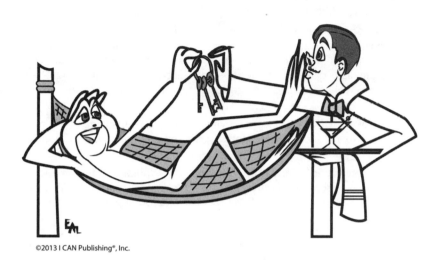

©2013 I CAN Publishing®, Inc.

R educes stiffness, spasms, pain in muscles

E valuate liver function tests

L imit driving, operating machinery because of drowsiness, dizziness

A void taking relaxants with antidepressants

X out alcohol

Mr. Frog has hopped one too many times, and now needs to "RELAX" with some Muscle relaxants.

ADDERALL

Action: Norepinephrine from nerve endings is released. CNS and respiratory stimulation, vasoconstriction. Mydriasis (pupillary dilation). Increased motor activity and mental alertness. Decrease fatigue in narcoleptic clients.

Indications: Narcolepsy. ADHD.

Warnings: Hyperexcitable states including hyperthyroidism; Psychotic personalities; Suicidal tendencies. Glaucoma; Structural cardiac abnormalities (may increase the risk of sudden death). Caution with cardiovascular disease, hypertension, diabetes mellitus; Tourette's syndrome. Geriatrics or debilitated clients may be more susceptible to undesirable effects.

Undesirable Effects: Hyperactivity, insomnia, restlessness, tremor, dizziness; palpitations, tachycardia; anorexia, constipation, cramps, diarrhea, dry mouth, metallic taste, nausea, vomiting.

Other Specific Information: Use with MAO Inhibitors or meperidine can result in hypertensive crisis. Increase in adrenergic effects with other adrenergics or thyroid preparations. Sodium bicarbonate or acetazolamide alkalinize urine resulting in a decrease in the excretion and an increase in the effects. Drugs that acidify urine (ammonium chloride), large doses of ascorbic acid increase excretion, decreasing the effects. Beta blockers taken with these drugs can increase the risk for hypertension and bradycardia. Digoxin taken with these amphetamine mixtures may contribute to arrhythmias. St. John's Wort may increase serious undesirable effects. Fruit juices can increase the effect of amphetamines.

Interventions: Monitor blood pressure, heart rate, and respirations. May provide a false sense of euphoria. Has a high dependency and abuse potential. Tolerance occurs quickly; do not increase the dose of this medication. Monitor weight biweekly and notify provider of care for significant loss. May be taken without regard to food. Assess attention span, impulse control, and interaction with others.

Education: Advise to take as ordered. Instruct to take medication 6 hours prior to going to bed. Review importance for good mouth care. Advise not to take in excess amount of caffeine. Advise client to use caution when driving and report undesirable effects. Take periodic holidays from the drug to assess progress and decrease dependence. Instruct not to alter dose without consulting with provider of care.

Evaluation: Client will have an improved attention span and a decrease in narcoleptic symptoms.

Drugs: amphetamine mixtures (Adderall, Adderall XR, Amphetamine Salt)

ADDERALL
"ADD + HER + ALL = ADDERALL"

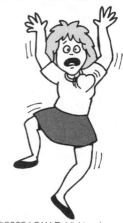

A DHD—indication

D ilaton of pupils

D oes not sleep—indication

©2009 I CAN Publishing, Inc.

H yperactivity—undesirable effect

E valuate for palpitations & tachycardia

R emind client never to alter dose without consultation

A void MAOI, caffeine, stimulants

L oss of weight and other undesirable effects

L ook for a false sense of euphoria

While a client may have an improvement in their attention span, there are many risks to theses drugs. It is IMPERATIVE that significant weight losses and caridac symptoms are reported to the provider of care. Clients should be advised to take periodic holidays from the drug to assess progress and decrease dependence.

CENTRAL NERVOUS SYSTEM STIMULANT: RITALIN

Action: Increases release of norepinephrine, dopamine in cerebral cortex to reticular activiting system.

Indications: Attention deficit hyperactivity disorder, narcolepsy.

Warnings: Hypersensitivity to any component in the drug; history of Tourette's disorder; history of agitation, anxious, glaucoma; caution if client has a history of depression, hypertension, drug dependency.

Undesirable Effects: Nervousness, headache, hypertension, tachycardia, insomnia, dizzy, anorexia, dry mouth, bruising (rare).

Other Specific Information: CNS stimulants may have addictive effect. MAO inhibitors may increase effect. Decreased effect of guanethidine. Increased effects of tricyclics, anticonvulsants, SSRIs. Increased stimulation with caffeine. Increased stimulation with ephedra, cola nut, guarana.

Interventions: Do not crush or allow client to chew sustained release dosage form. Administer at least 6 hr before hs to avoid sleeplessness (regular release); at least 10 hr (SR, ER). Discontinue drugs or decrease dose if paradoxical return of attention deficit disorder. Monitor B/P. Monitor CBC, urinalysis, in diabetes: blood sugar, urine sugar; insulin changes may need to be made due to a decrease in eating. Monitor height, growth rate q 3 months. Monitor mental status. Monitor for undesirable effects.

Education: Review how to take med and the appropriate time of the day. Decrease caffeine consumption. Avoid OTC preparations unless approved by provider. Taper off slowly or depression, lethargy, and increased sleeping may occur. Avoid driving if experiencing blurred vision. Avoid alcohol. Get needed rest; client will be more tired at the end of the day. Review and report undesirable effects. Dry mouth—sugarless gum, sips of tepid water.

Staff Education: Do not confuse methylphenidate with methadone. Follow standards of care when administering a Controlled Substance Schedule II medication.

Evaluation: Client will have a decrease in hyperactivity (ADD or ADHD) or ability to stay awake (narcolepsy).

Drugs: methylphenidate (Ritalin, Ritalin SR, Concerta, Metadate CD, Metadate ER, Methylin, Methylin SR, PMS-methylphenidate, Methidate, PMS-Methylphenidate, Riphenidate; dexmethylphenidate (Focalin); dextroamphetamine (Dexedrine)

RITALIN

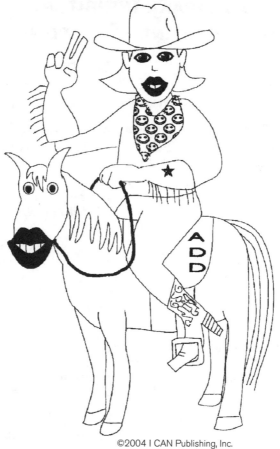

©2004 I CAN Publishing, Inc.

Avoid caffeine

Do not break, crush or chew time-released

Dopamine in cerebral cortex is increased

TexRita is on her horse ADD. Ritalin is given for attention deficit disorder.

NOREPINEPHRINE SELECTIVE REUPTAKE INHIBITOR: ATOMOXETINE (STRATTERA)

Action: Blocks reuptake of norepinephrine at synapses in the CNS.

Indications: Attention-Deficit/Hyperactivity Disorder (ADHD)

Warnings: Use cautiously in clients with cardiovascular disease. Contraindicated in concurrent or within 2 week therapy with MAO inhibitors; Angle-closure glaucoma.

Undesirable Effects: Appetite suppression, weight loss, growth reduction; nausea and vomiting; suicidal ideation (in children and adolescents); hepatotoxicity; dizziness, fatigue, insomnia; hypertension, orthostatic hypotension, dry mouth, constipation; urinary retention.

Other Specific Information: Concurrent use of MAOIs may result in hypertensive crisis. Increased risk of cardiovascular effects with albuterol or vasopressors (use cautiously). Drugs which inhibit the CYP2D6 enzyme pathway (quinidine, fluoxetine, paroxetine) will increase blood levels and effects; it is recommended that the dose be ↓.

Interventions: Assess the client's weight, height, and growth and compare to baseline. Monitor blood pressure and pulse routinely during therapy. Administer immediately prior to meals. Encourage healthy eating and avoid unhealthy food and snacks. Advise to take with some food if nausea occurs. Monitor for signs of depression. Review importance of having client report a change in mood, agitation, irritability, and excessive sleeping. Report signs of liver damage (flu-like symptoms, jaundice, abdominal pain). Avoid using MAOIs. Notice any change in child related to dosing and timing of medication. Administer in a daily dose in the AM or in two divided doses, morning and afternoon.

Education: Instruct client that it may take at least one week for effect to fully develop.

Evaluation: Client will experience an improvement of symptoms of ADHD such as ability to focus.

Drug: atomoxetine (Strattera)

ATOMOXETINE (STRATTERA)

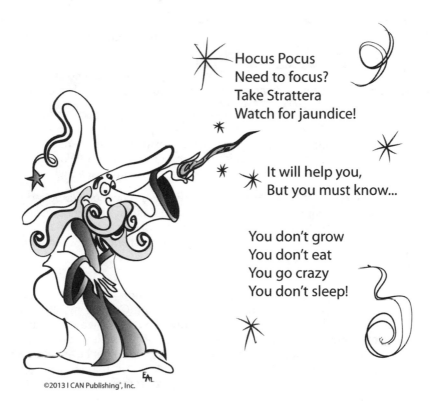

Hocus Pocus
Need to focus?
Take Strattera
Watch for jaundice!

It will help you,
But you must know...

You don't grow
You don't eat
You go crazy
You don't sleep!

©2013 I CAN Publishing®, Inc.

Remember, if any of these symptoms start occuring, call heathcare provider to intervene, so these will stop reoccuring.

NEUROMUSCULAR BLOCKERS

Action: Inhibits transmission of nerve impulses by binding with cholinergic receptor sites, antagonizing the action of acetylcholine.

Indications: Facilitates endotracheal intubation, skeletal muscle relaxation during mechanical ventilation, surgery, or general anesthesia.

Warnings: **HIGH ALERT DRUG** Hypersensitivity to bromide ion (Pavulon). Cardiac disease, children < 2, electrolyte imbalances, dehydration, neuromuscular disease, respiratory disease. History of malignant hyperthermia.

Undesirable Effects: Bradycardia; tachycardia; increased or decreased blood pressure; ventricular extrasystoles. Prolonged apnea, bronchospasms, cyanosis, respiratory depression. Weakness to prolonged skeletal muscle relaxation. Rash, pruritus. Anaphylaxis.

Other Specific Information: Increased neuromuscular blockade with aminoglycosides, clindamycin, enflurane, isoflurane, lincomycin, lithium, local anesthetics, opioid analgesics, polymyxin anti-infectives, quinidine, thiazides. If taken with theophylline the client may experience dysrhythmias.

Interventions: Concurrent sedation is required because of anxiety related to immobility; the client can feel, but not respond to pain. Total physical care, including ventilatory support. Cardiac monitoring including HR, BP, and ECG. Eye lubrication to prevent corneal abrasions. Interact appropriately with client and close to client since hearing is not impaired. During recovery, respirations must be assessed carefully. Neostigmine (Prostigmin) is antidote for nondepolarizing agents. Need DVT prophylaxis. Train of Four monitoring for ICU continuous infusion paralysis.

Education: Reassure client and / or family that the paralysis is only temporary. Repeat explanations about procedures and equipment due to high anxiety level.

Evaluation: The client will be paralyzed.

Drugs: atracurium (Tracrium), doxacurium (Nuromax), pancuronium (Pavulon), pipecuronium (Arduan), vecuronium (Norcuron)

RAGGEDY ANNE

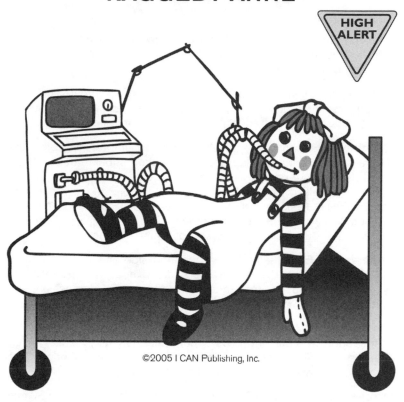

©2005 I CAN Publishing, Inc.

Raggedy Anne needs a cure. She is not unconscious but her arms and legs are falling off the table due to skeletal muscle relaxation. She can't breathe without the help of her ventilator. She has received a neuromuscular blocking agent. Many of these drugs have "curonium" in them.

ANESTHETICS–LOCAL

Action: (General) Act on the CNS to produce tranquilization and sleep before invasive procedures. Anesthetics (local) inhibit conduction of nerve impulses from sensory nerves.

Indications: General anesthetics are used to premedicate for surgery, induction and maintenance in general anesthesia. For local anesthetics, refer to individual product listing for indications.

Warnings: Persons with CVA, increased intracranial pressure, severe hypertension, cardiac decompensation should not use these products, since severe adverse reactions can occur. Use in caution with the elderly, clients with cardiovascular disease (hypotension, bradydysrhythmias), renal disease, liver disease, Parkinson's disease, children < 2 yr, and pregnant women. Clients allergic to lidocaine, novocaine or bupivacaine, use chloroprocaine (Nesacaine).

Undesirable Effects: The most common side effects are dystonia, akathisia, flexion of arms, fine tremors, drowsiness, restlessness, and hypotension. Also common are chills, respiratory depression, and laryngospasm.

Other Specific Information: Metabolized in the liver and excreted in the urine. MAOIs, tricyclics, phenothiazines may cause severe hypotension or hypertension when used with local anesthetics. CNS depressants will potentiate general and local anesthetics.

Interventions: Assess VS q 10 min during IV administration, q 30 min. after IM dose. Administer anticholinergic peroperatively to decrease secretions. Administer only with crash cart, resuscitative equipment nearby. Provide a quiet environment for recovery to decrease psychotic symptoms.

Evaluation: Maintenance of anesthesia, decreased pain.

Drugs: (Injectionables only): *Local anesthetics:* lidocaine (Xylocaine), procaine (Novocaine), tetracaine (Pontocaine)

FEELINGLESS FIFI

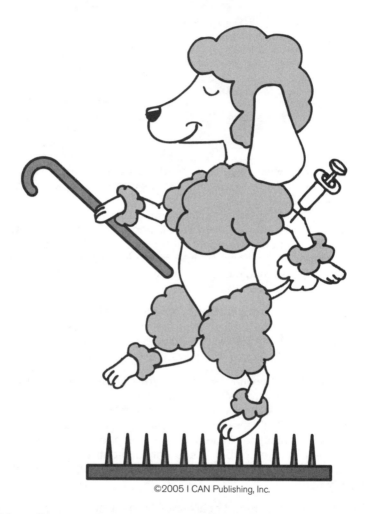

Fifi is walking across a bed of nails carrying her "caine" and feeling nothing. She has had an injection of a local anesthetic. Many of these anesthetics have the word **caine** in them.

GENERAL ANESTHETIC: PROPOFOL

Action: General anesthesia/sedation

Indications: Procedures requiring conscious sedation for children and adults; continuous sedation in intubated, ventilated clients.

Warnings: **HIGH ALERT DRUG** Med-risk for significant harm if used incorrectly! Do not use with egg and soybean allergies. Caution with burns, sepsis, seizure disorders, cardiovascular or respiratory disease.

Undesirable Effects: Anaphylaxis; over-sedation; respiratory depression or apnea; hypotension (dose dependent); bradycardia; fever; metabolic acidosis; rash; myoclonus,twitching or pain. Be aware of Propofol Infusion Syndrome in prolonged, high doses: metabolic acidosis and multi-organ failure. Causes rapid sedation effect (less than 30 seconds after administration) and wears off quickly—within 5-10 minutes. An effective agent for short-term sedation needs such as procedures—MRIs, bone marrow biopsies, etc. Drug "holidays" to prevent build up of medication and allow assessment of mental status if using for multiple days continuously.

Other Specific Information: Additive CNS and respiratory depression when taken with alcohol, antihistamines, opioid analgesics, and sedative/hypnotics (dosage reduction may be necessary). Serious bradycardia can occur with concurrent use of fentanyl in children.

Interventions: Continuous cardiac/respiratory monitoring and airway management a must! If not intubated, need to monitor ability to protect airway. Have mask and ambu-bag, suction, and artificial airway equipment at bedside. IV injection is painful—give IV lidocaine before or with this medication. Monitor ABGs, electrolytes, renal function during treatment. Remember this is only a sedative; pain medication needed too! **Do not confuse Diprivan (propofol) with Diflucan (fluconazole).**

Education: Confirm report of allergies (especially egg and soybean!) and past anesthesia reactions at every hospitalization. Review with family the effects of sedation and the monitoring needs post-procedure.

Evaluation: Client will tolerate procedure without adverse effects from undersedation, pain, or oversedation. Client's airway and breathing will be maintained during administration of Propofol.

Drug: propofol (Diprivan)

PROPOFOL (DIPRIVAN)

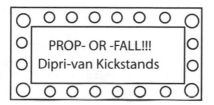

PROP- OR -FALL!!!
Dipri-van Kickstands

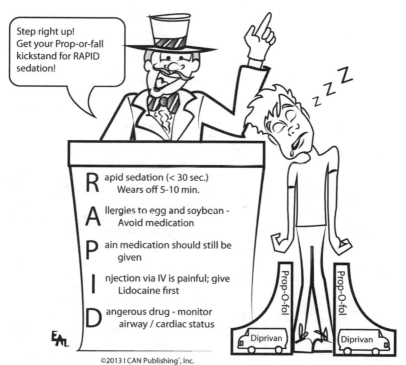

Step right up!
Get your Prop-or-fall
kickstand for RAPID
sedation!

R apid sedation (< 30 sec.)
Wears off 5-10 min.

A llergies to egg and soybean -
Avoid medication

P ain medication should still be
given

I njection via IV is painful; give
Lidocaine first

D angerous drug - monitor
airway / cardiac status

©2013 I CAN Publishing®, Inc.

NONOPIOID ANALGESIC: PREGABALIN (LYRICA)

Action: Binds to calcium channels in CNS tissues which regulate neurotransmitter release. Does not bind to opioid receptors.

Indications: Pain due to diabetic peripheral neuropathy, postherpetic neuralgia, fibromyalgia. Adjunctive therapy of partial-onset seizures in adults. Schedule V.

Warnings: Contraindicated in clients with myopathy (known or suspected). Use cautiously in renal impairment (dose alteration recommended for CCr < 60 ml / min); Elderly clients due to age-related decrease in renal function; CHF; History of drug dependence / drug-seeking behavior; Children (safety not established).

Undesirable Effects: Hypersensitivity; dizziness, drowsiness, altered concentration; Edema, blurred vision; dry mouth, constipation, ↑ appetite, vomiting, weight gain. May cause an elevation in the creatinine kinase levels. May cause a decrease in the platelet count.

Other Specific Information: Concurrent use with thiazolidinediones (pioglitazone, rosiglitazone) may increase risk of fluid retention. Increase risk of CNS depression with other CNS depressants including alcohol, benzodiazepines, opioids, or other hypnotics / sedatives.

Interventions: Diabetic Peripheral Neuropathy, Post-herpetic Neuralgia, and Fibromylagia: Assess characteristics, location, and intensity of pain/ discomfort throughout therapy. If administered for seizures, assess location, duration, and characteristics of seizure. May be administered without regard to food. Pregabalin should be slowly discontinued over at least 1 week. Abrupt stopping may result in nausea, insomnia, headache, and diarrhea when used for pain and may result in increase seizures when treating seizures.

Education: Advise client to take as directed. Do NOT discontinue abruptly. May cause dizziness and drowsiness and blurred vision, so do not operate any equipment or engage in any activity that may require alertness until cognitive response has been determined. Notify provider for any visual changes. Discontinue if myopathy is diagnosed or if elevated creatinine kinase levels occur. Review with client that weight gain and edema may occur. Instruct to notify provider if pregnant or suspected. Inform male clients who plan to father a child of the risk of male-mediated teratogenicity. Review regimen of medication prior to treatment. Recommend to carry an identification describing disease process and medication regimen at all times.

Evaluation: Client will experience a decrease in the intensity of the chronic pain. Client will experience a decrease in the frequency or cessation of seizures.

Drug: pregabalin (Lyrica)

LYRICA

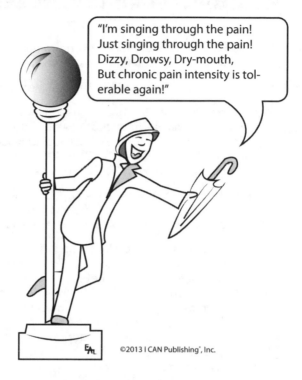

"I'm singing through the pain!
Just singing through the pain!
Dizzy, Drowsy, Dry-mouth,
But chronic pain intensity is tolerable again!"

©2013 I CAN Publishing®, Inc.

P ain due to diabetic peripheral neuropathy; postherpetic neuralgia; fibromyalgia.

A djunctive therapy of partial-onset seizures in adults.

I f myopathy is diagnosed or if creatinine kinase levels are elevated, discontinue and call provider.

N otify provider for any visual changes. Notify client that weight gain and edema may occur.

Some classic "Lyricas"

INSOMNIA AGENT–(MELATONIN RECEPTOR AGONISTS): ROZEREM

Action: Activates melatonin receptors, which promotes maintenance of the circadian rhythm, a component of the sleep-wake cycle.

Indications: Insomnia characterized by difficult sleep onset.

Warnings: Contraindicated in hypersensitivity; severe hepatic disease; concurrent fluvoxamine. Pediatrics–safety not yet determined. Use cautiously in depression or history of suicidal ideation; Moderate hepatic impairment; Concurrent use of CYP3A4 inhibitors, such as ketoconazole; Concurrent use of CYP2C9, such as fluconazole; OB.

Undesirable Effects: Abnormal thinking, behavioral changes, syncope, fatigue, headache, insomnia (worsened), sleep–driving. Increases prolactin levels and decreases testosterone levels.

Other Specific Information: Blood levels and effects are increased by fluvoxamine, potent inhibitor of the CYP1A2 enzyme system; concurrent use is contraindicated. Levels and effects may be decreased by rifampin. Concurrent use of CYP3A4 inhibitors, such as ketoconazole may increase levels and effects; use carefully. Concurrent use of CYP2C9 inhibitors, such as fluconazole may increase levels and effects. Increased risk of excessive CNS depression may occur with other CNS depressants including alcohol, benzodiazepines, opioids, and other sedatives/hypnotics.

Interventions: Assess patterns of sleep prior to and during therapy. Do not administer after a high fat meal; recommend taking on an empty stomach. Prior to admitting, reduce external stimuli and provide comfort measure to facilitate rest.

Education: Instruct to take as prescribed, 30 minutes prior to going to bed and to decrease activities to those preparing for sleep. Caution client not to drive after taking due to it causing sleep. Review the importance of not taking in any alcohol or other CNS depressants.

Evaluation: Client will be able to sleep and be relieved of insomnia.

Drug: ramelteon (Rozerem)

ROZEREM (MELATONIN)

I ndication: Insomnia characterized by difficult sleep onset

N ot given if client has severe hepatic disease

S yncope, fatigue, headache, insomnia may worsen, abnormal thinking, behavioral changes (undesirable effects)

O ther CNS depressants may interact and result in ⬆ CNS depression

M easures to promote rest (e.g., reduce external stimuli)

N o driving after taking Rozerem due to causing lethargy

I nstruct to not take after a high fat meal; recommend taking on an empty stomach

A dminister 30 minutes prior to going to bed

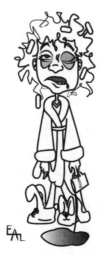

EAL
©2013 I CAN Publishing®, Inc.

CENTRAL NERVOUS SYSTEM STIMULANTS: MODAFINIL (PROVIGIL)

Action: Produces CNS stimulation.

Indications: To improve wakefulness in clients with excessive daytime drowsiness due to narcolepsy, shift work sleep disturbances, or sleep apnea.

Warnings: Contraindicated in hypersensitivity; History of left ventricular hypertrophy or ischemic ECG alterations, dysrhythmia, chest pain, or other significant changes of mitral valve prolapsed in association with CNS stimulant use. Use cautiously in clients with a history of MI or unstable angina; Hepatic impairment that is severe including clients with or without cirrhosis; Use of MAO inhibitors; Geriatric clients; Pregnancy, lactation, or children < 16 years of age (safety not established).

Undesirable Effects: Headache, amnesia, anxiety; Rhinitis, abnormal vision, pharyngitis; dyspnea, lung disorder; nausea, abnormal liver function; anorexia, diarrhea; dry skin, herpes simplex, hyperglycemia. May cause elevated liver enzymes.

Other Specific Information: May decrease the metabolism and increase the effects of diazepam, phenytoin, propranolol, or tricyclic antidepressants. May increase metabolism and decrease effects of hormonal contraceptives, cyclosporine, and theophylline (dosage adjustments or additional methods of contraception may be necessary). Stimulant effect may be increased if used with caffeine-containing herbs (cola nut, tea, coffee).

Interventions: Observe and document frequency of narcoleptic occurrences. Monitor liver enzymes per protocol. Monitor as a single dose in the morning for clients with narcolelpsy or sleep apnea. Administer one hour prior to the start of work shift for clients with shift work sleep disturbances.

Education: Instruct to take as prescribed. Review importance of not driving due to potential alteration in judgment. Nonhormonal methods of contraception should be used during and for 1 month following discontinuation of therapy. Notify provider if pregnancy is suspected or planned or if breastfeeding. Instruct to avoid taking OTC or other meds without consulting provider. Limit alcohol. Notify provider if rash, hives or other allergic reactions occur.

Evaluation: Client will experience a decrease in narcoleptic symptoms and an increased ability to stay awake.

Drugs: modafinil (Provigil)

MODAFINIL (PROVIGIL)

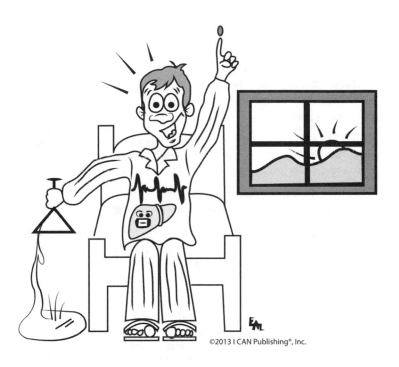

©2013 I CAN Publishing®, Inc.

A Arrhythmias, ECG changes – do not administer

W Wakefulness in clients with narcolepsy

A AST/ALT – monitor

K Know to take a single dose in the AM

E Eliminate alcohol

MIOTICS

Action: Stimulates pupillary and ciliary sphinceter muscles resulting in pupillary constriction.

Indications: Decrease IOP in glaucoma; surgical procedures on the eye.

Warnings: Retinal detachment, ocular inflammation; avoid systemic absorption of drug with coronary artery disease, GI/GU obstruction, asthma, epilepsy.

Undesirable effects: Blurred vision, myopia, eye pain; headache; nausea, vomiting; muscle tremors; hypertension, tachycardia; retinal detachment; long term: bronchospasm.

Other Specific Information: Avoid using carbachol with pilocarpine. ↓ antiglaucoma effects with belladonna alkaloids.

Intervention: Baseline vital signs. Monitor for postural hypotension. Assess breath sounds; may develop rales or rhonchi from bronchospasm and increase bronchial secretions. Press inner canthus for a minute or two to minimize systemic absorption.

Education: Instruct client not to rinse the dropper; do not place dropper on any surface. Do not use discolored solution. Advise client not to take any atropine-like medications due to the potential increase in IOP. Instruct client and family how to safely administer eye drops. Have a return demonstration. Remember the importance of WASHING HANDS. Instruct client that long-term therapy is a possibility.

Evaluation: Intraocular pressure will return to therapeutic range.

Drugs: carbachol (Carboptic); pilocarpine (Isopto Carpine); pilocarpine nitrate (Ocusert Pilo-20, Pilo-40)

MIOTICS: CONSTRICT EYES

MIOTICS
   O
   NO ATROPINE!!
   S
   T
   R
   I
   C
   T

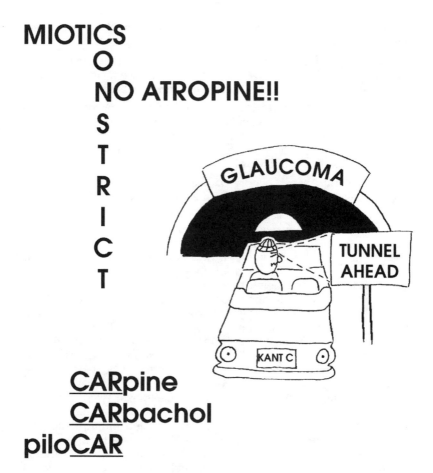

CARpine
CARbachol
pilo**CAR**

BOTOX

Action: A temporary reduction in wrinkles is caused when the nerve activity is blocked in the muscles.

Indications: To treat cervical dystonia, hyperhidrosis, and certain eye muscle conditions caused by nerve disorders. Lessens the appearance of facial wrinkles only temporarily.

Warnings: Allergies to botulinum toxin, heart disease, ALS, myasthenia gravis, or Lambert-Eaton syndrome.

Undesirable Effects: Drooping eyelids, vision problems, trouble breathing (weak or shallow), talking or swallowing, severe muscle weakness, flu like symptoms, chest pain, and nausea.

Other Specific Information: Aminoglycosides, or other agents interfering with neuromuscular transmission (e.g., curare-like nondepolarizing blockers, lincosamides, polymyxins, quinidine, magnesium sulfate, anticholinesterases, succinylcholine chloride) may potentiate the effects of Botox.

Interventions: Assess history of client to determine any potential risks for having this procedure. Monitor for undesirable effects.

Education: Instruct client to seek immediate medical attention if swallowing, speech or respiratory disorders arise. If receiving Botox injections for an eye muscle condition, instruct client that they may need to use eye drops, ointment, or a special contact lens or other device to protect the surface of the eye. Follow the physician's instructions. If client is being treated for excessive sweating, instruct client to shave the underarms about 24 hours prior to receiving the injection. Instruct regarding the importance of not applying underarm antiperspirants or deodorants for 24 hours prior to receiving the injection. Avoid exercise and hot foods or beverages within 30 minutes before the injection. It may take up to 2 weeks after injection before neck muscle spasm symptoms begin to improve. Clients may notice the greatest improvement at 6 weeks after injection. It may take only 1 to 3 days after injection before eye muscle spasm symptoms begin to improve. Clients may notice the greatest improvement at 2 to 6 weeks after injection. The effects of a Botox injection are temporary. Symptoms may return completely within 3 months after an injection. After repeat injections, it may take less and less time before symptoms return, especially if the body develops antibodies to the Botox. Do not seek Botox injections from more than one medical professional at a time. If client changes healthcare providers, it is important to inform the new provider how long it has been since the last Botox injection.

Evaluation: Client will experience no undesirable effects from the injection and will have desirable effects from the procedure.

Drug: botulinum toxin type A (Botox)

BOTOX

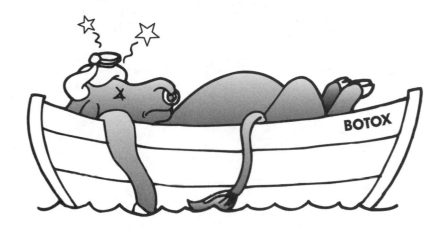

©2008 I CAN Publishing, Inc.

B otulinum

O ccasional headaches and nausea

T arget muscles relax

O pening of the eye may be affected

X out clients who have muscle weakness

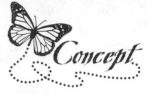

MIGRAINES

M edication administration when headache starts

I dentify triggers

G I complication with constipation with verapamil (Calan) and amitriptyline (Elavil)—increase fluids!

R eview importance of lying down in a quiet, dark room

A lchohol is to be avoided since it is a trigger. Assess pain, location, duration, intensity and associated symptoms.

I mportant not to drive until level of cognitive response from med has been determined

N otify provider of care of signs and symptoms

E valuate HR and BP prior to administering verapamil (Calan)

S timuli in room needs to be reduced—quiet, dark to decrease complications

MIGRAINES

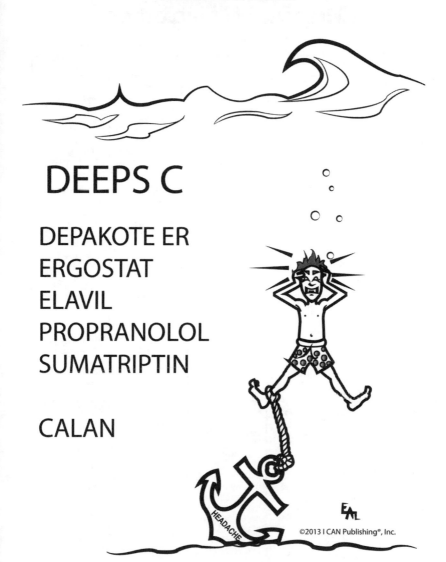

DEEPS C

DEPAKOTE ER
ERGOSTAT
ELAVIL
PROPRANOLOL
SUMATRIPTIN

CALAN

HEADACHE

©2013 I CAN Publishing®, Inc.

A headache can make you feel like you're trapped
beneath the deep sea! (DEEPS C)

COMPARISON OF
MIGRAINE MEDICATIONS

Classification	Generic (Trade Name)	Warnings	Undesirable Effects	Nursing Interventions
Anticonvulsant	Divalproex (Depakote ER)	Liver disease; Neural tube defects;	Liver toxicity; Pancreatitis; abdominal pain; leukopenia; thrombocyto-penia	Use adequate contraceptives. Monitor AST/ALT. Report abdominal pain, nausea, vomiting and anorexia. DC med.
Ergot Alkaloids	Ergotamine (Ergostat)	Liver and/or renal dysfunction; sepsis, CAD	GI: nausea/vomiting; Ergotism (muscle pain; paresthesias in fingers and toes; cold, pale, pale extremities). Physical dependence.	Administer metoclopramide (Reglan). DC med; notify HCP immediately if symptoms occur. Inform clients regard-ing symptoms of withdrawal (headache, nausea, vomiting, restlessness) and instruct clients to notify provider if symptoms occur.
Tricyclic antidepres-sants	Amitriptyline (Elavil)	Recent MI or within 14 days of a MAO inhibitor. Use caution in clients with seizure history, urinary reten-tion, prostatic hypertrophy, angle-closure glaucoma, hyperthyroid-ism and others.	Anticholinergic effects (Can't pee, see, spit, and sh*t) tachycardia; hypotension; Drowsiness, dizziness	↑fluid and fiber intake, exercise. Administer stimulant laxa-tives, such as biscodyl (Dul-colax), to alter reduced bowel motility. Stool softeners, such as docu-sate sodium (Colace), to decrease constipation. Report blurred vision.

Classification	Generic (Trade Name)	Warnings	Undesirable Effects	Nursing Interventions
Beta-blockers	Propranolol (Inderal)	Greater than first degree heart block, bradycardia, bronchial asthma, cardogenic shock or CHF	Extreme fatigue and tiredness, depression, asthma exacerbation; bradycardia, hypotension	Notify provider if undesirable effects occur. Assess HR and BP. Advise client to take apical HR prior to dosage.
Calcium Channel Blockers	Verapamil (Calan)	Greater than first degree heart block, bradycardia, hypotension, left ventricle disease, atrial fibrillation or flutter or heart failure. Caution in clients with renal or liver impairment or increased intracranial pressure.	Orthostatic hypotension, bradycardia; constipation	Recommend client sit down if lightheaded or dizzy. Change positions slowly. Assist with ambulation as needed. Assess HR. ↑fluid, fiber, exercise. Administer stimulant laxatives, such as bisacodyl (Dulcolax) to assist with bowel motility or stool softeners, such as docusate sodium (Colace).
Serotonin receptor agonists (Triptans)	Sumatriptan (Imitrex)	Liver failure, ischemic heart disease, HX of myocardial infarction, uncontrolled hypertension, and other heart diseases.	Chest pressure (heavy arms or chest tightness); Coronary artery vasospasm/angina; dizziness or vertigo.	Used only DURING a migraine; not to prevent. Educate client about symptoms. Notify HCP for severe chest pain. If migraine symptoms return, a 2nd injection may be used. Allow at least 1 hr between doses, and do NOT use more than 2 injections in any 24-hr period.

DIVALPROEX (DEPAKOTE)

Action: Increase levels of GABA, an inhibitory neurotransmitter in the CNS. Decreased frequency of migraine headaches by preventing the inflammation and dilation of the intracranial blood vessels, thereby relieving migraine pain.

Indications: Prevention of migraine headaches. Stopping an acute migraine attack.

Warnings: Avoid use during pregnancy. Use adequate contraception during therapy due to the complication of neural tube defects. Contraindicated with liver disease. Use cautiously in bleeding disorders.

Undesirable Effects: Liver toxicity, pancreatitis. Abdominal pain, anorexia, diarrhea, indigestion, nausea, vomiting, constipation; weight gain; leukopenia, thrombocytopenia; tremor, ataxia.

Other Specific Information: Aspirin, chlorpromazine, and cimetidine may result in bleeding. Benzodiazepines, alcohol, opioid analgesics, MAO inhibitors, and sedative/hypnotics may cause CNS depression. Do not use these together. Divalproex may increase levels of phenobarbital and phenytoin.

Interventions: Medication should be administered at the first sign of a headache. Assess pain location, duration, intensity, and associated symptoms such as photophobia, phonophobia, nausea, and vomiting during migraine attack and frequency of attacks. Monitor levels per protocol. Do not use with benzodiazepines due to risk for CNS depression. Monitor AST, ALT, LDH, and bilirubin and serum ammonia prior to and during therapy. DC if hyperammonemia occurs. **Do not confuse Depakote ER and regular dosage forms.** (Refer to "**MIGRAINES**" on page 346 for general nursing care.)

Education: Advise clients who have migraines to avoid trigger factors that cause stress such as intake of alcohol, fatigue, and tyramine-containing foods (wine and aged cheese). Review the importance of lying down in a dark, quiet room (place) may decrease symptoms. Recommend that taking with food may reduce GI symptoms. Tablets or capsules take whole; do not crush, break, or chew. Client may experience dizziness or drowsiness, so it is important for client to avoid driving or engaging in activities that mandate alertness until cognitive response from med has been determined.

Evaluation: Relief of migraine attack.

Drugs: divalproex sodium (Depakote ER)

DIVALPROEX (DEPAKOTE ER)

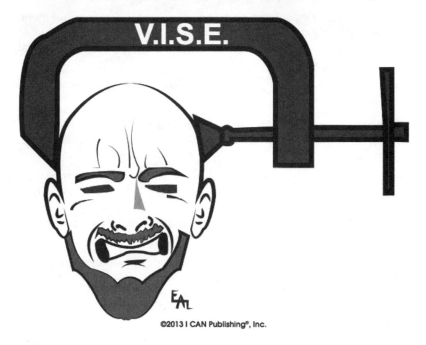

©2013 I CAN Publishing®, Inc.

Veer away from driving—med may cause dizziness and drowsiness

Inflamed/dilated intracranial blood vessels are relieved by this medication

Safely use med - avoid in pregnancy and don't use with aspirin or benzodiazepines

Early signs of migraine headache—give med immediately; eliminate with liver disease

ERGOTAMINE (ERGOSTAT)

Action: Prevents the dilation and inflammation of the intracranial blood vessels, resulting in relief of the migraine pain. Directly stimulates alpha-adrenergic and serotonergic receptors, producing vascular smooth muscle vasoconstriction.

Indications: Treatment of vascular headaches including migraine attacks with or without aura.

Warnings: Contraindicated with liver and/or renal complications, sepsis, CAD and during pregnancy. Use cautiously in clients with peripheral vascular pathology such as diabetes mellitus.

Undesirable Effects: Abdominal pain, nausea and vomiting; Ergotism (muscle pain; paresthesia in fingers and toes; cold, pale extremities) (*Refer to next page for the Undesirable Effect Song; sung to the tune of "Head, Shoulders, Knees and Toes!*); fetal abortion. Physical dependency on the medication.

Other Specific Information: Sumatriptan may lead to spastic reaction of the blood vessels. Several HIV protease inhibitors, antifungal medications, and macrolide antibiotics may increase ergotamine levels, resulting in an increased vasospasm. Do not use together.

Interventions: Administer metoclopramide (Reglan) if client experiences gastrointestinal discomfort such as nausea and vomiting. If client experiences any ergotism, discontinue medication immediately and notify provider of care. Review the importance of not exceeding the prescribed dose. Inform clients regarding symptoms of withdrawal (headache, restlessness, nausea, and vomiting). Discuss the importance of notifying the provider of care if symptoms do occur. (Refer to "**MIGRAINES**".)

Education: Review with clients who experience migraine headaches how to avoid trigger factors that may cause stress such as fatigue, alcohol, and tyramine-containing foods such as aged cheese and wine. Discuss lying down in a dark, quiet place may decrease complications from the migraine. Use adequate contraception during therapy.

Evaluation: Client will experience evidence that therapeutic effects have occurred by having decrease in frequency of migraine attacks and even a termination of the migraine headaches.

Drug: ergotamine (Ergostat)

ERGOTAMINE (ERGOSTAT)

The Side Effect Song
"Head, stomach, fingers and toes,
fingers and toes. Head, stomach, fingers
and toes, fingers and toes... Vo-mit-ing from
the mouth and nose... Head, stomach
fingers and toes."

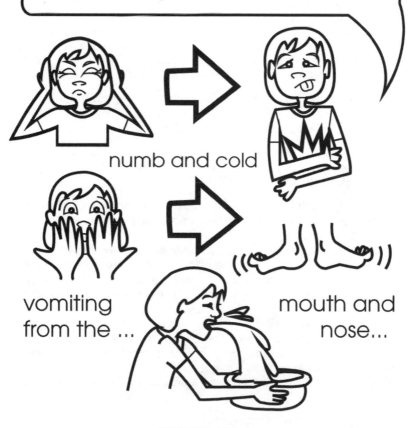

numb and cold

vomiting
from the ...

mouth and
nose...

TRICYCLIC ANTIDEPRESSANT AMITRIPTYLINE (ELAVIL)

Action: Prevents inflammation and dilation of the intracranial blood vessels, thereby relieving migraine pain.

Indications: Stopping an acute migraine attacks. Prevention of migraine attacks.

Warnings: Contraindicated in clients with recent MI or within 14 days of a MAO inhibitor. Use with caution in clients with seizure history, urinary retention, prostatic hypertrophy, angle-closure glaucoma, hyperthyroidism and others.

Undesirable Effects: Decreased blood pressure, drowsiness, dizziness; anticholinergic effects (dry mouth, constipation, urinary retention, blurred vision, tachycardia). Refer to **"Tina's Hat"** on the next page to help you remember these undesirable effects.

Other Specific Information: Barbiturates may cause increased CNS depression. Cimetidine may increase amitriptyline levels. MAOIs may increase CNS excitation or cause seizures.

Interventions: Monitor medication effects. Monitor undesirable effects. Do not administer amitriptyline within 2 weeks of stopping MAOIs. (Refer to **"MIGRAINES"**.)

Education: Teach to use caution in case client develops orthostative hypotension. Advise clients who have migraines to avoid trigger factors that cause stress such as intake of alcohol, fatigue, and tyramine-containing foods (wine and aged cheese). Review the importance of lying down in a dark, quiet room (place) may decrease symptoms. Instruct about the importance of avoiding driving or engaging in activities that mandate alertness until cognitive response from med has been determined. Increase fluid intake. Increase physical activity by routinely exercising. Administer laxative such as bisacodyl (Dulcolax), to assist with reduced bowel motility, or stool softeners, such as docusate sodium (Colace), to prevent constipation. Recommend client void routinely such as every 3-4 hours and report to HCP if any retention is occurring. Discuss the importance of reporting any blurred vision.

Evaluation: Relief of migraine attack.

Drugs: amitriptyline (Elavil)

AMITRIPTYLINE (ELAVIL)

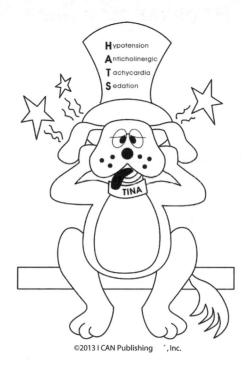

Hypotension
Anticholinergic
Tachycardia
Sedation

TINA

©2013 I CAN Publishing ˊ, Inc.

T urn down the lights to avoid triggers

I nflammation and dilation are prevented of the intracranial vessels

N ot give within 14 days of MAO inhibitors

A ngle-closure glaucoma—avoid administering

BETA BLOCKER:
PROPRANOLOL (INDERAL)

Action: Blocks stimulation of Beta$_2$ (vascular)–adrenergic receptor site, thereby relieving migraine pain.

Indications: Prevention of vascular headaches.

Warnings: Contraindicated in clients with greater than first degree heart lock, bradycardia; bronchial asthma; cardiogenic shock or heart failure. Use with caution in clients taking other antihypertensives, liver or renal impairment, or diabetes mellitus.

Undesirable Effects: Extreme tiredness, fatigue, depression, asthma exacerbation. Bradycardia and hypotension. Propranolol use can mask the hypoglycemic effect of insulin and prevent the breakdown of fat in response to hypoglycemia. (Refer to next page to "Road Blocks to Propranolol" to help remember undesirable effects.)

Other Specific Information: Verapamil (Calan) and diltiazem (Cardizem) have additive cardiosuppression effects. Diuretics and antihypertensive medications have additive hypotensive effects. Propranolol can mask the hypoglycemic effect of insulin and prevent the fat breakdown as a result of hypoglycemia.

Interventions: Medication should be administered at the first sign of a headache. Assess pain location, duration, intensity, and associated symptoms such as photophobia, phonophobia, nausea, and vomiting during migraine attack and frequency of attacks. Monitor heart rate, ECG, and blood pressure. **Do not confuse propranolol with pravachol. Do not confuse Inderal (a brand name of propranolol with Adderall (an amphetamine/dextroamphetamine combination drug).** Refer to next page to assist in remembering when to hold and NOT administer the medication.

Education: Teach client how to take apical pulse prior to taking propranolol. Advise clients who have migraines to avoid trigger factors that cause stress such as intake of alcohol, fatigue, and tyramine-containing foods (wine and aged cheese). Review the importance of lying down in a dark, quiet room (place) may decrease symptoms. Review to take with foods to increase absorption. Teach client how to take apical heart rate prior to dose. Notify provider of care of significant change. Caution client about the importance of not sharing medication with anyone due to risk involved. (Refer to "**MIGRAINES**".)

Evaluation: Prevention of vascular headaches.

Drugs: propranolol (Inderal)

BLOCKER

BRADYCARDIA
BLOOD PRESSURE—TOO LOW
BRONCHIAL CONSTRICTION
BLOOD SUGAR—MASKS LOW
BLOCKS (HEART) > 1st DEGREE

"BLOCKER" outlines undesirable effects of Beta Blockers.

CALCIUM CHANNEL BLOCKER: VERAPAMIL (CALAN)

Action: Preventing dilation of the intracraninal blood vessels, thereby relieving migraine pain.

Indications: Prevention of migraine headaches. Stopping an acute migraine attack.

Warnings: Contraindicated in clients with greater than first degree heart block, bradycardia, hypotension, left ventricle disease, atrial fibrillation or flutter or heart failure or flutter or heart block. Use cautiously with clients who have renal or liver impairment or increased intracranial pressure.

Undesirable Effects: Orthostatic hypotension, bradycardia, constipation.

Other Specific Information: Carbamazepine, digoxin may increase medication levels. Atenolol, esmolol, propranolol, and timolol may increase effects from Calan.

Interventions: Monitor medication levels and adjust dose as necessary. Monitor BP, HR. (Refer to "**MIGRAINES**".)

Education: Advise client who have migraines to avoid trigger factors that cause stress such as intake of alcohol, fatigue, and tyramine-containing foods (wine and aged cheese). Review the importance of lying down in a dark, quiet room (place) may decrease symptoms. Instruct about the importance of avoiding driving or engaging in activities that mandate alertness until cognitive response from med has been determined. Monitor BP, HR. Advise to sit or lie down if symptoms of lightheadedness or dizziness occur and to change positions slowly. Provide assistance with ambulation as needed. Increase fiber in diet. Increase physical activity by engaging in regular exercise. Administer stimulant laxatives, such as biscodyl (Dulcolax) to counteract decreased bowel motility, or stool softeners, such as docusate sodium (Colace) to prevent constipation. (Refer to "**MIGRAINES**".)

Evaluation: Relief of migraine attack.

Drugs: verapamil (Calan)

VERAPAMIL (CALAN)

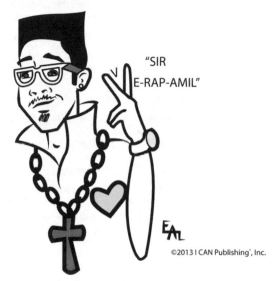

"SIR E-RAP-AMIL"

©2013 I CAN Publishing®, Inc.

R egular checks of B/P and HR may indicate...
orthostatic hypotension and bradycardia

A cute migraine attacks are trouble- treat with
Verapamil on the double

P umper Problems? Pump up the vibe, and be
sure to mention... Check client for a heart
condition

P osition changes should be slow. Orthostatic
hypotension can occur you know

E limination may be slow- prevent constipation...
so you can go (with laxatives and stool
softener)

R apping may be hard on ya'... check for Bradycardia.
Don't get in a tizzy... Calan may make you dizzy

SUMATRIPTAN (IMITREX)

Action: Prevents the dilation and inflammation of the intracranial blood vessels, resulting in relief of the migraine pain. Acts as a selective agonist of 5-HT1, resulting in vasoconstriction in the large intracranial arteries.

Indications: Stopping an acute migraine attack.

Warnings: Ischemic cardiac disease, history of myocardial infarctions, uncontrolled hypertension, and other heart diseases.

Undesirable Effects: Dizziness or vertigo; coronary artery vasospasm / angina; chest pressure (heavy arms or chest tightness); drowsiness.

Other Specific Information: Use of MAOIs with Sumatriptan may lead to MAO toxicity. Ergotamine may lead to spastic reaction of the blood vessels. SSRIs may result in weakness and hyper-reflexes when taken with Sumatriptan. Increased risk of serotinergic side effects including serotonin syndrome with St. John's Wort and SAMe.

Interventions: Give initial subcut dose under close observation to clients with potential for coronary artery disease including postmenopausal women, men > 40 years, clients with risk factors for CAD such as hypertension, hypercholesterolemia, obesity, diabetes, smoking, or family history. Evaluate blood pressure before and for 1 hr after initial injection. If angina occurs, monitor ECG for ischemic changes. If pain becomes continuous or severe, advise to notify provider of care. Do not administer Sumatriptan within 2 weeks of stopping MAOIs. Do not administer Ergotamine simultaneously when administering Sumatriptan. Monitor client closely for weakness and hyper-reflexes if taking SSRIs simultaneously. **Do not confuse sumatriptan with zolmitriptan.** Caution client to use adequate contraception during therapy.

Education: Inform client that sumatriptan should only be used during a migraine not to prevent or reduce the number of attacks. If migraine symptoms return, a 2nd injection may be used. Allow at least 1 hr between doses, and do not use more than 2 injections in any 24-hr period. Review with clients who experience migraine headaches how to avoid trigger factors that may cause stress such as fatigue, alcohol, and tyramine-containing foods such as aged cheese and wine. Discuss lying down in a dark, quiet place may decrease complications from the migraine. Advise not to drive or operate machinery until medication effect has been established. Consult health care provider prior to taking any additional medications. Instruct client regarding appropriate technique for loading, administering, and discarding the auto-injector. Client information pamphlet is provided. Inform that redness at site usually lasts less than 1 hr. (Refer to **"MIGRAINES"**.)

Evaluation: Client will experience evidence that therapeutic effects have occurred by having a relief of the migraine headache.

Drug: sumatriptan (Imitrex)

SUMATRIPTAN (IMITREX)

I schemic heart disease, history of M.I., high BP - use with caution

M AOI's may lead to MAOI toxicity

I nitial dose evaluate B/P 1 hr before and after administration

T each to use adequate contra-ception during therapy

R emind to allow 1 hr between doses; no > than 2 doses in 24 hrs

E valuate EKG for changes if angina occurs

X out a migraine headache- not just to prevent headaches

©2013 I CAN Publishing®, Inc.

This "Suma" (Sumo) wrestler is going to knock out your migraine HA. There is a lovely lady in the crowd who will remind him of the importance of using contraception during therapy.

ANTI-PARKINSON'S MEDICATIONS

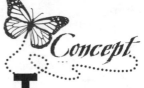

Concept

T herapeutic Use: the ability to perform ADLs; does NOT halt progression of Parkinson's disease!

R ecommend avoiding high protein meals and snacks

E ffects of these drugs may not be noticeable for several weeks to several months

M edication "holidays" may be indicated, but client must be in the hospital to be monitored

O bserve for dyskinesias with Dopaminergics and Dopamine agonists

R emember to notify provider if symptoms reoccur due to sudden loss of medication effects

S afety precautions due to risk for drowsiness and/or possible othostatic hypotension

PARK DARK

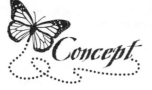

P ill rolling

A bout to fall

R igidity

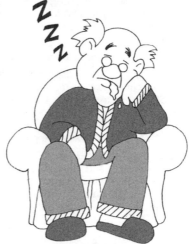

©2013 I CAN Publishing®, Inc.

K an't swallow/speak (drools)

Feels like a "**DOPE**" with these meds

D ecrease Parkinson's symptoms

O rthostatic hypotension

P sychosis (visual hallucinations, nightmares)

E ffects of drugs may be undesirable and result in nausea and/or dyskinesia

DOPAMINERGICS

Action: Decrease symptoms of Parkinson's disease that are related to depletion of dopamine in the corpus striatum. Administration of carbidopa with levodopa makes more levodopa, the metabolic precursor of dopamine, available for transport to the brain for conversion to dopamine.

Indications: Parkinson's disease, symptomatic parkinsonism which may follow injury to the nervous system by carbon monoxide and/or manganese intoxication. Not used for drug-induced extrapyramidal reactions.

Warnings: MAO inhibitors are contraindicated and must be discontinued at least two weeks prior to initiating therapy. Sinemet should not be used in clients with undiagnosed or suspicious skin lesions or a history of melanoma as Levodopa may activate a malignant melanoma. It should not be used in clients with a history of narrow-angle glaucoma.

Undesirable Effects: Dyskinesias such as choreiform, dystonic and other involuntary movements, and nausea. May report sudden urges for gambling, increased libdo. Symptomatic postural hypotension may occur when given with hypertensive medications. False positive reaction for urinary ketone bodies when test tape is used for determination of ketonuria.

Other Specific Information: Before starting Sinemet, clients who are being treated with levodopa, must discontinue levodopa at least 12 hours before therapy with Sinemet is initiated. MAO inhibitors may result in a hypertensive crisis when taken with dopaminergics. Phenothiazines, haloperidol, papervine, phenytoin, and reserpine may decrease effect of levodopa. Large doses of pyridoxine or foods ↑ in pyridoxine (*Refer to p. 466 for specifics on food and drug facts*) may decrease beneficial effects of levodopa. Antihypertensives administered with these meds may result in hypotension. Anticholinergics may ↓ absorption of levodopa. Kava-kava may ↓ levodopa effectiveness. Foods with large amounts of pyridoxine may ↓ the effects of levodopa.

Interventions: Give medication on assigned schedule as prescribed by the HCP without variation. Assess client for signs and symptoms of orthostatic hypotension if client is receiving antihypertensive drugs. False positive reaction for urinary ketone bodies when test tape is used for determination of ketonuria. Monitor Hgb, Hct, WBCs, AST/ALT, BUN, serum glucose. Assess for parkinsonian symptoms (*Refer to* "**PARK DARK**"). "On-off" phenomenon" may cause symptoms to appear or improve suddenly. Assess HR and BP frequently during period of dose adjustment. **Do not confuse levodopa with methylodopa.** In the carbidopa/levodopa combination, the number following the drug name represents the milligrams of each respective drug. Never crush controlled-release tablets.

Education: Instruct the client regarding the importance of taking the medication on a regular schedule as prescribed. Advise client that occasionally, a dark color (red, brown or black) may appear in the saliva, urine or sweat. The client should also be advised to the possibility of a sudden onset of sleep during daily activities, without warning, may occur. (Refer to "**TREMORS**" for medication management.) Refer to the "8 D's" on next page to summarize what to teach regarding safe medication administration.

Evaluation: Reduction in the tremor and muscle rigidity and ↑ mobility.

Drugs: Carbidopa/Levodopa (Sinemet)

DOPAMINERGICS "THE 8 D'S"

1) Dizziness/ Drowsiness/ avoid Driving
2) Dyskinesias/ Dreams (nightmares)
3) Decrease in reality due to hallucinations
4) Decrease in B/P from Orthostatic Hypotension
5) Decrease protein diet and eat shortly after
    taking med
6) Decrease Pyridoxine
7) Discoloration of sweat and urine are harmless
8) Decrease dry mouth with good hygiene

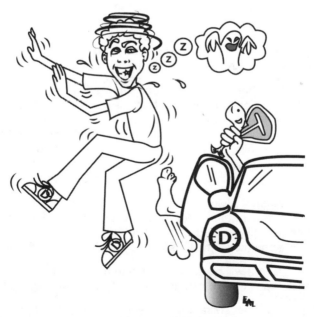

DOPAMINE AGONISTS

Action: Stimulate parts of the brain that are affected by dopamine. They may be taken alone or in combination with medications containing levodopa.

Indications: To manage the major symptoms of Parkinson's disease.

Warnings: Some studies have linked these medications to compulsive behaviors such as gambling and shopping. Use with caution with alcohol, anti-hypertensives, anti-psychotics and anti-depressants. Geriatric clients (increased risk of hallucinations); Renal impairment (Increased dosing interval recommended if CCr < 60 mL/min).

Undesirable Effects: Nausea, constipation; headache, hallucinations; hypotension, sedation (which may include sudden sleepiness). Dyskinesia, extrapyramidal syndrome; dry mouth. (Refer to "**RESTLESS**" on next page to assist in remembering these undesirable effects.)

Other Specific Information: Apomorphine (Apokyn), is a powerful fast acting injectable medication that relieves PD symptoms within minutes, but only is effective for 30-60 minutes. It is used for clients that experience sudden wearing-off spells, leaving them unexpectedly immobile. It can cause severe nausea. Concurrent levodopa increases risk of hallucinations, dyskinesia, and orthostatic hypotension. Effectiveness of dopamine agonists may be increased by cimetidine.

Interventions: Start with low dose of medication and increase gradually. Monitor for undesirable effects as dose is increased. Assess for drowsiness or sleep attacks. Drowsiness is a common side effect, but sleep attacks or episodes of falling asleep during activities may occur without warning. Assess for signs and symtoms of Parkinson's diseases such as ataxia, rigidty, tremor, muscle weakness prior to and throughout therapy. Administer with meals to decrease risk of nausea.

Education: Instruct client on the signs and symptoms of low blood pressure and the potential for sudden sleepiness. Review safety precautions to minimize falls. If the client is prescribed Apomorphine (Apokyn), an anti-emetic must also be taken with this medication.

Evaluation: Client will have a reduction in tremor and muscle rigidity symptoms and an improvement in quality of life activities.

Drugs: pramipexole (Mirapex), ropinirole (Requip), apomorphine (Apokyn), bromocriptine (Parlodel)

DOPAMINE AGONIST

R enal impairment

E xtrapyramidal symptoms

S eeing things (hallucinations)

T hirsty (dry mouth)

L ethargy

E xpress concern of falling - asleep during activity

S ickness (nausea)

S tuck-up (constipation)

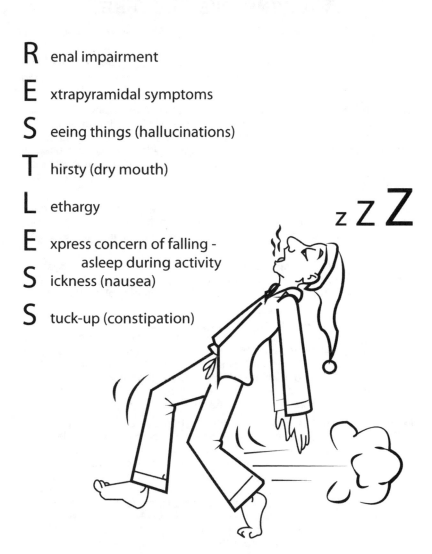

CENTRALLY ACTING ANTICHOLINERGICS: PARKINSON'S DISEASE

Action: Decrease the activity of acetylcholine, a neurotransmitter that regulates movement.

Indications: Secondary medication for the management of all forms of Parkinson's disease, including drug-induced extrapyramidal effects and acute dystonic reactions.

Warnings: Hypersensitivity. May impair mental and/or physical abilities required for performance of hazardous tasks, such as driving or working with complex equipment. Older clients are susceptible to confusion and hallucinations on anticholinergics, so they should not be used in clients over the age of 70. Angle-closure glaucoma; tardive dyskinesia; use cautiously in prostatic hypertension; seizure disorders; cardiac arrhythmias; OB, Lactation.

Undesirable Effects: Blurred vision, urinary retention, dry mouth, constipation; arrhythmias, hypotension, palpitations, tachycardia; confusion, depression, dizziness, hallucinations; headache, sedation, weakness.

Other Specific Information: Should not be used with antipsychotic (phenothiazines or haloperidol) or tricyclic antidepressants. Should be used with caution with alcohol, antihistamines. Antacids and antidiarrheals may ↓ absorption.

Interventions: Therapy should begin at low dose and increased gradually over a five or six day interval. Monitor for anticholinergic side effects: constipation, dry mouth, nausea, urinary retention, blurred vision. Monitor HR and BP closely and remain in bed for 1 hr after administration. Administer with food or immediately after meals to decrease GI distress. If client has difficulty swallowing, then drug may be crushed and administered with food. Do not double up on doses.

Education: Due to the long duration of action, it is particularly suitable for bedtime administration. Advise to change positions slowly to decrease risk of orthostatic hypotension. Safety precautions should be reviewed to minimize risk for falls. Teach client the importance of frequent rinsing of mouth, good oral hygiene and sugarless gum or candy may decrease dry mouth. Instruct to notify provider of care if presents with constipation, difficulty with urination, abdominal discomfort, rapid or pounding heart beat, confusion, eye pain, or rash occurs. Review the importance of eating foods high in fiber and increase fluid intake to 2 to 3 L/day. Advise to consult with provider of care prior to taking any OTC meds.

Evaluation: Client will have improvement in tremors and ease dystonia. Client will experience an improvement in gait and balance. Therapeutic effects are seen in 2-3 days after initiation of therapy.

Drugs: trihexyphenidyl (Artane), benztropine (Cogentin)

CENTRALLY ACTING ANTICHOLINERGICS: UNDESIRABLE EFFECTS

Can't pee: Monitor I & O; assess for urinary retention

Can't see: Safety precautions

Can't spit: Chew sugarless gum, ↑ fluids to 2–3 L/day

Can't sh*t: Eat foods high in fiber and ↑ fluids to 2–3 L/day

AND IS

DROWSY (Antihistamine effects): Safety precautions

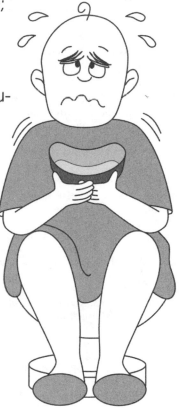

©2013 I CAN Publishing®, Inc.

&

VOMITING: Take medication with food

DOPAMINE RELEASER: ANTIVIRAL

Action: Used to stimulate the release of dopamine and prevent its reuptake.

Indications: Amantadine (Symmeteral) is a secondary medication that is a mild agent used early in the diagnosis of Parkinson's disease to reduce tremors muscle rigidity. Also, prophylaxis and treatment of influenza A viral infections.

Warnings: Use with caution with: alcohol, benztropine (Cogentin), orphenadrine (Disipal), levodopa (Sinemet), trihexyphenidyl (Artane). Hypersensitivity. Cautiously use in seizure disorders; Liver disease; Psychiatric problems; Congestive heart failure; Renal impairment (dosage reduction/increased dosing interval required if CCr $\leq$ 50 ml/min); May increase risk to susceptibility to rubella infections. Caution with Geriatrics.

Undesirable Effects: Nausea, dizziness, hypotension; insomnia; urinary retention; mottling, livedo reticularis, rashes; leukopenia, neutropenia.

Other Specific Information: Clients with a history of epilepsy or other seizures should be observed for potential increased seizure activity. Concurrent use of antihistamines, phenothiazines, quinidine, disopyramide, and tricyclic antidepressants may increase anticholinergic effects (dry mouth, blurred vision, constipation). Increased risk of undesirable CNS reactions with alcohol. Increased risk of CNS stimulation with other CNS stimulants.

Interventions: Assess client for orthostatic hypotension, mood/mental changes, swelling of extremities, difficulty urinating and or shortness of breath occur. Amantadine (Symmetrel) should not be discontinued abruptly because it may lead to a parkinsonian crisis, delirium, agitation, delusions, anxiety and slurred speech. Assess for diffuse red mottling of the skin (livedo reticularis), especially in the lower extremities or on exposure to cold. This will most likely disappear with continued therapy; however, it may not resolve until 2-12 weeks after therapy has been discontinued. Monitor intake and output closely in geriatric clients. May result in urinary retention. Report bladder distention. Do not administer last dose of medication near bedtime due to the risk of it producing insomnia in some clients. If client has difficulty swallowing, med may be mixed with food or fluids. For Parkinson's Disease assess rigidity, akinesia, tremors, and gait disturbances prior to and during therapy. If used for antiviral prophylaxis, administer in anticipation of contact to virus and continue for at least 10 days following exposure. For influenza prophylaxis or treatment, assess respiratory status and temperature periodically. **Do NOT confuse amantadine with rimantadine or ranitidine.**

Education: Inform client that blurry vision and/ or impaired mental acuity may occur with this medication. The client should also be informed of the importance of not abruptly discontinue taking this medication. Review importance of changing positions slowly due to $\downarrow$ BP. Dry mouth can be relieved by good oral hygiene. Report confusion, mood changes, difficulty urination, or an $\uparrow$ in the PD symptoms.

Evaluation: Client will experience a reduction in tremor and muscle rigidity. If used for influenza, there will be a decrease in symptoms.

Drugs: amantadine (Symmetrel)

DOPAMINE RELEASER (ANTIVIRAL)

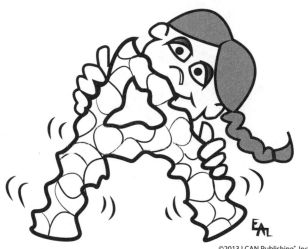

©2013 I CAN Publishing®, Inc.

Shake-off
Flu-A
"Lose the shakes
And prevent Flu A
Don't get too DRY
Like "mottling" clay"

Miss Amantadine is using "mottling" (modeling) clay to create a "Symmetrel" (symmetrical) letter A, to represent influenza A. She doesn't want it to DRY out by giving other medications which can create anticholinergic effects. Also, she can develop MOTTLING of the skin (livedo reticularis) as an undesirable effect. She needs to lose the shakes (prevent Parkinson's symptoms) in order to create her masterpiece!

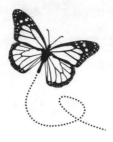

All men dream but not equally. Those who dream by night in the dusty recesses of their minds wake in the day to find that it was vanity; but the dreamers of the day are dangerous men, for they may act on their dream with open eyes to make it possible.

T. E. LAWRENCE

Anticonvulsant Agents

ANTICONVULSANT: DILANTIN

Action: Reduces motor cortex activity by altering transport of ions.

Indications: Grand mal and complex partial seizures.

Warnings: Hypersensitivity, heart block, psychiatric disorders.

Undesirable Effects: Nausea, vomiting, headache, diplopia, confusion, drowsiness, dizziness, ataxia, gingival hyperplasia, gingivitis, hepatitis, agranuloctyosis, red/brown discoloration of urine, male sexual dysfunction.

Other Specific Information: ↑ effects with cimetidine, chloramphenicol, isoniazid. ↓ effects of anticoagulants, antihistamines, corticosteroids, cyclosporin, dopamine, oral contraceptives, theophylline, quinidine, rifampin. *(There are numerous interactions; it is beyond the scope of this book to review all of them. We refer you to a Drug Handbook.)*

Interventions: Monitor serum drug levels (therapeutic range: 10–20 mcg/ml); labs related to renal and liver function. Provide safety during and after a seizure. If given in a suspension, shake well before pouring. If given intravenous (IV), it should be administered slowly due to potential hypotension and dysrhythmias. Administer only through a saline line. Do not mix with other drugs. Validate a good blood return.

Education: Instruct client regarding safety precautions while taking med. Inform provider of any undesirable effects. Women taking oral contraceptives may need to use an additional method of contraception. Advise female clients considering getting pregnant to consult with provider of health care since drug may have a teratogenic effect on the fetus. Do not abruptly stop the drug. Recommend preventative dental check-ups; use a soft toothbrush. Advise client that the urine may be red/brown. Discuss the importance of wearing an alert ID card and/or medic alert bracelet.

Evaluation: Client will experience less or no seizures. The serum drug level will remain therapeutic with no undesirable effects.

Drug: phenytoin (Dilantin)

DILANTIN
(DIAL AT TEN)

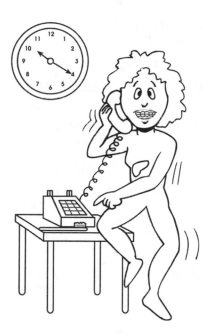

G ingival hyperplasia

U se alternate birth control

M outh care—
preventative
dental check-up

S oft tooth brush,
don't stop abruptly

©2001 I CAN Publishing, Inc.

The time is 10–20 on the clock to help you remember the therapeutic range for dilantin (10–20 mcg/ml).

ANTIEPILEPTIC AGENT: NEURONTIN

Action: Not fully understood; anticonvulsant action activity may be a result of its ability to prevent the polysynaptic responses and inhibit post-tetanic potentiation.

Indications: Combination therapy in managing partial seizures; amyotrophic lateral sclerosis. Unlabeled use: neuropathic pain.

Warnings: Hypersensitivity; lactation.

Undesirable Effects: Dizzy, insomnia, somnolence, ataxia, nervousness; nausea/vomiting; rhinitis; pruritis.

Other Specific Information: Neurontin levels will be decreased when taken with antacids.

Intervention: Arrange for support groups for epileptics.

Education: Instruct to take drug exactly as prescribed; do not abruptly make any changes without consulting provider. For nausea, recommend taking with food or milk; eat small frequent meals. Review the importance of wearing a medical alert tag identifying the medication and the fact client has epilepsy.

Evaluation: Client will experience no seizures and no undesirable effects from the drug.

Drug: gabapentin (Neurontin)

CAESAR

C NS: dizziness, insomnia—U E

A ntacids decrease

E at food with drug

S upport group for epileptics

A lert tag indicating specific drug

R eport U E

ANTICONVULSANT: VALPROIC ACID

Action: Increases levels of GABA in the brain which decreases seizure activity.

Indications: Seizures, manic episodes associated with bipolar disorder (delayed-release only); migraine headache prevention (delayed and extended release).

Warnings: Hypersensitivity, hepatic impairment, urea cycle disorders.

Undesirable Effects: Confusion, sedation, tremor, hepatotoxicity, nausea, vomiting, abdominal cramps, diarrhea, weight gain, rash, prolonged bleeding time.

Other Specific Information: Increased risk of bleeding with antiplatelet agents, including aspirin, NSAIDs, tirofiban, eptifibatide, and abciximab, cefamandole, cefoperazone, cefotetan, heparins, and thrombolytic agents or warfarin. Additive CNS depression with CNS depressants, alcohol, antihistamines, antidepressants, opioid analgesics, MAO inhibitors, and sedative / hypnotics.

Interventions: Monitor hepatic function (LDH, AST,ALT, and bilirubin) and serum ammonia concentrations, especially during initial 6 months of therapy; fatalities from liver failure have occurred. Discontinue if hyperammonemia occurs. Therapeutic levels range from 50–100 micrograms per mL. Monitor mental status, respiratory status. Tablets or capsules whole; do not crush, break, or chew. Elixir alone; do not dilute with carbonated beverage; do not give syrup to client on a sodium restriction. Give with food or milk.

Education: Review that physical dependency may result from extended use. Avoid driving and other activities that require alertness. Do not discontinue after long-term use; convulsions my result. Report undesirable effects to provider of care.

Evaluation: Client will experience decreased seizure activity or decreased manic behavior, or frequency of migraine headaches.

Drugs: valproic acid (Depakote, Depakote ER, Depakene, Epival)

VALPROIC ACID

D iscontinue if hyperammonemia occurs

E levate levels of GABA in brain

P rolonged bleeding if given with antiplatelet agents

A void CNS depressants and don't give
wth carbonated beverages

C
O
Y
O
T
E

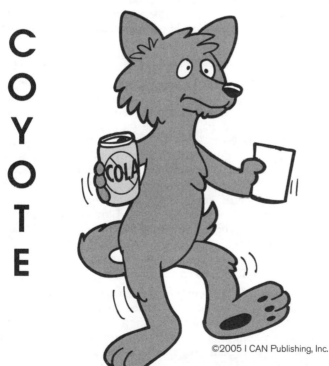

©2005 I CAN Publishing, Inc.

Coty Coyote may be shaking from mania, seizures or his head may be pounding from a migraine. Depakote treats these symptoms but should not be given with carbonated beverages. Milk helps prevent GI upset.

ANTICONVULSANT: CARBAMAZEPINE

Action: Inhibits nerve impulses by limiting influx of sodium ions into the motor cortex from across the cell membrane.

Indications: Tonic-clonic, complex-partial, mixed seiqures; trigeminal neuralgia, diabetic neuropathy. Mood stabilizers. Alternative to lithium or valproic acid or adjunctive treatment for bipolar disorder.

Warnings: Hypersensitivity to this category or tricyclics, bone marrow depression, MAOIs. Glaucoma, hepatic, renal or cardiac disease.

Other Specific Information: CNS toxicity when taken with lithium. Increased carbamazepine levels with cimetidine, clarithromycin, danazol, diltiazem, erythromycin, fluoxetine, fluvoxamine, isoniazid, propoxyphene, valproic acid, verapamil. Decreased effects of benzodiazepines, doxycycline, felbate, haloperidol, oral contracteptives, phenobarbital, phenytoin, primidone, theophylline, thyroid hormones, warfarin. Increased levels of desmopressin, lithium, lypressin, vasopressin. Fatal reaction with MAOIs. Increased peak concentration of carbamazepine with grapefruit juice.

Undesirable Effects: Anorexia, nausea, dizziness, sedation, headache, dry mouth, constipation, rash.

Interventions: For seizures, identify and document the character, duration, location, frequency, and presence of an aura. For trigeminal neuralgia document the characteristics of the facial pain. Monitor renal studies, ALT, AST, bilirubin. Blood studies (hgb, hct, RBC) should be evaluated q month. Maintain drug level between 4–12 micrograms/ml. Anorexia may indicate increased blood levels. Notify provider if mood, sensorium, affect or any behavioral changes occur. Monitor eyes by ophthalmic examinations before, during, and after treatment. Discontinue if client experiences purpura or a red raised rash. Blood dyscrasias may present with a sore throat, fever, bruising, rash, and/or jaundice. Report immediately. May take med with food, milk to reduce GI distress. Do not crush, break, or chew ext. rel. tab; chewable tabs: tell client to chew tab, not swallow it whole; ext. rel. cap may be opened and mixed with food.

Education: Carry emergency ID identifying client's name, drugs currently taking, condition, health care provider's name, phone number. Avoid driving or any activities that require alertness for a minimum of 3 days to determine the response from the medication. Do not quickly discontinue the medication after long-term use. Report any undesirable effects.

Evaluation: Client will experience decreased seizure activity.

Drug: carbamazepine (Apo-Carbamazepine, Atretol, Carbatrol, Epitol, Novo-Carbamaz, Tegretol, Tegretol CR, Tegretol-XR)

CARBAMAZEPINE

T rigeminial Neuralgia, Tonic-clonic seizures

E valuate for UE; anorexia, nausea, dizziness, sedation, headache, sore throat

G ive with food, milk to reduce GI distress

R eview levels, maintain—between 4–12 micrograms/ml

E valuate for anorexia—may indicate toxic levels

T ablet—chewable; do not swallow whole, chew. Take extended-release capsules whole—no crushing or breaking

O pen & mix with food—extended-release capsules

L ook for MANY drug/drug interactions

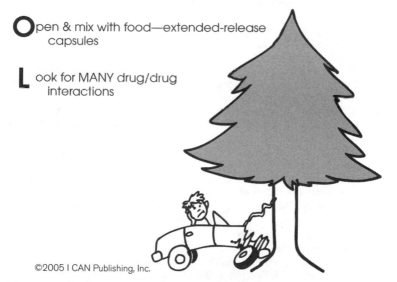

©2005 I CAN Publishing, Inc.

Remember the CAR BAMA (banged at) ZE (the) PINE tree. An undesirable effect of this drug could be sedation and dizziness. Before operating any dangerous equipment or driving an automobile, clients need to determine their response to the drug.

LAMICTAL

Action: Stabilizes neuronal membranes by inhibiting sodium transport.

Indications: Used as adjunct treatment of partial seizures in adults and children older than 2 years old. It is also used to delay mood episodes in clients with bipolar disorder.

Warnings: If taking this drug together with valporic acid or depakote a serious skin rash may be more likely. Clients should not take this drug if they are allergic to lamotrigine. A client should let their provider of care know if they have kidney, liver, or heart disease.

Undesirable Effects: Ataxia, dizziness, drowsiness, blurred vision, headache, nausea, vomiting, photosensitivity, rash, fever, sore throat, swollen glands, behavior changes, mood changes (depression, anxiety, feeling of agitation).

Other Specific Information: Concurrent use with carbamazepine may result in decreased levels of lamotrigine and increased levels of an active metabolite of carbamazepine. Lamotrigine levels are decreased by concurrent use of phenobarbital, phenytoin, or primidone. Concurrent use with valproic acid results in a twofold increase in lamotrigine levels, increase incidence of rash, and decrease in valproic acid level. Oral contraceptives may decrease serum levels of lamotrigine.

Interventions: Monitor labs for renal function, monitor of plasma levels of Lamictal (proposed therapeutic range is 1–5 mcg/ml. Client may have thoughts about suicide. Do not miss scheduled appointments with provider of care. Assess for skin rash during administration. Discontinue at first sign of rash. This may be life-threatening. Steven-Johnsons syndrome or toxic epidermal necrolysis may develop. Rash usually occurs during the initial 2–8 weeks of therapy and is more frequent in clients taking multiple antiepileptic agents, especially valproic acid. Clients < 16 are higher risk for this complication. Assess and monitor for hypersensitivity reactions. Assess seizures for location, duration, and characteristics. Assess mood, ideation, and behaviors frequently. Initiate suicide precautions as indicated. **Do not confuse lamotrigine (Lamictal) with terbinafine (Lamisil), diphenoxylate/ atropine (Lomotil), or lamivudine (Epivir).** PO may be administered without regard to food. Discontinue gradually. May swallow whole, chewed, or dispersed in water or dispersed in fruit juice. If chewed, follow with water or fruit juice to aid in swallowing. Only use whole tablets, do not attempt to administer partial quantities of dispersible tablets.

Education: This drug may impair your vision or your ability to react in situations/reaction time. Check with your provider of care or pharmacist about the multiple drug-drug interactions that are related with this drug. Do not discontinue abruptly. Notify provider of rash or other undesirable effects. Initiate safety precautions due to drowsiness, dizziness, and potential undesirable effect of blurred vision. Advise to use sunscreen.

Evaluation: Client will experience a decrease in the frequency or the cessation of seizures. There will also be a decrease in the incidence of mood swings in bipolar disorders.

Drug: lamotrigine (Lamictal)

THE SEIZING LAMB

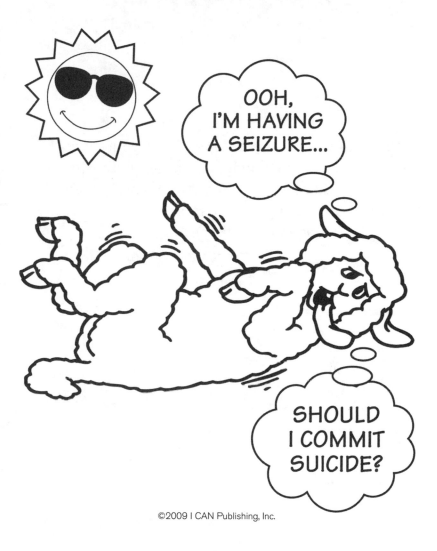

©2009 I CAN Publishing, Inc.

The lamb is having a seizure. Don't give Lamictal if client (Lamb) has suicidal tendencies.

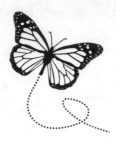

How far you go in life depends on your being tender with the young, compassionate with the aged, sympathetic with the striving, and tolerant of the weak and strong. Because someday in your life you will have been all of these.

GEORGE WASHINGTON CARVER

Anxiolytics, Antidepressants, and Antipsychotic Agents

ANTIANXIETY: BENZODIAZEPINES

Action: Appears to enhance action of gamma-aminobutyric acid (GABA inhibitory neurotransmitter). Depresses the limbic and subcortical CNS.

Indications: Anxiety, preoperative medication, and skeletal muscle relaxant. Versed is commonly used for induction of anesthesia and sedation prior to diagnostic tests and endoscopic exams. Klonopin is used primarily as an anticonvulsant. Ativan and Librium for alcohol withdrawal.

Warnings: Hypersensitivity, renal or hepatic dysfunction, mental depression, pregnancy, lactation, glaucoma, young children, addiction-prone, 14 days within a MAO inhibitor. Caution in the elderly, debilitated, or client with COPD. Ativan clearance less affected by hepatic dysfunction than other benzodiazepines.

Undesirable Effects: The 3 D's that most frequently occur are **d**rowsiness, **d**izziness, and **d**ecreased blood pressure. When taken alone, there is a low incidence of toxicity. Rare effects include: **d**ependence on drug, **d**epressed respirations, liver **d**ysfunction and blood **d**yscrasias (4 D's).

Other Specific Information: CNS depressants, especially alcohol, may result in ↑ sedation. ↑ effect with cimetidine, disulfiram, omeprazole, oral contraceptives.

Interventions: Monitor VS, cardiovascular status, mental status; liver function tests and blood counts with clients on long-term therapy. Assess for symptoms of leukopenia (i.e., fever, sore throat). Provide a restful environment if giving IV infusion. Consider for abuse and dependence. If given IV, have respiratory equipment available; keep client recumbent. Do not mix antianxiety drugs with other drugs in a syringe. Safety precautions for drowsiness. Flumazenil (Rocmazicon) is approved for benzodiazepine overdose. May cause physical or psychological dependence.

Education: Recommend small frequent meals. Encourage to rise slowly from supine position and dangle feet prior to standing. Avoid alcohol, smoking and other CNS depressants. Avoid activities needing good psychomotor coordination until CNS effects are known. Avoid abrupt discontinuation after prolonged use. Providers, including dentists should be advised that client is taking this medication. Review methods to control excess stress and anxiety. Advise client to wear medical alert indicating drug therapy.

Evaluation: Client will be less anxious and will be able to cope with the daily stressors in life.

Drugs: (C-IV controlled substance) alprazolam (Xanax); chlordiazepoxide (Librium); clonazepam (Klonopin); clorazepate (Tranxene); diazepam (Valium); lorazepam (Ativan); midazolam (Versed); oxazepam (Serax)

ANTIANXIETY

A void abrupt discontinuation after prolonged use

N ot give if ↑BP, renal/hepatic dysfunction or hx of drug abuse

X anax, Ativan, Serax—a few examples

I ncrease in 3Ds—drowsiness, dizziness, decreased BP

E nhances action of GABA (inhibitory transmitter)

T each to rise slowly from supine

Y es, alcohol should be avoided

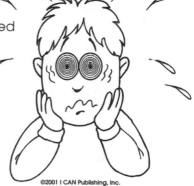

©2001 I CAN Publishing, Inc.

MISCELLANEOUS ANTIANXIETY AGENTS: NONBENZODIAZEPINES

Action: Interacts with serotonin and dopamine at presynaptic neurotransmitter receptors in the CNS, resulting in an antianxiety effect.

Indications: Short term relief management (up to 4 wks.) of anxiety and anxiety disorders. Nonaddicting: used to avoid benzodiazepines and barbiturates.

Warnings: Hypersensitivity to buspirone or any components. Renal/hepatic impairment, MAO inhibitor therapy; pregnancy/lactation.

Undesirable Effects: Dizziness, drowsiness, headache, nausea, fatigue. Insomnia, blurred vision, and confusion are experienced less frequently.

Other Specific Information: Alcohol or CNS depressants may ↑ sedation. MAO inhibitors may ↑ blood pressure. ↓ effects with fluoxetine when given with Buspar. Refer to tricyclic antidepressants for drug interactions with Sinequan.

Interventions: Monitor level of anxiety, mental status, neuromuscular coordination, and vital signs. Offer support for anxious client. Assist with ambulating if drowsy or dizzy.

Education: Inform client that it may take 1–2 weeks of therapy before the effects are present. Therapeutic effect generally takes 3–4 weeks of therapy. Avoid any task requiring alertness until established response of drug. Avoid alcohol and other CNS depressants (unless ordered by provider). Recommend taking medication with food. Do not abruptly discontinue this drug.

Evaluation: Client's behavior will reflect less anxiety with no undesirable effects from the medication.

Drugs: buspirone (Buspar); doxepin (Sinequan); meprobamate (Miltown, Equanil)

BUSPAR BUS

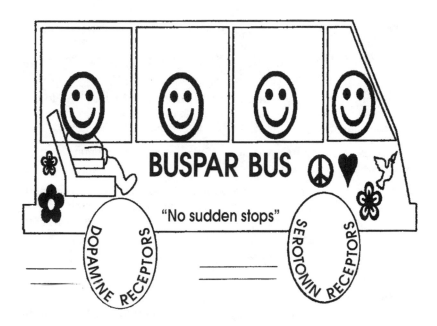

Get on the Buspar Bus to decrease ansiety. The seats recline for the undesirable effect of dizziness and drowsiness. Smiles can be seen after taking the drug for a week.

Concept: DEPRESSION

Driving is out until response to drug has been determined:
Since some of the undesirable effects from these medications include
sedation, drowsiness, hypotension, and blurred vision, instruct client
not to drive. Recommend that client determines the response of the
drug dose prior to operating hazardous machinery.

Effect has a delayed onset of 7–21 days: Client needs to be
informed that the effectiveness of these drugs may take 7–21 days.
Client may get frustrated prior to this, so it is important to share this
information.

Planning pregnancy–consult with provider of care: Due to the
potential teratogenic effects of the drug on the fetus, it is recommended
that the client not get pregnant while taking these medications.

Relieves symptoms, not a CURE: Recommend counseling to
assist with the depression.

Evaluate vital signs: Orthostatic hypotension is common.
Anticholinergic like symptoms may occur such as dry mouth, urinary
retention, blurred vision, increased heart rate, and constipation.
Evaluate weight several times a week.

Stopping drug abruptly is OUT: Client needs to understand the
importance of this.

Safety measures (i.e., change position slowly): Instruct the
client to come to a standing position slowly to avoid feeling faint from
orthostatic hypotension.

Instruct client to report undesirable effects: Inform client to
report anticholinergic effects of the drugs, such as dry mouth and
eyes, blurred vision, constipation, and urinary retention. Since dry
mouth is a common undesirable effect, encourage client to practice
good oral hygiene to prevent dental caries. Ice chips, breath mints,
and sugarless candies are also effective in promoting comfort.

Observe for suicidal tendencies: The risk of suicide is typically
higher near the end of the depression cycle. Client needs to be
monitored for suicidal tendencies.

No alcohol or CNS depressants: Instruct client to avoid alcoholic
beverages or other CNS depressants while taking antidepressants
because CNS depression may be increased.

ANTIDEPRESSANTS

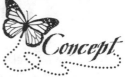

Concept

D riving is out until response to drug has been determined

E ffect has a delayed onset of 7–21 days

P lanning pregnancy—consult with provider of care

R elieves symptoms, not a CURE!

E valuate vital signs

S topping drug abruptly is OUT!

S afety measures (i.e., change position slowly)

I nstruct client to report undesirable effects

O bserve for suicidal tendencies

N o alcohol or CNS depressants

SELECTIVE SEROTONIN REUPTAKE INHIBITORS (SSRIs)

Action: Causes selective inhibition of serotonin uptake resulting in an antidepressant response.

Indications: Depression, obsessive-compulsive disorder, panic disorder, and appetite disorders.

Warnings: Renal or hepatic function impairments. Seizures, mania, cardiac disease, pregnancy/lactation, or within 14 days of MAOIs.

Undesirable Effects: "**CNS**" will help you recall these effects. **C**NS stimulation-headache, insomnia, nervousness, agitation. **N**ausea, anorexia, diarrhea, vomiting. **S**kin rash, sexual dysfunction. (SSRIs are **less** likely than the other antidepressants to cause anticholinergic effects, cardiotoxicity, sedation, seizures, as well as inducing mania in bipolar clients.)

Other Specific Information: Avoid use with highly protein-bound drugs (e.g., warfarin), within 14 days of MAOIs, alcohol, caution with CNS depressants. Antacids may ↓ absorption. Use cautiously with type IC antiarrhythmics due to potential drug interactions. ↑ risk of reaction if combined with St. John's Wort.

Interventions: For long-term therapy, liver/renal function tests should be monitored. Blood tests should be performed periodically. Monitor PT and INR with clients receiving concurrent warfarin therapy. Monitor BP, HR, weight, and stools for consistency. A rash, especially with a temperature, should be reported immediately. Monitor elderly for fluid and sodium imbalance. If client experiences dizziness, assist with ambulation.

Education: Advise client to take medication in the morning to avoid insomnia. To obtain maximum therapeutic response, it may require 3-4 weeks of therapy (in the elderly, it may take 10-12 weeks of therapy). Advise clients on warfarin therapy to promptly report signs of bleeding. (Refer to "**DEPRESSION**".)

Evaluation: Client has improvement in clinical state (i.e., appearance, behavior, interest, mood, speech patterns).

Drugs: citalopram (Celexa); fluoxetine (Prozac); fluvoxamine (Luvox); paroxetine (Paxil); sertraline (Zoloft), escitalopram (Lexapro)

PAXIL

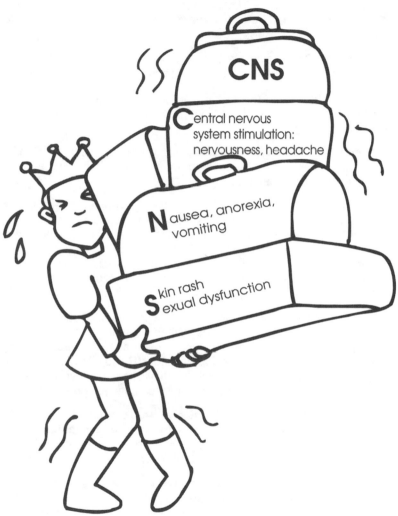

CNS

Central nervous system stimulation: nervousness, headache

Nausea, anorexia, vomiting

Skin rash sexual dysfunction

©2001 I CAN Publishing, Inc.

Paxil packs extra baggage when taking SSRIs. The baggage will help you remember some of the major undesirable effects from these medications.

TRICYCLIC ANTIDEPRESSANTS

Action: Blocks re-uptake of norepinephrine and serotonin into nerve endings.

Indications: Depression. Imipramine is also used for childhood enuresis. Clomipramine is used for obsessive-compulsive disorders.

Warnings: Epilepsy, glaucoma, cardiovascular disease, urinary retention, seizures, hyperthyroidism, pregnancy/lactation, within 14 days of receiving MAOIs.

Undesirable Effects: Manic signs in bipolar clients. Refer to**"HATS"** to help remember these effects. **H**ypotension, **A**nticholinergic effects, **T**achycardia, and **S**edation.

Other Specific Information: Oral contraceptives may alter tricyclic serum levels. ↑ effect of alcohol, CNS depressants, adrenergic agents, and anticholinergics. Antithyroid agents may ↑ risk of agranulocytosis. Phenothiazines may ↑ sedative effects. Cimetidine may ↑ toxicity. If taking sympathomimetics, may ↑ cardiac effect. If taking MAO inhibitors, may ↑ risk of hypertensive crisis, convulsion. Do not give TCAs with MAOIs.

Interventions: Monitor periodic blood cell counts, glaucoma tests, hepatic and renal function studies. When evaluating the drug level, blood samples should be taken immediately before the first morning dose or at least 8 hours after a dose. Monitor BP and HR at appropriate intervals. Manic or hypomanic episodes may occur with cyclic types of disorders. May need to discontinue tricyclics until episode is relieved.

Education: Instruct client if sedation is problematic, a single dose at bedtime may be beneficial. Due to adverse interactions with anesthetic agents, instruct client to discontinue the TCAs 2–3 days prior to surgery. (Refer to **"DEPRESSION".)**

Evaluation: Client has improvement in clinical state (i.e., appearance, behavior, effects, interest, mood, speech patterns).

Drugs: amitriptyline (Elavil); amoxapine (Asendin); clomipramine (Anafranil); desipramine (Norpramin); doxepin (Adapin, Sinequan); imipramine (Tofranil); nortriptyline (Aventyl, Pamelor); protriptyline (Vivactil); trimipramine (Surmontil)

TINA TRICYCLE

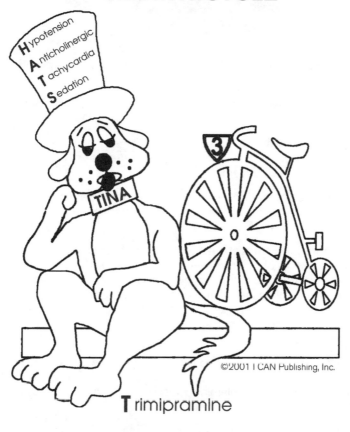

Hypotension
Anticholinergic
Tachycardia
Sedation

©2001 I CAN Publishing, Inc.

T rimipramine

I mipramine

N ortriptyline

A mitriptyline

Tina Tricycle is sitting on the curb as she is sleepy and can't pee, can't see, can't spit nor can't sh*t. Obviously she should not be driving "heavy machinery" while taking tricyclic antidepressants. The 3 wheels of the ticycle will help you remember that the therapeutic effects may have a 3 week delay of onset. After her body adjusts to the meds she may be able to ride again. "HATS" are some of the other undesirable effects she may experience.

MONOAMINE OXIDASE INHIBITOR (MAOI)

Action: Inhibits the enzyme (MAO) that breaks down norepinephrine and serotonin.

Indications: Second or third line drugs for the depression. These are effective, but are more dangerous than others.

Warnings: Alcoholism, congestive heart failure, pheochromocytoma, history of headache, uncontrolled hypertension, hepatic/renal impairment. Do not give Demerol.

Undesirable effects: Orthostatic hypotension. Hypertensive crisis if food containing tyramine is eaten. CNS effects: agitation, headache. Anticholinergic effects. Photosensitivity.

Other Specific Information: Hypertensive crisis within several hours of ingestion of a tyramine-containing product. Parnate is the most likely drug to cause this problem and the onset is rapid. Avoid foods containing tyramine such as aged cheese, beer, ale, red wine, pickled foods, smoked or pickled fish, beef or chopped liver, avocados, or figs. Tricyclic antidepressants, fluoxetine, and trazodone may cause serotonin syndrome.

Interventions: Monitor periodic liver function tests and ongoing VS. Assess for needed emotional support. Discontinue immediately with hypertensive crisis. Phentolamine mesylate (Regitine) should be on hand to control a severe hypertension reaction.

Education: After stopping the MAOI, instruct client to wait 2–3 weeks prior to taking another antidepressant. Review products high in tyramine. Administer in AM to avoid insomnia. Notify provider for signs of hypertensive crisis. Recommend wearing a medical identification band indicating MAOI therapy. Inform provider about the MAOI if dental or emergency care is needed. Usually discontinue MAOIs 10 days prior to surgery. (Refer to "**DEPRESSION**".)

Evaluation: Client has improvement in clinical state (i.e., appearance, behavior, interest, mood, speech patterns).

Drugs: isocarboxazid (Marplan); phenelzine (Nardil); tranylcypromine (Parnate)

THE "TYRANT" KING

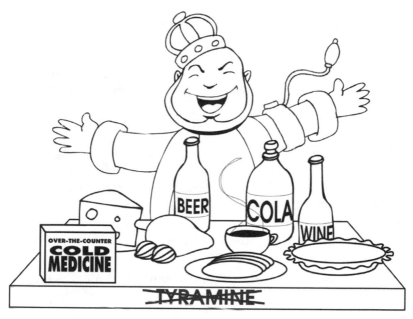

©2001 I CAN Publishing, Inc.

The "tyrant" king loves good food, but can develop a life threatening hypertensive crisis if he eats or drinks products containing **TYRAMINE** while taking MAO inhibitors. The "tyrant" is **N**o **P**opular **M**an (**N**ardil, **P**arnate, **M**arplan (this will help you remember MAO inhibitors).

OTHER ANTIDEPRESSANTS

Action: Inhibits reuptake of dopamine, serotonin, norepinephrine.

Indications: Depression, Wellbutin also is used for smoking cessation.

Warnings: Convulsive disorders, prostatic hypertrophy, severe renal, hepatic, cardiac disease depending on the type of medication. Use cautiously in suicidal clients, severe depression, schizophrenia, hyperactivity, diabetes mellitus, and the elderly.

Undesirable Effects: Dizziness, drowsiness, diarrhea, dry mouth, decrease urinary output (from retention), and decrease in the blood pressure from orthostatic hypotension. **"GOATS"** on the next page will assist you in remembering the major undesirable effects. They are minimal, however, in comparison to the other categories of antidepressants. GI effects are actually the major effects with these drugs.

Other Specific Information: Refer to individual monographs since interactions vary widely among products.

Interventions: Monitor B/P (lying, standing), pulse q 4 h; if systolic B/P drops 20 mm HG, hold drug, notify provider. Monitor blood studies, AST, ALT, bilirubin, creatinine, weight. Monitor for EPS in elderly clients. Monitor mental status, urinary retention, constipation. Do not discontinue abruptly. If alcohol is consumed hold drug until AM. Increase fluids for urinary retention and bulk in diet if constipation occurs. If GI symptoms occur, administer with food or milk. Gum, hard candy or frequent sips of water for dry mouth. Assistance with ambulation while beginning therapy. Safety measures including side rails primarily in elderly. Check to see if PO medication is swallowed.

Education: Teach that therapeutic effects may take 2–3 weeks. Use caution with driving due to drowsiness, dizziness or blurred vision. Avoid alcohol or other CNS depressants. Do not discontinue quickly.

Evaluation: Client will have a decrease in depression.

Drugs: amoxapine (Asendin), bupropion (Wellbutrin, Wellbutrin SR), maprotiline (Ludiomil, Novartis), mirtazapine (Remeron Organon), nefazodone (Serzone), trazodone (Desyrel, Trialodine), venlafaxine (Effexor/Effexor XR)

GOATS

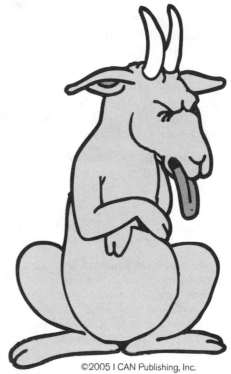

©2005 I CAN Publishing, Inc.

G I distress

O rthostatic hypotension

A nticholinergic effects (can't see, pee, spit, shit)

agi **T** ation/insomnia

S edation
   exual dysfunction

The goat is sitting to prevent falling from low blood pressure. His expression indicates his agitation, but he doesn't have enough energy to run.

CYMBALTA

Action: SSNIR drug: Inhibits serotonin and norepinephrine reuptake in the CNS. Both the antidepressant and pain inhibition are centrally mediated.

Indications: Major depressive disorder. Management of peripheral neuropathic pain for a diabetic client. Generalized anxiety disorder. Unlabeled uses: Fibromyalgia. Neuropathic pain / chronic pain. Stress urinary incontinence.

Warnings: MAO Inhibitor therapy. Uncontrolled angle-closure glaucoma; end stage renal disease. Chronic hepatic impairment or alcohol abuse may result in hepatitis. History of suicide attempt.

Undesirable Effects: Seizures, fatigue, drowsiness, insomnia, decrease in appetite, constipation, dry mouth, nausea, dysuria; increase sweating; increase in blood pressure.

Other Specific Information: Use with MAO inhibitors may result in a fatal reaction (do not use within 14 days of discontinuing MAOI). Wait at least 5 days after stopping duloxetine to start MAOI. Chronic alcohol abuse may result in hepatotoxicity. Tramadol, linezolid, and triptans may increase the risk of serotonin syndrome. Drugs that inhibit CYP1A2 or CYP2D6 increase risk of adverse reactions. Thioridazine may result in increase arrhythmias. St. John's wort may increase the serotonin syndrome.

Interventions: Assess for sexual dysfunction. Monitor blood pressure, appetite, weight, mental status, and suicidal tendencies. Assess characteristics of pain. Monitor ALT, AST, bilirubin, CPK, and alkaline phosphatase. May be taken without regard to meals. Capsules should be swallowed whole.

Education: Instruct to take as directed. Report undesirable effects. Avoid driving or other activities that require alertness until response to medication is evaluated. Advise not to take any alcohol. Recommend a support group.

Evaluation: Client will experience an increased sense of well being. If taking drug for diabetic peripheral neuropathy, the client will have a decrease in neuropathic pain.

Drug: duloxetine (Cymbalta)

CYMBALTA

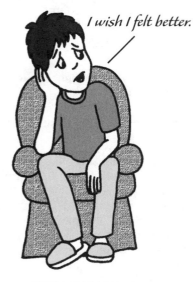

I wish I felt better.

©2009 I CAN Publishing, Inc.

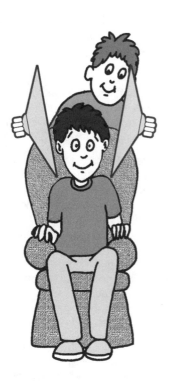

The cymbals will assist you in remembering the desired effect from Cymbalta, which is increasing a client's sense of well-being.

ANTIMANIC MEDICATION

Action: Inhibits release of norepinephrine and dopamine. Alters sodium transport in nerve and muscle cells.

Indications: Manic episodes of manic-depressive (Bipolar) disorder.

Warnings: Cardiovascular disease, renal disease, severe dehydration, thyroid disease, elderly.

Undesirable Effects: *Minor toxicity:* nausea, vomiting, diarrhea, GI upset, fine hand tremors, thirst, polyuria. *Mild to moderate toxicity:* coarse tremors, confusion, ataxia, blurred vision, diluted urine, severe polydipsia, tinnitus. *Life threatening:* Cardiac dysrhythmias, circulatory collapse.

Other Specific Information: ↑ risk of toxicity when given with thiazide diuretics, methyldopa, and NSAIDS. ↓ lithium levels with excess sodium and antacids. ↑ CNS toxicity with haloperidol. There is a narrow therapeutic index. (0.6–1.2 mEq/L: therapeutic), (> 1.5mEq/L: toxic), (2.0mEq/L: lethal).

Interventions: Therapeutic levels for maintenance are 0.6–1.2 mEq/L. Long term levels should be maintained below 0.9 mEq/L. Evaluate levels every 3–4 days during initial phase of therapy, every 1–2 months thereafter, and weekly if no improvement of mania or undesirable effects continue to occur. Blood samples taken just before the AM dose when there is a maximum stabilization of the serum concentration. Monitor fluid status, serum electrolytes, and renal function. Pre-treatment exam—thyroid, kidney function testing and EKG. Assess serum lithium levels daily with severe renal or cardiovascular disease, dehydration, and debilitation. Supervise suicidal risk. Monitor for undesirable effects. Management of lithium toxicity: osmotic diuretic.

Education: Teach symptoms of lithium toxicity. Avoid tasks requiring psychomotor coordination until CNS effects are known. Maintain a steady salt and fluid intake (2.5 to 3 liters per day; especially in summer). Administer with meals. Avoid caffeine.

Evaluation: Client is free of manic-depressive disorder as demonstrated by an improved mental status.

Drugs: Lithium Carbonate (Eskalith, Lithobid, Lithonate)

BIPOLAR CLOWN

L evel—therapeutic (0.6–1.2 mEq/L)

I ncreased urination

T hirst increased

H eadache and tremors

I ncrease fluids

U nsteady

M orton's Salt—adequate intake

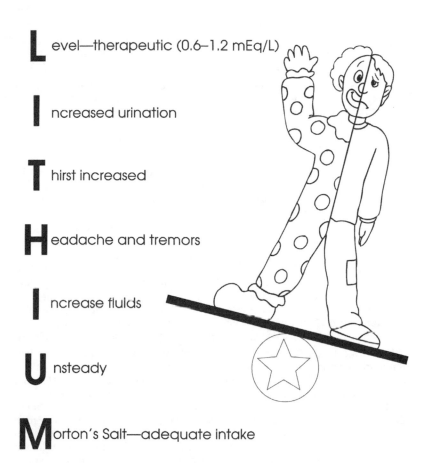

ANTIPSYCHOTICS

Action: Blocks dopamine receptor sites in the brain. There is a depression of the limbic system and cerebral cortex that controls aggression. Antiemetic effects by inhibiting the chemoreceptor trigger zones in the medulla. May initiate anticholinergic, antihistamine and/or sedative effects.

Indications: Schizophrenic disorders; mania; agitated organic disorders; delusional disorders. Antiemetic; intractable hiccups. Preoperative sedation (i.e., Compazine, Phenergan).

Warnings: Alcoholism, or other CNS depression; hepatic, renal, or coronary disease; cerebral insufficiency; severe hypotension; glaucoma; bone marrow depression; blood dyscrasias; young children. Use cautiously in elderly and debilitated clients.

Undesirable Effects: "**STANCE**" on the next page will help you remember these effects.

Other Specific Information: Alcohol, CNS depressants may ↑ CNS and respiratory depression. Tricyclics and MAO inhibitors may ↑ sedation, hypotensive and anticholinergic effects. ↓ levodopa effects. Lithium, antacids, and antidiarrheals may ↓ absorption.

Interventions: Monitor periodic liver function studies, WBCs, serum glucose, VS, and psychological assessments during therapy. Orthostatic hypotension is likely to occur; rise slowly with assistance and initiate safety measures. Suicidal precautions if necessary. Do not mix parenteral solutions with other drugs in same syringe. Give deep IM injection. Following parenteral route, remain in supine position for at least 30 minutes. Liquid should be protected from light and should be diluted with fruit juice before administering. Avoid skin contact with oral suspension solution. Treat extrapyramidal symptoms with anticholinergics (i.e., Cogentin). Discontinue at least 48 hours before surgery.

Education: Teach that urine may turn pink or reddish brown. Advise that the medication may take 6 wks or longer to achieve a full therapeutic effect. Instruct to give daily dose 1–2 hours before bedtime. Oral concentrate must be diluted in 2–3 oz. of liquid (water, fruit juice, carbonated drink, milk, or pudding). Avoid sun exposure (use sun block). Caution against driving a car or operating machinery. Explain the importance of reporting a sore throat, fever, or symptoms of infection. Undesirable effects usually subside within approximately 2 weeks of therapy or decrease by dose adjustment. Inform other providers when taking these drugs. Advise client to wear an ID bracelet indicating the medication therapy.

Evaluation: The client is able to cope with and perform activities of daily living independently.

Drugs: *Phenothiazines:* chlorpromazine (Thorazine); fluphenazine (Prolixin); mesoridazine (Serentil); perphenazine (Trilafon); prochlorperazine (Compazine); promazine (Sparine); thioridazine (Mellaril); trifluoperazine (Stelazine); triflupromazine (Vesprin); *Nonphenothiazines:* clozapine (Clozaril); haloperidol (Haldol); loxapine (Loxitane); molindone (Moban); olanzapine (Zyprexa); pimozide (Orap); quetiapine (Seroquel); risperidone (Risperdal); thiothixene (Navane)

STANCE

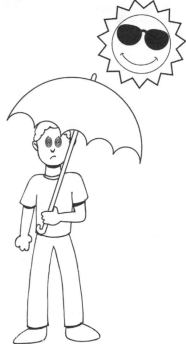

S edation
unlight sensitivity

T ardive dyskinesia
achycardia
remors

A nticholinergic
granulocytosis
ddiction

N euroleptic malignant syndrome

C ardiac arrhythmias (orthostatic hypotension)

E xtrapyramidal (akathesia)
ndocrine (change in libido)

STANCE will help you remember the undesirable effects of Antipsychotics

ATYPICAL ANTIPSYCHOTIC

Action: Atypical antipsychotic/neuroleptic. Benzisoxazole derivative. Exact mechanism unknown. Dopamine and serotonin receptor antagonists.

Indications: More effective for negative symptoms of schizophrenia (amotivation, affect, isolation).

Warnings: Hypersensitivity, lactation, seizure disorders, renal disease, hepatic disease, children, pregnancy, and the elderly.

Undesirable Effects: Newest agent in class (as such, minimal published clinical trial data); transient nausea, vomiting possible; anxiety and insomnia also reported; minimal to no prolactin elevation, QT prolongation, or weight gain. While the image on the next page is the same as the image for the typical antipsychotics, the undesirable effects in "STANCE" are very low for this drug.

Other Specific Information: Increased effects of aripiprazole: CYP3A4 inhibitors (ketoconazole), CYP2D6 inhibitors (quinidine, fluoxetine, paroxetine); reduce dose of aripiprazole. Increased sedation: other CNS depressants and alcohol. Increased EPS with other antipsychotics, lithium. Decreased effects of aripiprazole: CYP3A4 inducers (carbamazepine), increased dose of aripiprazole. Increased CNS depression with kava.

Interventions: Assess mental status prior to initiating drug. I&O. Monitor bilirubin, CBC, LFTs every month. Assess affect, LOC, gait, sleep pattern, etc. Monitor blood pressure standing and lying; also heart rate, respirations. Report drops of 30 mmHg in B/P; assess for ECG changes. Monitor dizziness, faintness, tachycardia on rising. Monitor EPS, including akathesia, tardive dyskinesia (bizarre movements of the jaw, mouth, tongue, extremities), pseudoparkinsonism. Assess for neuroleptic malignant syndrome; hyperthermia, increased CPK , altered mental status, muscle rigidity. Assess skin turgor daily along with constipation, urinary retention. Supervise ambulation until client is stabilized on the med. Decrease stimulus by dimming lights and avoiding loud environmental sounds.

Education: Advise client about orthostatic hypotension and how to handle rising from sitting or lying. Recommend avoiding hot tubs, hot showers, tub baths due to hypotension. Avoid abruptly withdrawing the drug. EPS may result. Withdraw slowly. Avoid OTC preparation unless approved by provider of care. Avoid hazardous activities if drowsy or dizzy. Report impaired vision, tremors, muscle twitching. In hot weather, take precautions to remain cool.

Evaluation: Client will experience a decrease in emotional excitement, hallucinations, delusions, paranoia. There will be evidence of a reorganization of patterns of thought and speech.

Drug: aripiprazole (Abilify)

STANCE

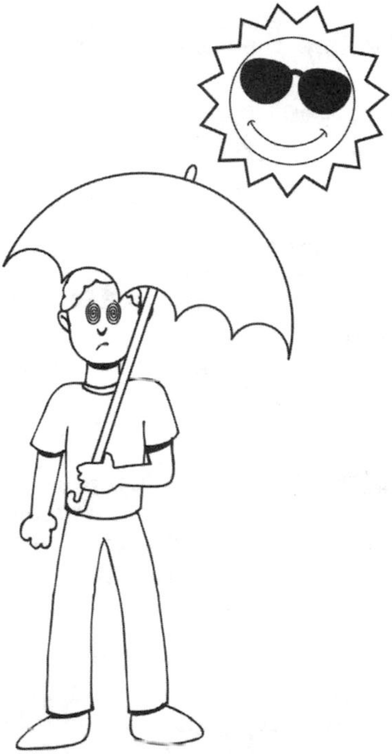

S edation
   unlight sensitivity

T ardive dyskinesia
   achycardia
   remors

A nticholinergic
   granulocytosis
   ddiction

N euroleptic malignant syndrome

C ardiac arrhythmias (orthostatic hypotension)

E xtrapyramidal (akathesia)
   ndocrine (change in libido)

GEODON

Action: Unknown: may be mediated through both dopamine type 2 (D2) and serotonin type 2 (5-HT2) antagonism. Benzisoxazole derivative.

Indications: Antipsychotic/neuroleptic. Schizophrenia, acute agitation.

Warnings: Hypersensitivity, lactation, seizure activity.

Undesirable Effects: EPS, pseudoparkinsonism, akathesia, dystonia, tardive dyskinesia; drowsiness, insomnia, agitation, headache, seizures, neuroleptic malignant sydrome, dizzy, tremor. Orthostatic hypotension, tachycardia, sudden death. Anorexia, constipation, weight gain, dry mouth, rhinitis.

Other Specific Information: Increased sedation with other CNS depressants, alcohol. Increased EPS with other antipsychotics, lithium. Increased excretion of ziprasidone: carbamazepine. Increased ziprasidone with ketoconazole. Increased hypotension with antihypertensives. Increased CNS depression with chamomile, kava, skullcap, or valerian.

Interventions: Assess mental status prior to initiating the drug. Assess I&O; palplate bladder if urinary output is low. Every month monitor Bilirubin, CBC, LFTs. Assess affect, orientation, LOC, etc. Assess B/P standing and lying; also heart rate, respirations. Monitor for undesirable effects. Decrease stimuli by dimming lights; provide a quiet environment. Supervise ambulation until client is stabilized on the medication. Increase fluids to decrease constipation.

Education: Instruct to take capsule whole and do not open or crush. Advise to take with food. Review the importance of rising from sitting or lying position gradually due to orthostatic hypotension. Avoid hot baths. Advise not to abruptly withdraw the drug due to EPS. Withdraw drug slowly. Avoid OTC preparations of cold, cough, hay fever medicine, alcohol, and CNS depressants. Report undesirable effects. In hot weather, take precautions to remain cool.

Evaluation: Client will have a decrease in emotional excitement, hallucinations, delusions, paranoia; reorganization of thinking process and speech.

Drug: ziprasidone (Geodon)

STANCE

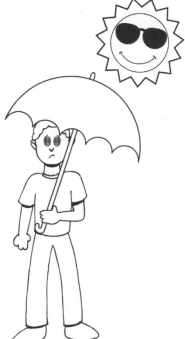

S edation
unlight sensitivity

T ardive dyskinesia
achycardia
remors

A nticholinergic
granulocytosis
ddiction

N euroleptic malignant syndrome

C ardiac arrhythmias (orthostatic hypotension)

E xtrapyramidal (akathesia)
ndocrine (change in libido)

©2001 I CAN Publishing, Inc.

Notice Stance has a doubled up fist because he is agitated. This drug may cause sensitivity to sun light. Geodon will help control this feeling.

ABSTINENCE MAINTENANCE (FOLLOWING DETOXIFICATION): ReVia

Action: Opioid antagonist that suppresses the effects of alcohol (also used for opioid withdrawal). Naltrexone oral is a special narcotic drug that blocks the effects of other narcotic medicines and alcohol.

Indications: Alcohol or narcotic addiction

Warnings: Contraindicated if any history of hypersensitivity; pregnancy; an addiction to narcotics; a history of drug or alcohol use in the last 7-10 days; or drug or alcohol withdrawal symptoms. Do not use narcotic drugs or alcohol while taking naltrexone oral. Use with caution if client has any renal or hepatic impairment, or a bleeding disorder such as hemophilia.

Undesirable Effects: Anxious, restless, irritable, lightheaded; increased thirst; muscle or joint aches; insomnia; decrease in libido. Notify provider of care and discontinue if any of the following occur: blurred vision or eye problems; tachycardia; mood changes (hallucinations), thoughts of hurting self; nausea, stomach pain, low fever, loss of appetite, dark urine, clay-colored stools, jaundice (yellowing of the skin or eyes); tinnitus; pruritus; wheezing

Other Specific Information: Do not use alcohol or narcotics. Do not take in any substance that has alcohol in it such as mouth wash, cough syrups, etc.

Interventions: Overdose symptoms may include nausea, stomach pain, dizziness, or seizure (convulsions). Notify provider of care. Use naltrexone oral exactly as it was prescribed. Administer the naltrexone oral tablet with a full glass of water and food to decrease stomach upset. Store naltrexone oral tablets at room temperature away from moisture and heat.

Education: Recommend client carry an ID card or wear a medical alert bracelet stating that they are using naltrexone, in case of emergency. Any doctor, dentist, or emergency medical care provider who treats should know that client is using this medication. Additional forms of counseling and/ or monitoring may be recommended during treatment with naltrexone oral. Recommend monthly IM injections for clients with difficulty adhering to the recommended regimen. If mediciation is missed, recommend taking the medication as soon as client remembers. If it is almost time for the next dose, skip the missed dose and wait until next regularly scheduled dose. Do not take extra medicine to make up the missed dose.

Evaluation: Client will be successful in abstinence from alcohol and/or opioids and will participate on a regular basis in a self-help group.

Drugs: naltrexone (ReVia)

NALTREXONE (REVIA)

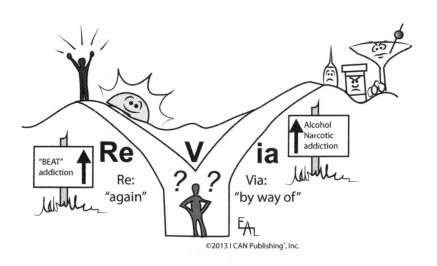

Re: "again"
??
Via: "by way of"

"BEAT" addiction

Re:

Via:

Alcohol Narcotic addiction

©2013 I CAN Publishing®, Inc.

"BEAT" addiction again, by way of Revia!

B leeding disorder, Hepatic or Renal impairment use with caution

E ducate to avoid alcohol containing products (mouthwash, cough syrups...)

A ddiction to alcohol or narcotics is the indication to take this medication

T ake tablet with a full glass of water and food to decrease stomach upset

ABSTINENCE MAINTENANCE (FOLLOWING DETOXIFICATION): ANTABUSE

Action: Disulfiram used with alcohol will result in acetaldehyde syndrome.

Indications: Management of chronic alcoholism in clients who require or desire an enforced state of sobriety. Disulfiram is a daily oral medication that is a type of aversion therapy.

Warnings: Contraindicated if hypersensitive to disulfiram or other thiurams (including those used in rubber vulcanization and pesticides); Significant cardiovascular disease; Psychosis; Any recent use of metronidazole, paraldehyde, or any alcohol or products containing alcohol. Use cautiously with client who has diabetes; epilepsy, hyperthyroidism, cerebral problems; hepatic/renal impairment; pregnant, or a child.

Undesirable Effects: Nausea, vomiting, weakness, sweating; hypotension, palpitations, and hepatic toxicity. Acetaldehyde syndrome may progress to respiratory arrest, cardiovascular suppression, seizures, death.

Other Specific Information: Avoid products that contain alcohol (cough syrups, aftershave, lotion, etc.)

Interventions: Administer one time a day. This is a type of aversion therapy for alcohol. Assess for undesirable effects from the medication such as acetaldehyde syndrome. This can progess to respiratory depression, cardiovascular suppression, seizures, and death. Monitor liver enzymes and assess for hepatic toxicity.

Education: Instruct client regarding the risk of drinking any alcohol. Review the importance of wearing a medical alert braclet. Discuss the need to attend a 12-step self-help program. Review that medication effects (risk for acetaldehyde syndrome) may persist for 2 weeks after discontinuation of the disulfiram.

Evaluation: Client will be successful in abstinence from alcohol and participate on a regular basis in a self-help group.

Drug: disulfiram (Antabuse)

ANTABUSE "ANT-ABUSE"

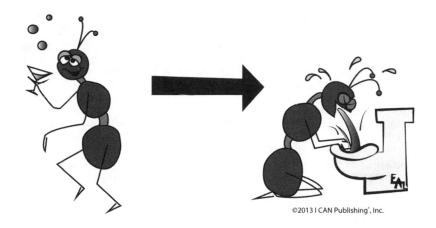

©2013 I CAN Publishing®, Inc.

B racelet- medical alert bracelet should be worn;
(UE: N/V, weakness, sweating, liver toxicity)

A cetaldehyde syndrome may occur. Watch for:
respiratory arrest, cardiovascular suppression,
seizures, death

R emind client to avoid products containing alcohol (e.g., mouth wash, cough syrup, after
shave)

F ollow up with a 12 step self-help program

SUBSTITUTION THERAPY FOR OPIOID WITHDRAWAL: METHADONE

Action: Opioid agonist that replaces the opioid to which the client is addicted. Methadone works to treat pain by changing the way the brain and nervous system respond to pain.

Indications: Withdrawal and long-term maintenance for clients addicted to heroin or other opioids. It is a narcotic pain reliever, similar to morphine.

Warrnings: Contraindicated: Hypersensitivitiy to any narcotic medicine including: morphine, Oxycontin, Darvocet, Percocet, Vicodin, Lortab, and many others); an asthma attack or has a paralytic ileus; head injury, a brain tumor, a stroke, or any other condition that caused high pressure inside the skull; irregular heartbeat; urethral stricture (narrowing of the tube that carries urine out of the body), enlarged prostate (a male reproductive gland), or any other condition that causes difficulty urinating; Addison's disease; mental illness; chronic obstructive pulmonary disease (COPD); sleep apnea; hypokalemia or low magnesium; or thyroid , heart, liver, or kidney disease.

Undesirable Effects: Undesirable effects that can be more serious: refer to **"HURTS"** on next page. Symptoms of overdose may be remembered by **"SLOW"**: **S**hallow breathing, small pinpoint pupils, **L**imp muscles, **O**btunded (deteriorating LOC), and **W**hite to blue skin color, cool and clammy). Remember, dependence may be transferred from the illegal opioid to methadone.

Other Specific Information: There are numerous drug-drug interactions that may occur when taking methadone. **"THE MAD WAR"** in the front of the book will also assist you in organizing some of the key players involved in drug-drug interaction. The KEY is to always review with the provider the other meds client is taking in order to decrease risk of drug–drug interaction. Risk of interactions with antidepressants, antifungals, buprenorphine, butorphanol, calcium channel blockers, diuretics, erythromycin, laxatives, anti-anxiety meds, anti-HIV meds. It is beyond the scope of this book to review each one, but remember there are NUMEROUS interactions, and it is always a great idea to either check with provider of care or look these up in the drug book.

Interventions: Ongoing assessments for undesirable effects. Refer to next page for signs of undesirable effects and signs of toxicity. Intervene prior to an overdose, but if unable to and in case of overdose, have emergency equipment available.

Education: Inform client that methadone dose must be slowly tapered to produce detoxification. May be habit forming. Never share methadone with another person, especially someone with a history of drug abuse or addiction. Keep the medication in a place where others cannot get to it. In case of overdose, call local poison control center. If the client has collapsed or is not breathing, call local emergency services at 911. Encourage client to participate in a 12-step- self-help program. Inform client that methadone must be administered from an approved treatment center.

Evaluation: Client will be successful in abstinence from opioids and will participate on a regular basis in a self-help group.

Drug: methadone (Dolophine)

METHADONE
(UNDESIRABLE SIDE EFFECTS)

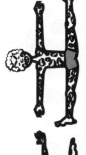 **IVES**

 RTICARIA

 ASH

 HE RR↓

 EIZURES

WITHDRAWAL/ABSTINENCE FROM OPIOIDS

Action: Binds to opiate receptors in the CNS. Changes the perception of and response to painful stimuli while at the same time producing generalized CNS depression. Has partial antagonist properties that may result in opioid withdrawal in physical dependent clients.

Indications: Opioid detoxicaton. SL: Suppression of withdrawal symptoms during detoxification and maintenance from heroin or other opioids by decreasing feelings of craving.

Warnings: `HIGH ALERT DRUG` Contraindicated in hypersensitivity. Use cautiously in increased intracranial pressure; severe hepatic, renal, or pulmonary disease; hypothyroidism; adrenal insufficiency; alcoholism; debilitated clients (may need to reduce dose); prostatic hyperplasia; abdominal pain. For geriatrics, there must be a reduction in the dose.

Undesirable Effects: Confusion, dysphoria, hallucinations, sedation, dizziness, euphoria, floating feeling, unusual dreams; respiratory depression; hypertension, hypotension, palpitations; nausea, constipation, dry mouth; sweating, clammy; physical dependence, tolerance. May cause ↑ serum amylase and lipase levels. Complications: jaundice, dark urine, light stools.

Other Specific Information: Use with caution with client receiving MAO inhibitors; ↑ CNS depression with alcohol, antidepressants, antihistamines, and sedative / hypnotics. May ↓ effectiveness of other opioid analgesics. Inhibitors of the CYP3A4 enzyme system including azole antifungals (itraconazole, ketoconazole), erythromycin protease inhibitor antiretrovirals (ritonavir, indinavir, saquinavir) ↑ blood levels and effects. Inducers of the CYP3A4 enzyme system including carbamazepine, rifampin, or phenytoin ↓ blood levels and effects. Concurrent abuse of IV buprenorphine and benzodiazepines may result in a coma and death. Concurrent use of kava kava, valerian, or chamomile can ↑ CNS depression.

Interventions: Do not confuse Buprenex (buprenorphine) with Bumex (bumetanide). Accidental overdosage of opioid analgesics has resulted in fatalities. Prior to administering, clarify all ambiguous orders; have second nurse independently check original order, dose calculations, route of administration, and infusion pump programming if being used. Sublingual (SL) is the route of administration during detoxification. Usually takes 2-10 min. to dissolve. Place under the tongue and do not chew or swallow. Assess client for signs and symptoms of opioid withdrawal prior to and during therapy. Monitor liver function tests prior to and during therapy. If an opioid antagonist is required to reverse respiratory depression or coma, naloxone (Narcan) is the antidote.

Education: Instruct client in the correct use of medication; must be administered from an approved treatment center. Medication must be used on a regular basis, not occasionally. If a dose is missed, take when remembered unless it is close to time for next dose. Do not take 2 doses at once. Do not DC without consulting with provider. It may cause withdrawal symptoms. If medication is discontinued, flush unused tablets down the toilet.

Evaluation: Client will be successful in abstinence from heroin or other opioids and will participate on a regular basis in a self-help group.

Drugs: buprenorphine (Buprenex, Subutex)

BUPRENORPHINE (FOR OPIATE DEPENDENCE)

HIGH ALERT

C ravings are decreased

H eroin and other Opioids

A drenal insufficiency, alcoholism, abdominal pain - use cautiously

I ncrease in CNS depression with alcohol, antidepressants, and sedatives/ hypnotics

N arcan is the antidote

S ublingual is the route of administration during detox

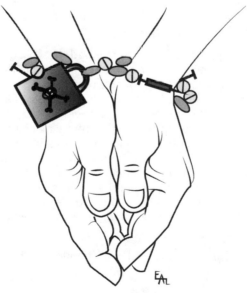

©2013 I CAN Publishing®, Inc.

NICOTINE AGONIST: CHANTIX

Action: Selectively binds to alpha$_4$, beta$_2$ nictotinic acetylcholine receptors, acting as a nicotine agonist; prevents binding of nicotine to receptors.

Indications: Smoking cessation

Warnings: Contraindicated with hypersensitivity; Pregnancy/OB; children. Use cautiously with clients who have severe renal impairment; Geriatric clients due to decline in renal function.

Undesirable Effects: Anxiety, decrease in attention span, depression, irritability, restless, insomnia; diarrhea, nausea, gingivitis; elevation in the liver function tests; flushing, hyperhydrosis; arthralgia, back pain, musculoskeletal pain.

Other Specific Information: Smoking cessation may decrease metabolism of warfarin, insulin and theophylline resulting in increased effects. Risk of undesirable effects (i.e., dizziness, nausea, vomiting, fatigue, headache) may be increased with nicotine replacement therapy (nicotine transdermal patches).

Interventions: Treatment is started one week prior to planned smoking cessation. Assess for desire to stop smoking. Assess for nausea; usually dose dependent. May result in anemia. Administer after eating with a full glass of water.

Education: Instruct to take as prescribed. Establish a date to stop smoking and start medication one week prior to this date. Encourage and support client with process of stopping even if they have had early lapses after the date for the goal to stop smoking. Caution never to share medication with others since it could be very harmful. Due to risk for dizziness, caution client not to operate machinery or drive until cognitive response has been evaluated. Review with the client that nausea and insominia may occur, but are usually temporary. Instruct to notify provider if symptoms continue and are bothersome, so dose may be reduced. Review importance of notifying provider of care prior to taking any meds while on the medication. After smoking cessation, some meds may need dose adjustments. Notify provider if pregnant or plan to become pregnant.

Evaluation: Client is successful with the identified goal for smoking cessation.

Drug: varenicline (Chantix)

NICOTINE AGONISTS (CHANTIX) CHAN "TICKS"

T emporary nausea and insomnia may occur

I rritability and restlessness may also occur

C essation may ⬇ metabolism of warfarin, insulin, and theophylline

K ick nicotine addiction

S electively binds to receptors, acting as a nicotine agonist

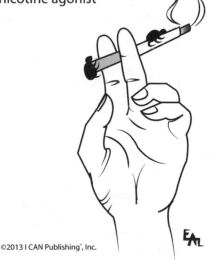

ZYBAN

Action: Decreases neuronal reuptake of dopamine in the CNS. Decreased neuronal uptake of serotonin and norepinephrine (less than tricyclic antidepressants). Decreases nicotine craving and symptoms of withdrawal.

Indications: Smoking cessation

Warnings: Contraindicated in hypersentisivity; history of bulimia, and anorexia nervosa. Concurrent MAO inhibitor or ritonavir therapy; lactation. Use cautiously in renal/hepatic impairment (decrease dose if recommended); Recent MI; History of suicide attempt / ideation. Use in geriatric clients could result in an accumulation of the drug. History of seizures, head trauma, or use of any meds that may decrease seizure threshold (such as antidepressants, antipsychotic, systemic corticosteroids, theophylline) require this med be used with extreme caution.

Undesirable Effects: Seizures, agitation, headache, insomnia, mania, psychoses; dry mouth, nausea, vomiting, change in appetite, weight gain or loss; hyperglycemia or hypoglycemia; tremors.

Other Specific Information: Increase risk of undesirable effects when used with amantadine, levodopa, or MAO inhibitor (concurrent use of MAO inhibitors is contraindicated). Increase risk of seizures when taken with antidepressants, phenothiazines, theophylline, corticosteroids, OTC stimulants/anorectics or if there is cessation of alcohol or benzodiazepines (avoid or decrease use of alcohol). Carbamazepine may decrease blood levels resulting in a decrease in effectiveness. Nicotine replacement used concurrently may result in hypertension. Warfarin may increase risk for bleeding.

Interventions: Do not confuse bupropion with buspirone. Do not confuse Zyban (bupropion) with Zagam (Sparfloxacin). Do not administer bupropion (Wellbutrin) with Zyban, which contains same ingredients. Administer doses in equally spaced time increments during day to decrease risk of seizures. Insomnia may be decreased by avoiding bedtime dose. May be administered with food to decrease GI irritation. Treat dry mouth by recommending client to chew gum or keep hard candy on hand, and to sip on small amounts of water or suck on ice chips. Review the importance of not taking any CNS stimulants or caffeine to control insomnia. Monitor mood changes and notify provider if client experiences an increase in anxiety, nervousness, or insomnia. Monitor renal and liver function.

Education: Instruct to take as prescribed. Missed doses for smoking cessation should be omitted. Do not double doses or take more than prescribed. Avoid alcohol during therapy and notify provider prior to taking any other meds with bupropion (Zyban). Review with client the need for frequent mouth rinses, good oral hygiene, and sugarless gum or candy to decrease dry mouth. Smoking should be stopped during the 2nd week of therapy to allow for the onset of bupropion and to maximize the goal of smoking cessation.

Evaluation: Client will successfully fulfill goal for smoking cessation.

Drugs: bupropion (Zyban)

ZYBAN (BUPROPION)

Zy "ban" smoking
from your life!

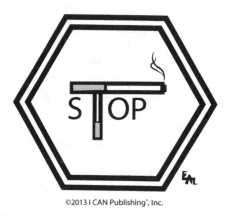

©2013 I CAN Publishing®, Inc.

S moking should stop the 2nd week of therapy

T he drug bupropion (Wellbutrin) should NOT be admin.
with Zyban, which contains same ingredients

O bserve for change in liver and/or renal function;
Omit CNS stimulants or caffeine to control insomnia

P revent seizures by giving doses in equally spaced time
increments. Put med with food; treat dry mouth
with chewing gum, water, hard candy

ANTI-ALZHEIMER'S AGENT: ARICEPT

Action: Elevates acetylcholine concentrations (cerebral cortex) by slowing degradation of acetylcholine released in cholinergic neurons. Reversible cholinesterase inhibitor.

Indications: Mild to moderate dementia in Alzheimer's disease.

Warnings: Hypersensitivity to donepezil or piperidine derivatives. Sick sinus syndrome, history of ulcers, GI bleeding, hepatic disease, bladder obstruction, asthma, COPD, seizures.

Undesirable Effects: Headaches, abnormal dreams, dizziness, drowsiness, depression, fatigue, insomnia, syncope, atrial fibrillation, hypertension, hypotension, vasodilation, diarrhea, nausea, anorexia, vomiting, frequent urination, hot flashes, ecchymoses, arthritis, muscle cramps.

Other Specific Information: Exaggerates muscle relaxation from succinylcholine. Increased drug-drug interactions with anticholinergics and theophylline. When taken with NSAIDs, there is an increased gastric acid secretion. Decreased donepezil effect: carbamazepine, dexamethasone, phenytoin, phenobarbital, rifampin.

Interventions: Monitor pulse during therapy due to risk of bradycardia. Caution client regarding the risk of dizziness. Advise client and caregiver to notify health care provider if nausea, vomiting, diarrhea, or changes in color of stool occur or if new symptoms occur. Administer between meals; may be given with meals for GI symptoms. Due to risk of dizziness, assist with ambulation during the beginning of therapy. If drug overdose occurs, withdraw drug, adminiter tertiary anticholinergics, provide supportive care.

Education: Advise client and/or family that dosage may be adjusted to response no more than q 6 weeks. Instruct to report undesirable effects such as nausea, vomiting, sweating, or twitching which indicates toxicity. Instruct regarding the importance of not to increase or abruptly decrease dose due to the serious consequences that may result. Family and client need to understand that the drug is not a cure; it only relieves symptoms. Recommend taking drug in the evening just before going to bed.

Evaluation: Client will experience decrease in confusion, improved mood.

Drug: donepezil (Aricept)

"A RICE PT"

A dminister in evening just prior to bedtime

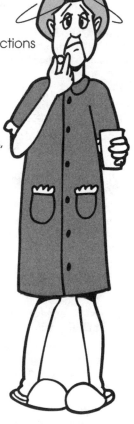

R ifampin may result in drug/drug interactions

I ndicated for Alzheimer's

C aution for the "dreaded 'd's'": dizziness, drowsiness, depression, diarrhea, deep muscle cramps

E levation in acetylcholine

P ulse may become bradycardia

T ake without regard to food

The client with Alzheimer's may need this medication. In early stages they may be very NICE. Later on, they may misinterpret their pill for a grain of RICE. "A RICE PT" will help you remember this Anti-Alzheimer's agent. Also remember "RICE" rhymes with "NICE".

ANTI-ALZHEIMER'S AGENT

Action: Enhances cholinergic function by reversible inhibition of cholinesterase. Cognitive enhancer.

Indications: Mild to moderate dementia of the Alzheimer's type.

Warnings: Hypersensitivity; severe hepatic or renal impairment. Use cautiously in clients with supraventricular cardiac conduction defects or concurrent use of drugs that may slow heart rate (increased risk of bradycardia). History of ulcer disease / GI bleeding or concurrent NSAID use. Severe asthma or obstructive pulmonary disease. Mild to moderate renal impairment (avoid use if CCr < 9 ml/min) ; Mild to moderate hepatic impairment (cautious dose titration recommended). Risk for cardiovascular mortality may be increased if using this drug.

Undesirable Effects: Fatigue, dizziness, headache, syncope. Bradycardia, chest pain. Anorexia, diarrhea, dyspepsia, flatulence, nausea, vomiting. Bladder outflow obstruction, incontinence. Tremor. Weight loss.

Other Specific Information: Will increase neuromuscular blockade from succinylcholine-type neuromuscular blocking agents. May increase effects of other cholinesterase inhibitors or other cholinergic agonists, including bethanechol. May decrease effectiveness of anticholinergic medications. Ketoconazole, paroxetine, amitriptyline, or fluvoxamine may increase blood levels.

Interventions: Assess cognitive function (memory, attention, judgment, decision making, language, ability to perform simple tasks) periodically during therapy. Monitor heart rate during therapy, since it may result in bradycardia. Client should be maintained on a stable dose for a minimum of 4 weeks prior to increasing dose. Restart at the lower dose if dose has been interrupted for several days. Administer twice daily, preferably with AM and PM meals and give with food. Antiemetic medications and ensuring adequate fluid intake may decrease nausea and vomiting. Razadyne XR can be opened and sprinkled on yogurt or applesauce; should be taken within 10 minutes.

Education: Review the importance of taking daily, as directed. Educate client and/or caregiver in correct use of pipette if using oral solution. Do not double dose; if miss a dose return to regular schedule the next day. Do not discontinue abruptly. Discuss fall prevention due to risk for dizziness. Notify healthcare provider if nausea or vomiting persists beyond seven days or if new symptoms occur or previously noted symptoms increase in severity. Discuss the importance of notifying healthcare provider of medication regimen prior to treatment or surgery. Review the importance of follow-up exams to monitor progress. Teach client and caregivers that improvements in cognitive functioning may take weeks to months to stabilize. Discuss with client and family that disease is not cured and degenerative process is not reversed.

Evaluation: Clients with Alzheimer's disease will experience an improvement in cognitive function (memory, attention, reasoning, language, ability to perform simple tasks).

Drugs: galantamine (Razadyne)

GALANTAMINE (RAZADYNE)

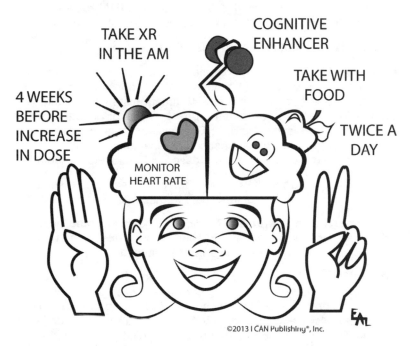

TAKE XR IN THE AM

COGNITIVE ENHANCER

TAKE WITH FOOD

4 WEEKS BEFORE INCREASE IN DOSE

TWICE A DAY

MONITOR HEART RATE

©2013 I CAN Publishing®, Inc.

M inimum of 4 weeks maintain prior to increasing dose

E xtended-release capsules in the AM, preferably with food

M ild to moderate dementia of the Alzheimer's type

O ral dose-administer twice daily; preferably with morning and evening meals

R easoning, memory, language and ability to perform simple tasks - Desired outcomes

Y es, heart rate must be monitored due to risk of developing bradycardia

ANTI-ALZHEIMER'S AGENT: NAMENDA

Action: Binds to CNS N-methyl-D-aspartate (NMDA) receptor sites, preventing binding of glutamate, an excitatory neurotransmitter.

Indications: Moderate to severe Alzheimer's dementia.

Warnings: Severe renal impairment it is contraindicated. Use cautiously in moderate renal impairment (consider decreasing dose); Concurrent use of other NMDA antagonists (i.e., amantadine, rimantadine, ketamine, dextromethorphan); Drugs or diets that cause alkaline urine should be avoided; Condition that increase urine pH including severe urinary tract infections or renal tubular acidosis may a lead to decrease in excretion and increase levels: OB and / or lactation.

Undesirable Effects: Dizziness, fatigue, headache, sedation, hypertension, rash, weight gain, urinary frequency

Other Specific Information: Medications that increase urine pH lead to decrease excretion and increase blood levels; some of these include carbonic anhydrase inhibitors or sodium bicarbonate.

Interventions: Assess cognitive function (attention, memory, reasoning, language, ability to perform activities of daily living) throughout therapy. Dose increases should occur no more frequently than weekly. May be administered without regard to food. Administer oral solution using syringe provided. Do not dilute or mix with other fluids. (Refer to AI on the next page to help you remember the general nursing care.)

Education: Review with the family that this medication does not cure disease and does not slow progression. It may take months for improvement to be observed. Review caregivers on how and when to administer medication. Caution that dizziness may occur, so initiate fall precautions.

Evaluation: A client with Alzheimer's disease will experience an improvement in cognitive function (memory, attention, language, ability perform activities of daily living).

Drugs: memantine (Namenda)

MEMANTINE (NAMENDA)

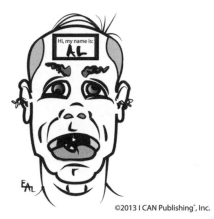

©2013 I CAN Publishing®, Inc.

N ot to be taken if one has severe renal
impairment; caution if taking drugs
or diets that cause alkaline urine

A ssess cognitive function (attention, memory,
reasoning, language, ability to perform
activities of daily living) throughout therapy

M ust not dilute or mix with other fluids

E ducate family / caregivers that med
does not cure disease

N ote: dizziness may occur, so initiate fall
prevention if necessary

D ose increases should occur no more
frequently than weekly

A dminister oral solution using syringe provided

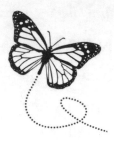

The difference between ordinary and extraordinary is that little extra.

JIMMY JOHNSON

Reproductive and Women's Health-Related Agents

OXYTOCINS

Action: Stimulates contraction of uterine muscle fibers.

Indications: Pitocin—Induction of labor contractions; Ergotrate/Methergine (E/M)—Control uterine atony after delivery of placenta.

Warnings: **HIGH ALERT DRUG** Cephalopelvic disproportion, fetal distress, anticipated nonvaginal delivery. E/M—hypertension, preeclampsia, history of CVAs.

Undesirable Effects: Pitocin—Nausea/vomiting; hypertension, cardiac arrhythmias; uterine hypertonicity, fetal bradycardia; water intoxication with convulsions and coma. E/M: Most frequent: nausea/vomiting; Less frequent: HTN, dizziness.

Other Specific Information: Use cautiously with dopamine, vasoconstrictors, and regional anesthetics.

Interventions: Baseline and ongoing maternal HR and BP, uterine activity, and fetal heart rate (FHR). Monitor I & O every 2 hrs. Maintain client in sitting or left lateral recumbent position. Be alert for signs of uterine rupture (very infrequent), which include decreased or absent FHR, sudden increased pain, absent contractions, hemorrhage, and the rapid development of hypov-olemic shock. Pitocin—IV administration under continuous observation. No bolus injection. Use infusion pump.

Education: Ergotrate—Instruct client to avoid smoking. Caution about exposure to cold. Alert client that discomfort may result form ergonovine-related contractions. Instruct about appropriate nonpharmacologic methods to decrease discomfort.

Evaluation: Positive uterine response; control of postpartum hemorrhage.

Drugs: ergonovine (Ergotrate); methylergonovine (Methergine); oxytocin (Pitocin, Syntocinon)

PITOCIN

P ressure is elevated

I ntoxication with water

T etanic contractions

O xygen decrease in fetus

C ardiac arrhythmia

I rregularity in fetal heart rate

N ausea and vomiting

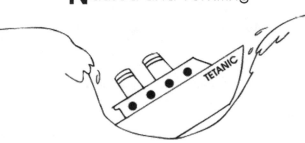

©2001 I CAN Publishing, Inc.

Oxytocin "squeezes" and contracts the uterus to initiate labor and stop hemorrage after delivery

MAGNESIUM SULFATE

Action: Reduces striated muscle contractions due to the depressant effect on the CNS. Blocks neuromuscular transmission.

Indications: Control of convulsions in preeclampsia or eclampsia.

Warnings: **HIGH ALERT DRUG** Do not give 2 hours preceding delivery because of risk of magnesium toxicity in neonate. Heart block, significant cardiac damage, or renal failure.

Undesirable Effects: Weakness, dizziness. Magnesium intoxication—flushing, sweating, hypotension, ↓ reflexes (patellar reflex is an indication regarding the depression of the CNS), ↓ respirations, flaccid paralysis, hypothermia, circulatory collapse, cardiac and CNS depression.

Other Specific Information: Neuromuscular blockade can be produced by neuromuscular agents such as gallamine, metocurine iodide, pancuronium, vecuronium.

Interventions: Monitor serum levels. Normal serum magnesium concentrations are 1.6 to 2.6 mEq/L. Monitor knee jerk reflex before repeated parenteral administration; maintain urine output at a level of 100 ml every 4 hours during parenteral administration. Antidote is calcium gluconate.

Education: Advise client to report undesirable effects such as sweating, flushing, muscle tremors, twitching, or inability to move extremities.

Evaluation: Convulsions will be controlled or prevented.

Drug: Magnesium Sulfate

A ROAD BLOCK TO PIH AND SEIZURES

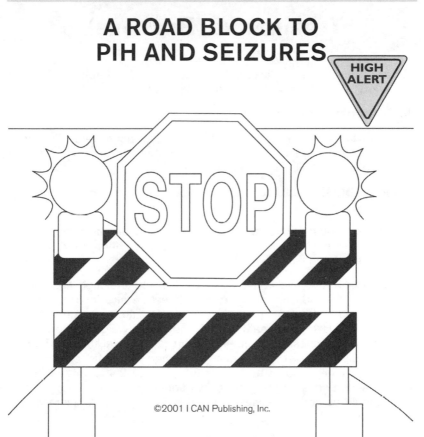

©2001 I CAN Publishing, Inc.

Magnesium sulfate, a CNS depressant, reduces or "stops" convulsions in the OB client.

Mag Sulfate
(sung to the tune of "Achy, Breaky Heart")

> Decreased BP
>
> Decreased Pee Pee
>
> These are toxic signs of mag sulfate.
>
> Drop in respiratory rate,
>
> Patellar reflex there ain't,
>
> Give antidote calcium gluconate!
>
> *(One more time)*

TERBULATINE (BRETHINE)

Action: Selectively activates Beta$_2$-adrenergic receptors (Beta$_2$-adrenergic agonist), resulting in uterine smooth muscle relaxation.

Indications: To delay preterm labor.

Warnings: Greater than 34 weeks gestation, acute fetal distress, severe pregnancy-induced hypertension or eclampsia, vaginal bleeding, cervical dilation greater than 6 cm.

Undesirable Effects: Tachycardia, palpitations, chest pain; tremors, anxiety, headache.

Other Specific Information: Use of adrenergic agonists can cause additive effects when taken with terbutaline. The effect of terbutaline can be decreased if used with beta blockers.

Interventions: Administered IV or SC due to the high first pass effect with oral administration. Assess injection site for infection if administered subcutaneously. Assess FHR, uterine contractions, maternal BP, HR, RR, breath sounds, and daily weights. If client is presenting with chest pain, maternal heart rate greater than 120/min, or presence of cardiac arrhythmias, hold med and notify provider of care. Fluid intake should be limited to 1,500 to 2,400 mL/24 hr. If contractions persist or increase in duration or frequency, provider of care should be notified. Assess for undesirable effects and intervene if appropriate.

Education: Instruct client to report any chest pain or a feeling of a racing heart. Review undesirable effects with client and advise to report if experiences any of them.

Evaluation: Contractions subsides and preterm labor discontinues.

Drug: terbutaline sulfate (Brethine)

TERBUTALINE SULFATE (BRETHINE)

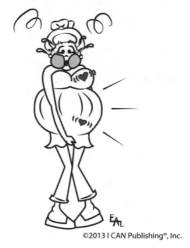

©2013 I CAN Publishing®, Inc.

B locks preterm labor contractions

R elaxes uterine smooth muscle

E valuate client's vitals, contractions and FHR

A mount of fluid intake should be limited to 1,500-2,400 mL / 24hrs

T achycardia, palpitations, chest pain, tremors, anxiety and headaches are undesirable side effects

H old medication and call provider of care if client has HR >120, cardiac arrhythmias or chest pain

RhoGAM

Action: Prevent production of anti-Rh (D) antibodies in Rh (D) negative clients who were exposed to Rh (D) positive blood. Prevention of antibody response and hemolytic disease of the newborn (erythroblastosis fetalis) in future pregnancies of women who have conceived a Rh (D) positive fetus. Prevention of Rh (D) sensitization following transfusion accident.

Indications: (IM, IV) Rh (D) negative clients who have been exposed to Rh (D) positive blood by pregnancy or delivery of a Rh (D) positive infant, abortion of Rh (D)positive fetus, fetal-maternal hemorrhage due to amniocentesis, or transfusion of Rh (D) positive blood or blood products to a Rh (D) negative client. (IV) Management of immune thrombocytopenic purpura (ITP).

Warnings: Prior hypersensitivity reaction to human immune globulin. Use cautiously in ITP clients with pre-existing anemia (decrease dose if Hgb < 10 g/dL). May also result in disseminated intravascular coagulation in ITP clients.

Undesirable Effects: Hypertension, hypotension, dizziness, headache, anemia, vomiting, diarrhea, anemia, arthralgia, pain at injection site.

Other Specific Information: May decrease antibody response to some live-virus vaccines (measles, mumps, rubella).

Interventions: For clients who have delivered a baby: type and cross-match of mother and newborn's cord blood must be performed to determine the need for medication. This should not be given to an infant, an Rh (D) positive individual, or to an Rh negative individual previously sensitized to the Rh (D) antigen. The IM injection must be given into the deltoid muscle. Dose should be given within 3 hours, but may be given up to 72 hours after an abortion, delivery, miscarriage, or transfusion. When using prefilled syringes, allow solution to reach room temperature before administering. Assess vital signs periodically during therapy if administered IV. For ITP, monitor client for signs and symptoms of intravascular hemolysis (IVH) (back pain, shaking chills, fever, hemoglobinuria), anemia, and renal insufficiency.

Education: Explain to the client that the purpose of the medication is to protect future Rh (D) positive infants which the client may have in the future. If administration is for ITP, explain the purpose of the drug to the client.

Evaluation: Future Rh (D)positive infants will not experience complications from erythroblastosis fetalis. Prevention of Rh (D) sensitization following incompatible transfusion. Decreased bleeding episodes in clients with ITP.

Drug: Rho (D) immune globulin (RhoGAM)

RHOGAM

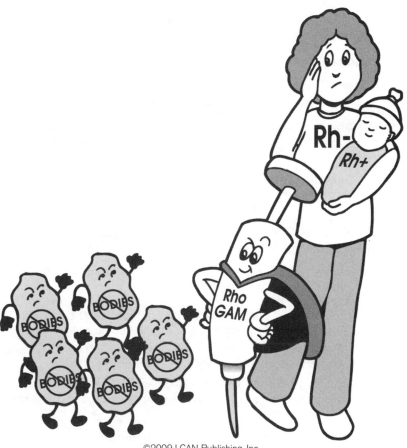

©2009 I CAN Publishing, Inc.

Rh (D) negative clients should receive RhoGam up to 72 hours after being exposed to Rh (D) positive blood after abortion, delivery, miscarriage or transfusion to prevent the production of anti-Rh (D) antibodies.

BIOPHOSPHONATES

Action: Inhibits normal and abnormal bone resorption, without reducing mineralization.

Indications: Osteoporosis, Paget's disease.

Warnings: Hypersensitivity; renal dysfunction; concurrent use of hormone replacement. Gastrointestinal diseases; pregnancy/lactation.

Undesirable Effects: Headache; abdominal pain (most frequent): nausea, abdominal distention, constipation/diarrhea, flatulence, heartburn; muscle pain. Overdosage may result in GI disturbances.

Other Specific Information: Food, beverages, and dietary supplements may interfere with absorption. IV ranitidine may ↑ level.

Interventions: Baseline and periodical bone density studies and calcium levels. Monitor electrolytes. Calcium and vitamin D deficiency must be corrected prior to therapy.

Education: Instruct regarding the importance of taking with 6–8 oz of water, first thing in the morning and at least 30 minutes prior to first beverage, food, or medication of the day. Do not lie down for at least 30 minutes after taking medication to reduce risk of esophageal irritation. Advise client to participate in supportive lifestyle changes, such as stopping smoking, no alcohol, regular weight-bearing exercises. Discontinue and notify provider if chest pain occurs.

Evaluation: The client will reflect a decrease in the progression of osteoporosis as evidenced by the bone density studies and calcium levels.

Drug: alendronate (Fosamax), risedronate (Actonel)

JOSEPHINE BONE-A-PART

B one mass rebuilds

O nly take with full glass of water, no food

N ausea—never lie down after taking

E sophageal irritation

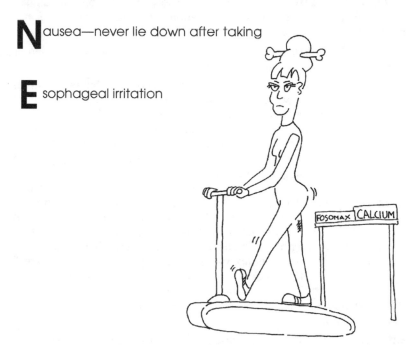

RECLAST

Action: Inhibits bone resorption. Inhibits increased osteoclast activity and skeletal calcium release induced by tumors.

Indications: Hypercalcemia of malignancy. Multiple myeloma and metastatic bone lesions from solid tumors. Paget's disease.

Warnings: Hypersensitive to zoledronic acid or other biphosphonates. Use cautiously in renal impairment. History of aspirin-induced asthma. Concurrent use of loop diuretics or dehydration. Concurrent dental surgery (may increase risk of jaw osteonecrosis).

Undesirable Effects: Agitation, anxiety, confusion, insomnia, hypotension, abdominal pain, constipation, diarrhea, nausea, vomiting, hypophosphatemia, skeletal pain, fever.

Other Specific Information: Concurrent use of aminoglycosides or loop diuretics may increase risk of hypocalcemia.

Interventions: Monitor I & 0. Hydrate vigorously. Maintain a urine output of 2 L per day during therapy. Do not over hydrate, but client must be hydrated very well. Observe for symptoms of hypercalcemia (nausea, vomiting, anorexia, weakness, constipation, thirst, cardiac arrhythmias). Observe for hypocalcemia (paresthesia, muscle twitching, laryngospasm, Chvostek's or Trousseau's sign). Assess for acute-phase reaction (fever, myalgia, flu-like symptoms, headache, arthralgia). Usually occur within 3 days of dose and resolve within 3 days of onset. It may take 7-14 days to resolve. Repeat dosing will decrease this incidence. Monitor serum creatinine prior to each treatment. Assess serum calcium, phosphate, and magnesium before and periodically during therapy. If hypocalcemia, hypophosphatemia, or hypomagnesemia occur, temporary supplementation may be required. Monitor CBC with differential and hemoglobin and hematocrit closely during therapy. Administration of acetaminophen or ibuprofen following administration may reduce the incidence of acute-phase reaction symptoms.

Education: Explain the purpose of the medication. Explain the importance of adequate hydration. Client should be instructed to drink at least 2 glasses of water prior to starting the medication. Advise to consult with provider prior to taking any prescription med, OTC, or herbal products with zoledronic acid. Recommend no dental surgery due to prolonged recovery. Reinforce the importance of monitoring lab tests to evaluate progress.

Evaluation: Decrease in calcium. Decrease in serum alkaline phosphatase.

Drugs: zoledronic acid (Reclast, Zometa)

RECLAST

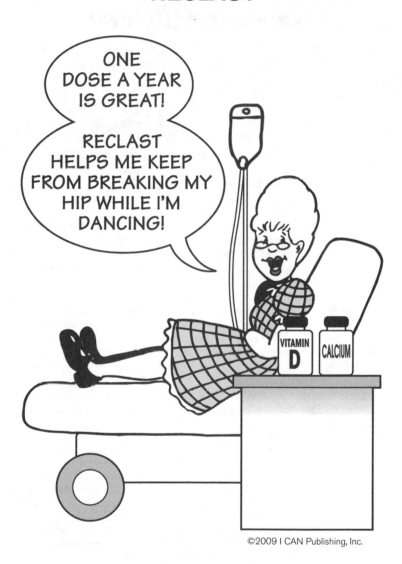

Bone Resorption Inhibitor
Ibandronate (Boniva)

Action: Inhibits resorption of bone by inhibiting osteoclast activity.

Indications: Postmenopausal osteoporosis treatment and/or prevention.

Warnings: Hypersensitivity; Uncorrected hypocalcemia; inability to stand/sit upright for at least 60 minutes; CCr < 30 ml / min. Use cautiously in geriatric clients; consider age-related decreases in body mass, renal and hepatic function, concurrent disease states and drug therapy. Concurrent use of aspirin or NSAIDS.

Undesirable Effects: Diarrhea, dyspepsia, esophagitis, gastric/ esophageal ulcer. Injection site reactions, pain in arms and/or legs.

Other Specific Information: Calcium, aluminum, magnesium, and iron-containing products, including antacids decrease absorption. To prevent this, ibandronate should be taken one hour before. There is an increase risk of gastric irritation if take concurrently with NSAIDS including aspirin. Milk and other foods may decrease the absorption. Mineral water, orange juice, coffee, and other beverages decrease absorption.

Interventions: Assess for low bone mass before and periodically during therapy. Assess serum calcium before and periodically during therapy. Hypocalcemia and vitamin D deficiency should be treated prior to initiating ibandronate therapy. May cause decrease total alkaline phosphatase levels. May cause hypercholesterolemia. Administer first thing in the AM with 6-8 oz. plain water 30 min. before other medications, beverages, or food. Once-a-month tablet should be administered on the same date each month. IV administration should not be administered if discolored or contains particulate matter. Do not administer with calcium-containing solutions or other IV drugs.

Education: Review the importance of eating a balanced diet and consult healthcare provider about the need for supplemental calcium and vitamin D. Wait at least 60 minutes after administration before taking supplemental calcium and vitamin D. Review the importance of participating in regular exercise and to modify behaviors that increase the risk of osteoporosis (e.g., stop smoking, reduce alcohol consumption). Notify healthcare provider if pregnancy is planned or suspected or if client is breastfeeding. Review the importance of taking as directed, first thing in the AM, 60 minutes prior to other medications, beverages, or food. Ibandronate should be taken with 6-8 oz. plain water (mineral water, orange juice, coffee, and other beverages decrease absorption). Do not chew or suck on tablet. Do not double up on dose if client forgets to take med. Caution client to remain upright for 60 min. following dose to facilitate passage to stomach and minimize risk of esophageal irritation.

Evaluation: Client will either decrease the progression of osteoporosis or prevent osteoporosis from occurring in postmenopausal women.

Drugs: ibandronate (Boniva)

BONIVA

B alanced Diet

A dminister 1st in AM (wait 1 hr. before
anything else)

L essen alcohol and stop smoking
(kick the habit!)

A fter menopause (assess serum Ca+)

N othing but water with med

C aution! Remain upright x 1 hr.
(balance Boniva!)

E xercise regularly

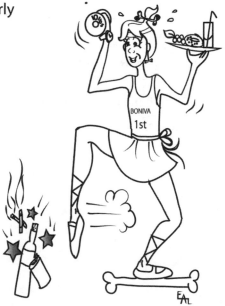

SELECTIVE ESTROGENT RECEPTOR MODULATOR (SERM)

Action: Has estrogen like effect on bone and lipid metabolism. Reduces resorption of bone and decreases overall bone turnover. Does not turn on breast or uterine receptors, (decreased risk of endometrial cancer).

Indications: Prevention of osteoporosis in postmenopausal women.

Warning: Pregnancy, blood clots.

Undesirable Effects: Hot flashes, leg cramps, infection. Rare: blood clots in the veins.

Other Specific Information: No increased risk of breast cancer and may be used in women with breast cancer.

Interventions: Discontinue 72 hours before and during prolonged immobilization; resume when fully ambulatory.

Education: Advise that medication may increase the risk of blood clots especially if there is a past history of clots in the legs, lungs, or eyes. May be taken with or without food at any time of the day. Avoid use with estrogen. Recommend that client also take a calcium supplement, vitamin D, stop smoking, and decrease alcohol intake.

Evaluation: Client's bone density studies will improve.

Drug: raloxifene (Evista)

SERM

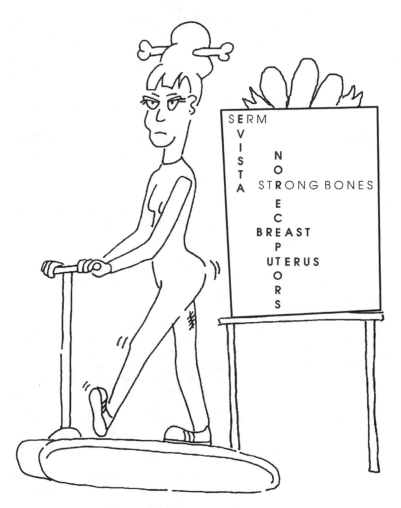

©2001 I CAN Publishing, Inc.

"SERM" is a gift to Josephine whose bones are coming "apart". **Selective Estrogen Receptor Modulators** are used to prevent osteoporosis in postmenopausal women. These drugs do not turn on breast or uterine receptors. The benefit "gift" is there is no increased risk of breast or endometrial cancer.

ESTROGEN

Action: Development and maintenance for adequate functioning of female reproductive system; affects release of pituitary gonadotropins; promotes adequate use in bone structures.

Indications: Moderate to severe vasomotor symptoms associated with menopause; postpartal breast engorgement, hormonal replacement therapy; prevention of osteoporosis and cardiovascular disease.

Warnings: Breast or reproductive cancer; estrogen dependent neoplasm; undiagnosed abnormal genital bleeding; thromboembolic disorders.

Undesirable Effects: Nausea, vomiting; headaches; breast tenderness; fluid retention, hypertension; leg cramps; break through bleeding; photosensitivity. Breast cancer, endometrial cancer. Gall bladder disease; mental depression; breast tenderness; change in libido; changes in vaginal bleeding pattern and alteration in bleeding and flow.

Other Specific Information: May ↓ effects of anticoagulant, oral hypoglycemic. ↓ effects with anticonvulsants, barbiturates, rifampin. Antibiotics ↓ the effects of estrogen. Toxicity with tricyclic antidepressants. ↑ effects of corticosteroids.

Interventions: Monitor blood pressure, weight, and serum glucose if client is a diabetic. Hepatic function studies should be done every 6 to 12 months for clients with hepatic dysfunction. Use lowest effective dose.

Education: Counsel client of childbearing age to use effective contraceptive method. Estrogens may cause congenital defects. Withdrawal bleeding may occur. Advise client to report severe headache, abdominal pain or mass, vomiting, breast lumps, dizziness, fainting, shortness of breath, blurred vision, or break through bleeding. Teach client self breast examination. Explain cyclic manner in which drug is usually administered. Instruct how to use the ordered form: oral, intravaginal, transdermal. Provide with package insert for drug to inform client how to safely use the med and specific warning signs to report. Warn against cigarette smoking and sun tanning. Instruct to report positive urine or blood sugar tests. If taking conjugated or esterified estrogens for osteoporosis prophylaxis, advise to increase the intake of calcium and vitamin D and to participate in regular weight-bearing exercises. Inform client regarding the importance of annual PAP smears, mammograms, and cholesterol series.

Evaluation: Client will demonstrate an improvement in the condition for which the medication was given without any undesirable effects.

Drugs: Esterified estrogens: (Estratab, Estratest, Menest); estradiol (Climara, Estrace, Estrace Vaginal Cream, Estraderm, Vivelle); estradiol cypionate (depGynogen, Depo-Estradiol, Dura-Estrin, E-Cypionate, Estro-Cyp, Estrofem, Estroject-LA); estradiol valerate (Delestrogen, Dioval 40, Dioval XX, Duragen-20, Duragen-40, Estra-L 40, Feminate, Femogex, Gynogen L.A., Menaval, Valergen-10, Valergen-20, Valergen-40); **Conjugated estrogens:** (Premarin, Premarin Intravenous, Premphase, Prempro)

"ESTER" ESTROGEN

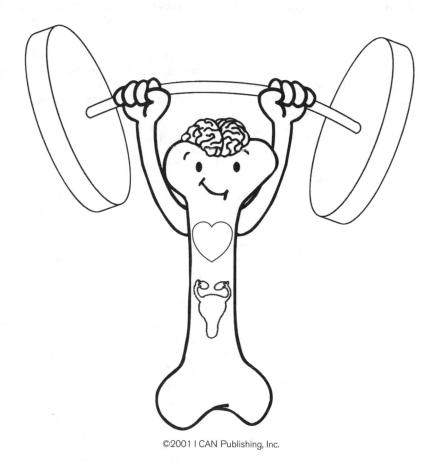

"Ester" Estrogen builds strength in bones (reducing bone loss) and protects the heart from cardiac disease. Estrogen also has been linked to the prevention of Alzheimer's. Estrogen helps maintain the functioning of the female reproductive system.

PROGESTERONES

Action: Progesterones induce favorable conditions for fetal growth and development and maintain pregnancy. Menstruation results from a decline in the progesterone levels.

Indications: Counters adverse effects of estrogen in hormone replacement therapy for treatment of: amenorrhea related to hormonal imbalance, dysfunctional uterine bleeding related to hormonal imbalance, endometriosis. Use with caution in clients with diabetes, migraine headaches, and seizure disorder.

Warnings: Contraindicated in Pregnancy; Undiagnosed vaginal bleeding; History of cardiovascular, cerebrovascular, or thromboembolic disease. History of breast cancer. History of smoking.

Undesirable Effects: Breast cancer; breakthrough bleeding, amenorrhea, breast tenderness; jaundice; edema; migraine headaches. Thromboembolic events (MI, pulmonary embolism, thrombophlebitis, cerebrovascular accident).

Other Specific Information: Decreases effectiveness of bromocriptine when used concurrently for galactorrhea / amenorrhea. Carbamazepine (Tegretol), phenobarbital, phenytoin (Dilantin), or rifampin may decrease contraceptive effectiveness. Smoking may increase risk for the development of thrombophlebitis.

Interventions: Assess for pain, swelling, warmth, or erythema of lower legs. Notify provider of chest pain or shortness of breath. Monitor the BP, I&O, and weight gain. Monitor for signs of jaundice such as yellowing of the sclera of the eyes and skin. Monitor liver enzymes. Notify provider of care for a severe headache.

Education: Encourage regular self-breast examinations, mammograms, and Pap smears. Discourage smoking. Review the importance to report any vaginal bleeding that is abnormal. Review the importance of using additional contraceptive measures with concurrent use of these meds. (Tegretol, Dilantin, Rifampin). Do not use bromocriptine (Parlodel) with progesterone. Discuss importance of reporting any undesirable effects to provider of care.

Evaluation: Client will experience regular menstrual periods and a decrease in endometrial hyperplasia in post-menopausal women receiving concurrent estrogen.

Drugs: medroxyprogesterone acetate (Provera), megestrol acetate (Megace), norethindrone (Micronor)

PROGESTERONES

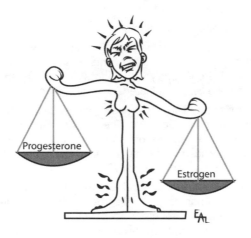

H ormone regulation - Balance of
estrogen and progesterone

O ccurence of breast cancer is an
undesirable effect

R isk of jaundice

M igraine headache is an undesirable
effect

O nset of lactation is an undesirable
effect

N otify provider of signs of a thrombolytic
event

E dema

HORMONAL CONTRACEPTIVES

Action: Oral contraceptives prevent conception by preventing ovulation. They also thicken the cervical mucus and change the endometrial lining to decrease the chance of fertilization.

Indications: Pregnancy prevention.

Warnings: Pregnancy. Contraindicated for clients who have history of thrombophlebitis and cardiovascular events. Risk factors or family history of breast cancer. Use cautiously with clients who are > 35 years of age, smoke, and who have hypercholesterolemia and diabetes mellitus.

Undesirable Effects: *Minor:* Breast tenderness, nausea, bloating, edema, and weight gain. *Serious:* The **4 B's**: **B**reast cancer, **B**lood pressure (high), **B**reakthrough or abnormal uterine bleeding, **B**lood clots: Thromboembolic events such as pulmonary embolism, MI, thrombophlebitis and cerebrovascular accident.

Other Specific Information: Oral contraceptives are less effective when taken with carbamazepine (Tegretol), phenobarbital, phenytoin (Dilantin), and rifampin. Oral contraceptives decrease the effects of warfarin (Coumadin) and oral hypoglycemics.

Interventions: Refer to **"PREVENT"** on next page.

Education: Teach about administration. Take pills at the same time each day. Instruct to take for 21 days followed by 7 days of no medication (or inert pill). Start the sequence on the fifth day after the onset of the menses. For one missed dose, teach clients to take 2 together at the next scheduled dose. For two missed doses, educate client to double up for 2 days. For three missed doses, due to the risk of ovulation and resulting pregnancy, advise client to use an additional form of birth control and to begin a new cycle of medications after waiting 7 days. Encourage an annual pelvic exam and Pap smear. Discourage smoking. Advise client to report warmth, edema, tenderness, and/or pain in lower extremities. Monitor the blood pressure and intervene if necessary to maintain normal blood pressure. Discuss the importance of recording duration and time frame of breakthrough bleeding. Evaluate the possibility of pregnancy if two or more menstrual cycles are missed. Oral contraceptives may increase growth of a pre-existing breast cancer. Do not give to women with breast cancer.

Evaluation: Client will present with no evidence of pregnancy.

Drugs: Combination oral: Ethinyl estradiol and norethindrone (Ovcon 35, Necon 1/35); Transdermal patch: Ethinyl estradiol and norelgestromin (Ortho Evra); Vaginal contraceptive ring: Ethinyl estradiol and etonogestrel (NuvaRing); and Parenteral: depot medroxyprogesterone acetate (DMPA) available as Depo-Provera for IM use and Depo-subQ for subcutaneous use.

ORAL CONTRACEPTIVES
(THE 4 BAD B'S)

P ressure (blood) needs to be monitored and
maintained in normal range

R eport swelling or redness in legs, shortness of
breath or severe headaches

E ncourage clients to quit smoking

V erify if pregnant prior to starting and if misses
2 or more menstrual periods

E ncourage client to record duration and frequency of breakthrough bleeding and notify
provider

N o oral contraceptives due to an increase
growth of a pre-existing breast cancer

T each about administration. Take pills at the same
time each day (Refer to: "Educate" on left page)

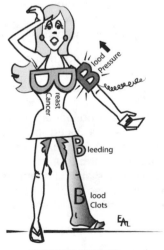

CLOMIPHENE (CLOMID)

Action: Ovulatory stimulant. Clomid stimulates the release of hormones necessary for ovulation to occur.

Indications: Female infertility. Also sometimes used to treat male infertility, menstrual abnormalities, fibrocystic breasts, and persistent breast milk production.

Warnings: Hypersensitivity. Long-term use of clomiphene may increase the risk of ovarian cancer. Clomiphene should not be used for more than about six cycles. Liver disease, ovarian cysts (except those from polycystic ovary syndrome), uterine fibroids, abnormal vaginal bleeding, a pituitary tumor, or thyroid or adrenal disease. Lactation; pregnant.

Undesirable Effects: Blurred vision; multiple pregnancies; flushing (feeling of warmth), upset stomach, vomiting, breast discomfort, headache, abnormal vaginal bleeding. These are uncommon, but if occur, provider of care must be notified: blurred vision, visual spots or flashes, diplopia, stomach or lower stomach pain, stomach swelling, weight gain, shortness of breath. Long-term use may increase risk of ovarian cancer.

Other Specific Information: No known drug interactions. Advise client to refer to provider of care prior to taking any additional meds.

Interventions: Assess for undesirable effects. Use Clomid exactly as directed by provider. Take each dose with a full glass of water. Clomid is usually taken in 5 day cycles and typically no more than 6 cycles.

Education: Clomiphene should not be used for more than 6 cycles. Keep this medication in the container it came in, tightly closed, and out of reach of children. Store it at room temperature and away from excess heat and moisture (not in the bathroom). Throw away any medication that is outdated or no longer needed. Advise to keep a list of any medication that client is taking for provider of care to review. Do not allow anyone else to take the medication. Use caution when driving, operating machinery, or performing other hazardous activities. Notify provider of care immediately if client develops any visual side effects and recommend to use caution when performing hazardous activities, especially under conditions of variable lighting.

Evaluation: Client will become pregnant.

Drug: clomiphene (Clomid)

CLOMID

Watch for "BAD" undesirable effects!

B lurred vision, bleeding
A bdominal discomfort, abdominal swelling
D yspnea, diplopia

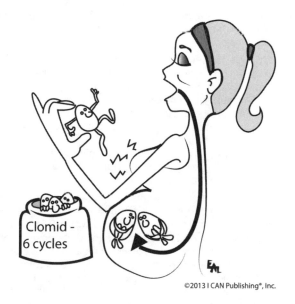

Clomid - 6 cycles

©2013 I CAN Publishing®, Inc.

Clomid is used to induce egg production in women who do not produce eggs. Clomid shouldn't be used for more than 6 cycles. Clomid can increase the likelihood of becoming pregnant with multiples. Breast discomfort is an undesirable side effect.

MIACALCIN

Action: Inhibits osteoclastic bone resorption and promotes renal excretion of calcium.

Indications: (IM, Subcut)—Treatment of Paget's disease of bone. Adjunctive therapy for hypercalcemia. (IM, Subcut, Intranasal)—Management of postmenopausal osteoporosis.

Warnings: Hypersensitivity to calcitonin, salmon protein, or gelatin diluents (in some products).

Undesirable Effects: Nasal only—headaches, rhinitis, epistaxis, arthralgia, back pain. IM, subcut—nausea, vomiting, injection site reactions. Facial flushing.

Other Specific Information: Previous bisphosphonate therapy, including alendronate, risedronate, etidronate, ibandronate, or pamidronate, may decrease response to calcitonin.

Interventions: Observe for signs of hypersensitivity (skin rash, fever, hives, anaphylaxis, serum sickness). Keep epinephrine, antihistamines, and oxygen nearby in the event a reaction occurs. Assess for signs of hypocalcemic tetany (nervousness, irritability, paresthesia, muscle twitching, tetanic spasms, seizures) during the first several doses of calcitonin. Have calcium gluconate available in case of complication from parenteral calcium. If taking intranasal, assess nasal mucosa, septum, turbinates and mucosal blood vessels periodically during therapy. DC drug if ulceration occurs. Monitor serum calcium and alkaline phosphatase periodically during therapy. Prior to therapy, perform a skin test if anticipate a sensitivity to calcitonin.

Education: Instruct that injection and unopened nasal spray bottle be stored in refrigerator. Nasal spray bottle in use can be stored at room temperature. Advise to take as directed. If miss and remembers within 2 hours of correct time, then take the missed dose. If scheduled for daily dose, take only if remembered that day. Do not double dose. Review the importance of reporting signs of hypercalcemia relapse (deep bone or flank pain, renal calculi, anorexia, nausea, vomiting, thirst, lethargy) or allergic response promptly. Reassure that client understands that flushing and warmth following the injection are transient and usually last about 1 hour. Recommend client to follow low-calcium diet if recommended by provider. Women with postmenopausal osteoporosis should adhere to a diet high in calcium and vitamin D. Intranasal: Demonstrate how to administer. Before first use activate pump by holding upright and depressing white side arms down toward bottle 5 times until a full spray is emitted. Following activation, place nozzle firmly in nostril with head in an upright position and depress the pump toward the bottle. The pump should NOT be primed before each daily use. Discard 30 days after first use. Review how exercise has been found to arrest and reverse bone loss.

Evaluation: Decrease in bone pain. Lowered serum calcium levels. Slowed progression of postmenopausal osteoporosis.

Drugs: calcitonin (Fortical, Miacalcin)

MIACALCIN

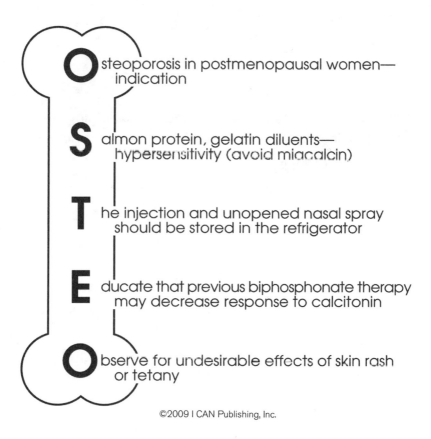

O steoporosis in postmenopausal women—indication

S almon protein, gelatin diluents—hypersensitivity (avoid miacalcin)

T he injection and unopened nasal spray should be stored in the refrigerator

E ducate that previous biphosphonate therapy may decrease response to calcitonin

O bserve for undesirable effects of skin rash or tetany

©2009 I CAN Publishing, Inc.

Miacalcin will slow progression of postmenopausal osteoperosis.

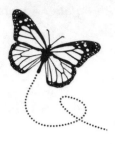

What is most beautiful in virile men is something feminine. What is most beautiful in feminine women is something masculine.

SUSAN SONTAG

Men's Health-Related Agents

FLOMAX

Action: Decreases contractions in smooth muscle of the prostatic capsule by binding to alpha 1-adrenergic receptors. Decreased symptoms of prostatic hyperplasia (urinary urgency, hesitancy, nocturia). Relaxes muscle in the prostate and bladder neck making it easier to urinate.

Indications: Management of outflow obstruction in male clients with prostatic hyperplasia.

Warnings: Clients at risk for prostate carcinoma (symptoms may be similar).

Undesirable Effects: Dizziness, headache, impaired thinking or reactions, orthostatic hypotension, insomnia.

Other Specific Information: Cimetidine may elevate blood levels resulting in toxicity. When taken with other peripherally acting anti-adrenergics (doxazosin, prazosin, terazosin), there is an increased risk for hypotenion.

Interventions: Assess for symptoms of prostatic hyperplasia (urinary hesitancy, feeling of incomplete bladder emptying, interruption of urinary stream) prior to and during therapy. Assess for first dose orthostatic hypotension and syncope. Monitor I & O, daily weight, and edema. Report weight gain or edema. **Do not confuse Flomax (tamsulosin) with Fosamax (alendronate).** Administer the daily dose 30 min. after the same meal daily.

Education: Review the appropriate way to take the medication. Review safety precautions in case client does present with dizziness. Change position slowly to minimize orthostatic hypotension. Notify provider of care before taking any cough, cold, or allergy medications. Inform client that flomax may cause the undesirable effects that may impair thinking or reactions, drive with care. Avoid drinking alcohol as it may increase dizziness. Take with a full glass of water and swallow whole.

Evaluation: Client will experience a decrease in urinary symptoms of benign prostatic hyperplasia.

Drugs: tamsulosin (Flomax)

FLOMAX

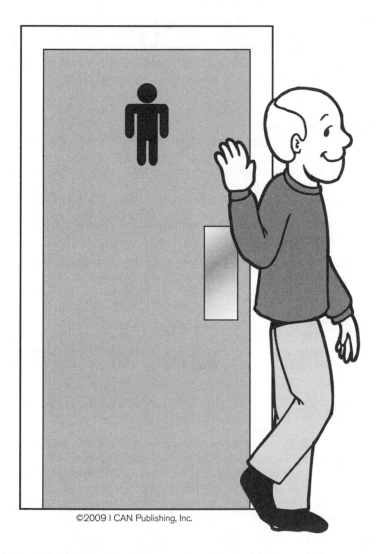

Using Flo"max" makes it so much easier for MAX to urinate, so that he has time to do other things.

VIAGRA

Action: Enchances effects of nitric oxide released during sexual stimulation. Nitric oxide activates guanylate cyclase, which produces increased levels of cyclic guanosine monophosphate (cGMP). cGMP produces smooth muscle relaxation of the corpus cavernosum, which promotes increased blood flow and subsequent ererction.

Indications: Erectile dysfunction

Warnings: Cardiac risk, renal or hepatic impairment. Use in caution with clients that have any anatomical deformation of the penis or clients that have sickle cell anemia, leukemia, or multiple myeloma. Use with caution in clients who have serious underlying cardiovascular disease including a history of MI, stroke, or serious arrhythmia within 6 months, history of CHF, uncontrolled hypertension or hypotension.

Undesirable Effects: Headache, flushing of skin, dyspepsia. Sudden death, cardiovascular collapse.

Other Specific Information: Increased risk of life-threatening hypotension with nitrates in any form or the drug ritonavir; concurrent use is contraindicated because of the risk of serious and potentially fatal hypotension. Blood levels and effects, including the risk of hypotension may be increased by enzyme inhibitors such as cimetidine, erythromycin, tacrolimus ketoconazole, itraconazole and protease inhibitor antiretrovirals. Increased risk of hypotension with antihypertensives (especially alpha-blockers) or substantial alcohol. Use cautiously with glipizde.

Interventions: May be administered 30 min. to 4 hours before sexual activity. Lasts for 4 hours.

Education: Clients need to be educated to take the medication approximately 1 hour before sexual activity and not more than once per day. Seek immediate medical care if erection last longer than 4 hours. There is no indication for this drug in women. May be taken without regard to food. **Emphasize the importance of not taking with nitrates!**

Evaluation: Male erection sufficient to allow intercourse.

Drug: sildena**fil** (Viagra), tadala**fil** (Cialis), vardena**fil** (Levitra)

VICK VIAGRA

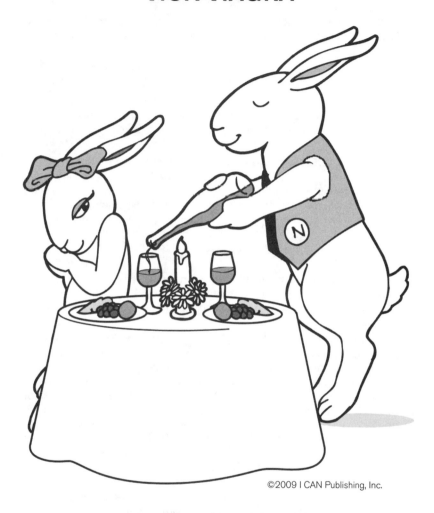

Vick Viagra is half filling the glass in preparation for a romantic evening without acute alcohol ingestion. His plate is filled with low fat food, so the drug will be more effective. High fat meals decrease the absorption. Note that all of the drugs utilized to treat erectile dysfunction, end in **fil**. Detect his **nitroglycerine patch**. This drug could cause sudden **hypotensive effects** if the user is taking nitroglycerine in any form including the nitro patch.

TESTOSTERONE

Action: Development of sex traits in men and the production and maturation of sperm. Increase in synthesis of erythropoietin. Increase in skeletal muscle.

Indications: Hypogonadism in males; delayed puberty in boys. Post menopausal breast cancer; androgen replacement in testicular failure.

Warnings: Contraindicated in pregnancy; men with prostate or breast cancer; clients who have hypercalcemia, and older adult clients. Use with caution in clients with heart failure, hypertension, cardiac, renal, or liver disease.

Undesirable Effects: Androgenic effects: women–irregularity or cessation of menses, hirsutism, weight gain, acne, lowering of voice, growth of clitoris, vaginitis, and baldness. In boys/men–acne, priapism, increased body and facial hair, and penile enlargement. Hypercholesterolema; increase in risk of prostate cancer; polycythemia; high potential for abuse. Edema from salt and water retention. Epiphyseal closure–premature closure of epiphysis in boys may decrease mature height. Cholestatic hepatitis, jaundice.

Other Specific Information: Androgens may alter effects of oral anticoagulants. Androgens may effect insulins and antidiabetic agents. Androgens taken along with hepatotoxic medications may increase result in hepatotoxicity.

Interventions: Advise clients regarding undesirable effects. Report effects. Medication may need to be discontinued to prevent permanent changes. Monitor epiphysis with serial X-rays. Assess for jaundice such as yellowing of the sclera of the eyes. Monitor liver enzymes and cholesterol levels. Advise to adjust diet to reduce cholesterol levels. Monitor for prostate cancer. Do not give if client has prostate cancer. Monitor hemoglobin and hematocrit. Identify high-risk groups for abuse problems. Inject into a large muscle and rotate sites. Monitor women for signs of masculinization (baldness, facial hair, deep voice, acne). Advise to use a barrier method of birth control. Montior PT, INR, glucose level and adjust dosages.

Education: Instruct to monitor for weight gain and swelling of the extremities and report to provider. Advise to reduce cholesterol in diet and to use a barrier method of birth control. Advise to adjust diet to reduce cholesterol levels.

Evaluation: Boys will experience puberty, and there will be evidence that testosterone will be increased in men. There will be a decrease in the progression of breast cancer. Medication will produce expected results with minimal side effects.

Drugs: Testosterone (Andronaq-50, Testred)

ANDROGENS (TESTOSTERONE)

G lucose, INR, and PT should be monitored

O ver-use/ abuse can occur

N ot to be given when the client has prostate
or breast cancer, hypercalcemia or is elderly

A cne, priaprism, increased hair and penis
growth can occur

D iet and cholesterol should be monitored

S top to prevent permanent development of
male characteristics in women

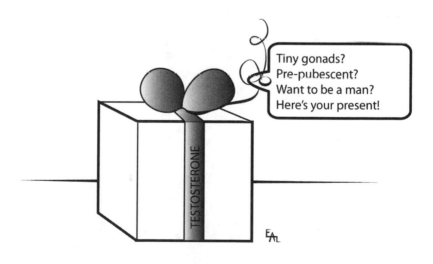

Tiny gonads?
Pre-pubescent?
Want to be a man?
Here's your present!

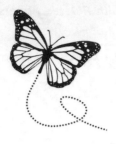

It is not work that kills a person, it is worry. Work is healthy; you can hardly put more on a person than he/she can bear. But worry is rust upon the blade. It is not movement that destroys the machinery, but friction.

HENRY WARD BEECHER

We are what we repeatedly do. Excellence, therefore, is not an act but a habit.

ARISTOTLE

Vitamins, Minerals, and Electrolytes

VITAMIN B6: PYRIDOXINE

Action: A coenzyme necessary for many metabolic functions affecting carbohydrate, lipid, and protein utilization in the body.

Indications: Pyridoxine deficiency.

Warnings: Pregnancy. IV therapy in cardiac clients.

Undesirable Effects: Rare. Occasional stinging at IM injection site.

Other Specific Information: Pyridoxine decreases effect of levodopa and can lead to serious toxic effects. Isoniazid (INH) may antagonize pyridoxine (may cause anemia/peripheral neuritis).

Interventions: Monitor for improvement of nervous system abnormalities (anxiety, depression, insomnia, peripheral numbness, and tremors) and skin lesions (glossitis, seborrhea like lesions around eyes, mouth, nose).

Education: Discomfort may occur at IM site. Foods rich in pyridoxine include avocado, bananas, bran, eggs, hazelnuts, legumes, organ meats, shrimp, tuna, wheat germ.

Evaluation: The client will maintain an appropriate intake of pyridoxine, intact mucous membranes and skin, and normal mental and neurologic status.

Drug: pyridoxine (vitamin B6)

B6

I N H (Isoniazid)
N
C
R
E
A
S
E

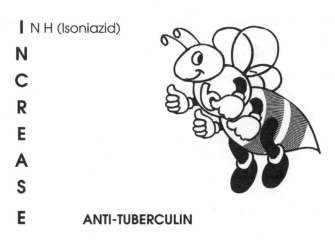

ANTI-TUBERCULIN

L evadopa
O
W
E
R

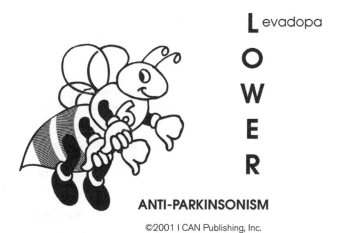

ANTI-PARKINSONISM

©2001 I CAN Publishing, Inc.

Our "B6" is telling you that, with his thumbs up, B6 should be increased when taking INH.

"B6"'s thumbs down with Levadopa. B6 should be lowered to prevent toxicity.

VITAMIN B9: FOLIC ACID

Action: Stimulates production of red and white blood cells and platelets. This is essential for nucleoprotein synthesis and the maintenance of normal erythropoiesis.

Indications: Megaloblastic, macrocytic anemia associated with pregnancy, infancy, childhood, inadequate dietary intake.

Warnings: Anemias (pernicious, aplastic, normocytic, refractory).

Undesirable Effects: Allergic hypersensitivity occurs rarely with parenteral form. Oral folic acid is nontoxic.

Other Specific Information: May decrease effects of hydantoin anticonvulsants. Analgesics, anticonvulsants, carbamazepine, estrogens may increase folic acid requirements. Antacids, cholestyramine may decrease absorption. Methotrexate, triameterene, trimethoprim may antagonize effects. May decrease vitamin B12 concentration.

Interventions: Pernicious anemia should be ruled out by Schilling test and vitamin B 12 blood level before therapy is initiated (may produce irreversible neurologic damage). Resistance to treatment may occur if decreased hematopoiesis, alcoholism, antimetabolic drugs or deficiency of vitamin B6, B12, or E is evident. Evaluate for improvement of vitamin deficiency such as: improved sense of well-being, relief from iron deficiency symptoms (fatigue, shortness of breath, sore tongue, headache, pallor).

Education: Folic acid should only be taken as prescribed. Foods high in folic acid should be encouraged such as fruits, vegetables, and organ meats. Hives or rash should be reported to provider of care immediately.

Evaluation: Client will present with a normal folic acid with no symptoms of anemia.

Drug: Folic Acid (Vitamin B9)

FOLIC ACID

F ood—bran, yeast, dried beans, nuts, fruits, fresh vegetables, asparagus

Gr **O** wth and production of erythrocytes

L iver disease, alcoholism, renal disease, pregnancy—issues

I nteraction—lowers metabolosm with anticonvulsants

C holestyramine may decrease absorption of folic acid

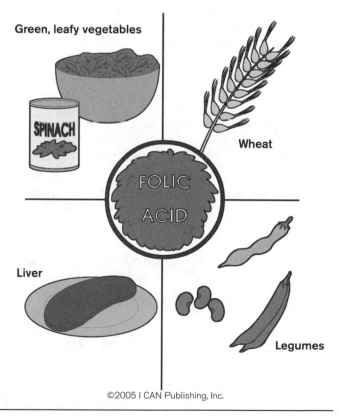

Green, leafy vegetables

SPINACH

Wheat

FOLIC ACID

Liver

Legumes

VITAMIN B12

Action: Coenzyme for metabolic functions (fat, carbohydrate metabolism, protein synthesis). Necessary for growth, cell replication, hematopoiesis, and myelin synthesis.

Indication: Prophylaxis, treatment of pernicious anemia, vitamin B12 deficiency, thyrotoxicosis, hemorrhage, and renal and/or hepatic disease.

Warnings: History of allergy to cobalamin, folate deficient anemia, hereditary optic nerve atrophy. Use cautiously if client has heart disease, history of gout, pulmonary disease, undiagnosed anemia.

Undesirable Effects: Occasional diarrhea, itching. Rare allergic reaction generally due to impurities in the preparation. May produce peripheral vascular thrombosis, hypokalemia, pulmonary edema, CHF.

Other Specific Information: Alcohol, colchicines may decrease absorption. Ascorbic acid may destroy vitamin B 12. Folic acid in large doses may decrease concentration.

Interventions: Assess for CHF, pulmonary edema, hypokalemia in clients with cardiac disease receiving SubQ/ IM therapy. Monitor potassium levels (3.5–5mEq/L), serum B 12 (200–800 mg/ml), rise in reticulocyte count (peaks in 5-8 days). Assess for reversal of deficiency symptoms: hyporeflexia, loss of positional sense, ataxia, fatigue, irritability, insomnia, anorexia, pallor, palpitation on exertion. Therapeutic response to treatment usually within 48 hours.

Education: Lifetime treatment may be imperative for clients with pernicious anemia. Instruct client to report symptoms of infection. Encourage foods rich in vitamin B 12 such as organ meats, clams, herring, oysters, red snapper, muscle meats, fermented cheese, egg yolks, and dairy products.

Evaluation: The client will be asymptomatic of clinical signs of a low vitamin B 12.

Drug: cyanocobalamin (vitamin B 12)

VITAMIN B12

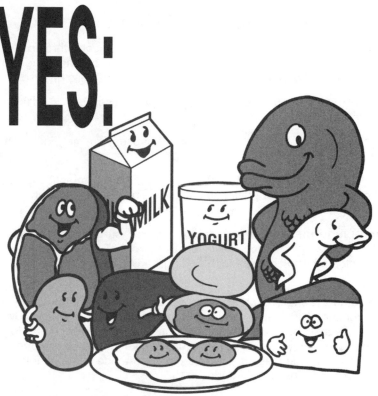

©2005 I CAN Publishing, Inc.

NO Ascorbic Acid High Doses of B 9 (Folic Acid)

Foods at the top of this image are high in vitamin B12 and should be encouraged to be eaten. Ascorbic acid and high doses of folic acid may decrease or destroy vitamin B12.

VITAMIN K (AQUAMETHYTON)

Action: Needed for adequate blood clotting factors (II, VII, IX, X)

Indications: Vitamin K malabsorption, hypoprothrombinemia, prevention of hypoprothrombinemia caused by oral anticoagulants. Prevention of newborn complications with hemorrhagic disease.

Warnings: Hypersensitivity. Severe hepatic disease. Avoid IV use if possible. Give SQ or IM.

Undesirable Effects: Headache, nausea, hemolytic anemia, hyperbilirubinemia, rash.

Other Specific Information: Decreased action of oral anticoagulants. Decreased action of phytonadione when taken with cholestyramine, mineral oil.

Interventions: Assess for bleeding: emesis, stools, urine. Assess PT during treatment (2-sec. deviation from control time, bleeding time, and clotting time); monitor for bleeding, heart rate, and blood pressure.

Education: *Review foods high in vitamin K:* liver (beef), spinach, tomatoes, coffee, asparagus, broccoli, cabbage, lettuce, greens. Recommend not to take other supplements unless directed by provider of care. Instruct to avoid IM injections, use soft tooth brush, do not floss, use electric razor until coagulation defect has been corrected. Report signs of bleeding. Discuss the importance of frequent lab test to monitor coagulation factors.

Evaluate: Client will experience a decrease in bleeding tendencies, decreased PT, and decrease in the clotting time.

Drug: phytonadione (AquaMEPHYTON)

VITAMIN K

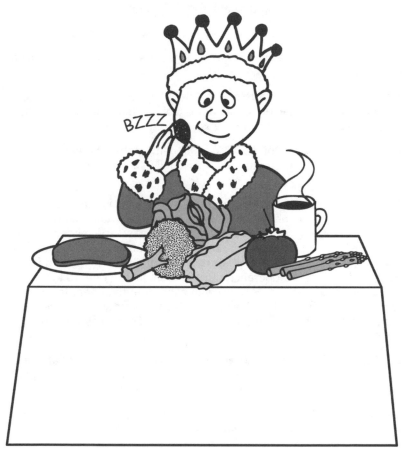

MINERAL: IRON

Action: Operates as an oxygen carrier in hemoglobin.

Indications: Prevents and treats iron deficiency anemia.

Warnings: Hemolytic anemia, peptic ulcer, ulcerative colitis.

Undesirable Effects: Nausea, vomiting, constipation, and abdominal cramps.

Other Specific Information: ↑ effect of iron with vitamin C; ↓ absorption with antacids, cimetidine. Coffee, tea, milk, eggs, whole grain breads and cereals ↓ iron absorption.

Interventions: Monitor RBC count, hemoglobin, hematocrit, iron level, and reticulocyte count. Administer IM injection by the Z-track method.

Education: Instruct to take drug between meals with at least 8 oz. of juice (vitamin C enhances absorption of iron) or water. Instruct client to take liquid iron with a straw. If GI distress is experienced, advise to take with food. Swallow whole tablet or capsule. Do not take drug within 1 hour of taking antacid or milk. Recommend increasing fluids, fiber, and exercise to decrease constipation. Instruct not to leave iron within reach of children. Review with client that treatment for anemia is generally < 6 months. Review diet high in iron such as liver, lean meats, legumes, green vegetables, and fruit. Stool may turn black or dark green.

Evaluation: The client will participate in activities with no fatigue or shortness of breath. The hemoglobin, hematocrit, reticulocyte count, and plasma iron values will remain in normal range.

Drugs: ferrous fumarate (Feostat, Ferrous fumarate); ferrous gluconate (Fergon, Ferralet); ferrous sulfate (Feosol, Fer-Iron)

IRON

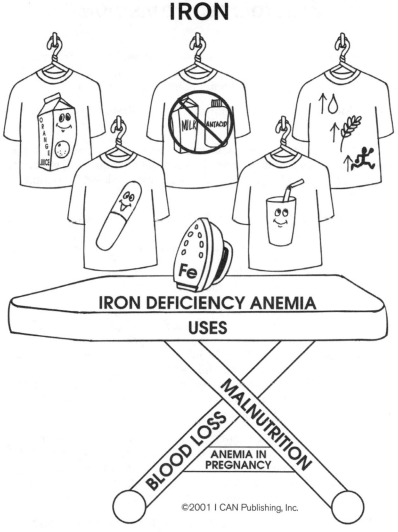

©2001 I CAN Publishing, Inc.

Iron improves iron deficiency anemia, anemia in pregnancy, malnutrition and blood loss.

When administering iron, the 5 hangers will assist you in remembering the priority teaching tips. Starting from left to right: take iron with vitamin C, swallow whole tablet or capsule (do not crush), do not take with milk or antacid, take liquid iron with a straw, and increase fluid, fiber and exercise.

ELECTOLYTE: POTASSIUM

Action: Necessary for many cellular metabolic processes; primary action is intracellular. Conducts nerve impulses; contracts cardiac, skeletal, smooth muscle. Maintains normal renal function.

Indications: Correct potassium deficiency. Strengthen cardiac and muscular activities.

Warnings: Addison's disease, cardiac/renal insufficiency, hyperkalemia, acidosis, burns, potassium-sparing diuretics, ACE inhibitors. Never push K CL. Always dilute. Solutions more diluted for peripheral vs. central line.

Undesirable Effects: Nausea, vomiting, diarrhea, abdominal discomfort, rash (rare), hyperkalemia manifested as cold skin, paresthesia of extremities, hypotension, confusion, cardiac arrhythmias.

Other Specific Information: ↑ serum potassium level with ACE inhibitors, potassium-sparing diuretics, and salt substitutes using potassium.

Interventions: Monitor serum potassium level (therapeutic 3.5–5.0 mEq/L), vital signs, ECG, and signs of hyper or hypokalemia. Assess signs of digitalis toxicity. Give IV infusions as diulte solution infuses slowly. Observe IV site for infiltration so tissue necrosis will not occur. **Potassium should never be given as an IV bolus or push.** Potassium CANNOT be given IM. Monitor urine output. 80–90% of potassium is excreted in the urine.

Education: Recommend client to have serum potassium level checked at regular intervals. Instruct to take oral preparation with at least 6–8 oz. of water or juice and at mealtime. Medical follow-up to the health related problem and medication are important. Review foods rich in potassium (i.e., bananas, canteloupes, oranges, raisins, potatoes).

Evaluation: Client's potassium level will remain in normal range.

Drugs: potassium acetate (Potassium acetate); potassium chloride (Kaochlor, K-Dur, K-Lor, Klotrix, K-Lyte/Cl, Slow-K); potassium gluconate (Kaon)

POTASSIUM

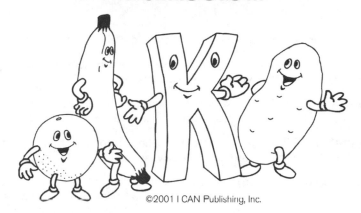

©2001 I CAN Publishing, Inc.

P otassium sparing diuretics—monitor K⁺

O utput—monitor closely

T ake with food

A ce Inhibitors—monitor K⁺

S igns of digitalis toxicity if K⁺ is ↓

S erum potassium level —3.5–5.0 mEq/L

I V potassium HIGH ALERT

U ndesirable Effects: N/V, cardiac arrhythmias

M edical follow-up

SUPPLEMENT: CALCIUM

Action: Promotes strong bones and teeth growth.

Indications: Prevents osteoporosis. Corrects calcium deficiency. Hyperacidity associated with peptic ulcer disease.

Warnings: Hypercalcemia, digitalis toxicity, renal calculi, ventricular fibrillation, renal, cardiac, or respiratory disorders.

Undesirable Effects: Nausea, vomiting, constipation; pain, headache; slowed heart rate; peripheral vasodilation.

Other Specific Information: Decreased effect of verapamil and decreased serum levels of oral tetracyclines, salicylates, and iron salts. Decreased absorption of oral calcium when taken with oxalic acid (found in rhubarb and spinach), phytic acid (bran and whole cereals), and phosphorus (milk and dairy products).

Interventions: Observe for anorexia, nausea, vomiting, and headache. Monitor serum calcium. Record consistency of stools.

Education: Instruct to take oral calcium supplements with food. Administer calcium carbonate antacid 1 and 3 hours after meals and at bedtime. Take other oral medications at least 1–2 hrs after calcium carbonate. Chew antacid tablets completely prior to swallowing; drink 1 full glass of water or milk after swallowing tablet. If taking suspension, shake and take with a small amount of water. Review foods high in calcium; protein and vitamin D are necessary to enhance calcium absorption. Avoid overuse of antacids and laxatives. For clients who are treating osteoporosis, review the importance of engaging in weight bearing exercises. Recommend that client discuss with provider of care about the pros and cons of estrogen supplement.

Evaluation: The calcium level will be within normal limits, and client will experience no signs of hypo or hypercalcemia. If being treated for osteoporosis, the bone density will be normal.

Drugs: calcium carbonate (Caltrate, Chooz, Equilet, OsCAL, Oystercal, Tums)

CALCIUM

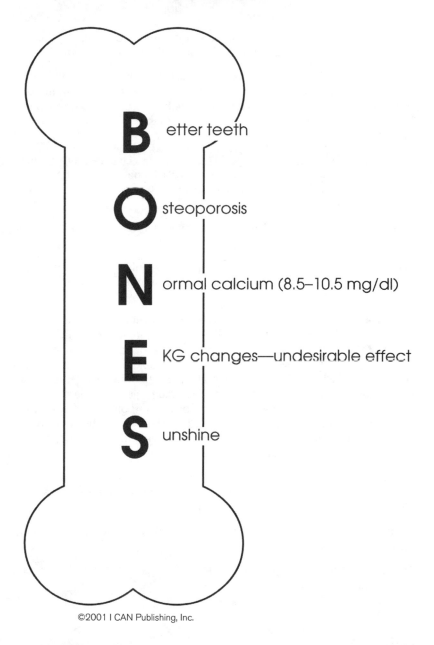

B etter teeth

O steoporosis

N ormal calcium (8.5–10.5 mg/dl)

E KG changes—undesirable effect

S unshine

©2001 I CAN Publishing, Inc.

MAGNESIUM SULFATE

Action: Activates many intracellular enzymes and plays a role in regulating skeletal muscle contractility and blood coagulation.

Indications: Hypomagnesemia: magnesium level less than 1.3 mEq/L. Oral preparations are used to prevent low magnesium levels. Parenteral magnesium is used for clients with severe hypomagnesemia. IV magnesium sulfate is used to stop preterm labor. (Refer to "Women's Health-related Agents")

Warnings: **HIGH ALERT DRUG** Pregnancy. Use cautiously with clients who have AV block, rectal bleeding, nausea/vomiting and abdominal pain. Use cautiously with clients who have renal and / or cardiac disease.

Undesirable Effects: Diarrhea; neuromuscular blockade and respiratory depression.

Other Specific Information: Magnesium sulfate may decrease the absorption of tetracyclines. Evaluate the therapeutic effect to determine if absorption has been affected.

Interventions: IV administration requires careful monitoring of the cardiac and neuromuscular status. Monitor the serum magnesium levels. Monitor for loss from the diarrhea. Monitor for dehydration by evaluating I & O. Monitor magnesium, calcium and phosphorus. Assess BP, HR, and RR when taking IV. Assess deep tendon reflexes and if absent this is a sign of toxicity. Calcium gluconate is given for toxicity. Always have an injectable form of calcium gluconate available when administering magnesium sulfate by IV. Review with client foods high in magnesium such as whole grain cereals, nuts, legumes, green leafy vegetables, bananas.

Education: Review with client foods high in magnesium such as whole grain cereals, nuts, legumes, green leafy vegetables, bananas. Review the undesirable effects with client.

Evaluation: Serum magnesium levels within expected reference range: 1.3 to 2.1 mEq/L.

Drugs: Parenteral: Magnesium sulfate, Oral: Magnesium gluconate, Magnesium hydroxide

MAGNESIUM SULFATE
(TO TREAT HYPO-MAGNESEMIA)

HIGH ALERT

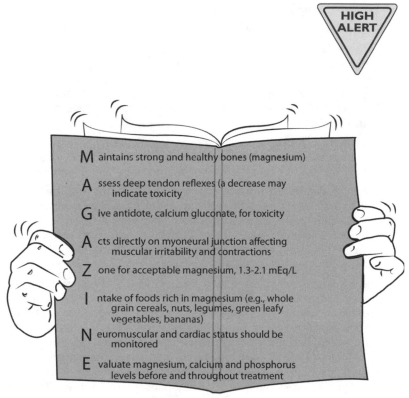

M aintains strong and healthy bones (magnesium)

A ssess deep tendon reflexes (a decrease may indicate toxicity

G ive antidote, calcium gluconate, for toxicity

A cts directly on myoneural junction affecting muscular irritability and contractions

Z one for acceptable magnesium, 1.3-2.1 mEq/L

I ntake of foods rich in magnesium (e.g., whole grain cereals, nuts, legumes, green leafy vegetables, bananas)

N euromuscular and cardiac status should be monitored

E valuate magnesium, calcium and phosphorus levels before and throughout treatment

There is something wrong with his skeletal muscle contractility. He can't even hold up his MAG azine! Time to give some magnesium sulfate!

KAYEXALATE

Action: Decreases serum potassium level by exchanging sodium ions for potassium ions in GI tract. (Each 1 g of sodium is exchanged for 1 mEq of potassium.)

Indications: Hyperkalemia

Warnings: Don't use with possible intestinal obstruction or perforation; hypernatremia; hypokalemia. Caution in severe CHF, hypertension, and edema. If severe hyperkalemia, may need faster-acting agents to reduce potassium. Not appropriate as treatment for constipation. In life-threatening hyperkalemia, more immediate interventions should be instituted.

Undesirable Effects: Hypokalemia, hypocalcemia, hypomagnesemia, hypernatremia, GI effects (nausea, vomiting, constipation, diarrhea). Especially be aware of electrolyte imbalance potential in renal failure.

Other Specific Information: Enema route is faster; oral route has greater overall effect over several hours. Don't use with laxatives or other medications that speed GI transit time (sorbitol). Hypokalemia may increase effects of digoxin. Administration with calcium or magnesium-containing antacids may decrease resin-exchanging ability and increase risk of systemic alkalosis.

Interventions: Monitor electrolyte levels before and following doses, especially potassium, sodium, calcium, magnesium. Monitor for symptoms of electrolyte imbalance, including arrhythmias on ECG. Evaluate effects of each dose, should be ordered one dose at a time or with a scheduled number of doses (not an unlimited or open-ended order)! Oral/NG doses can be mixed with water or syrup. Enema doses can be diluted in water. Never mix in citrus juice. It does not correct hyperkalemia immediately (may take hours to days). Monitor the bowel activity and stool consistency daily (fecal impaction may occur, especially in elderly clients).

Education: For those with renal failure or other chronic issue, teach about recognizing signs of electrolyte imbalances. Hold enema doses in colon as long as possible (up to several hours) to increase medication effects. Reinforce compliance with chronic care for renal failure, including diet and dialysis, to prevent repeat episodes of hyperkalemia.

Evaluation: Client's potassium level will decrease to a normal level (3.5-5.0 mEq/L) within 2-24 hours. Client will not experience adverse events due to abnormal potassium level.

Drugs: Sodium Polystyrene Sulfonate (Kayexalate)

KAYEXALATE

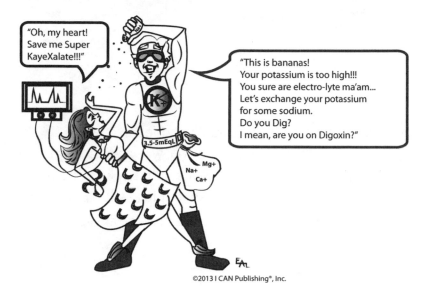

©2013 I CAN Publishing®, Inc.

K ayexalate should be ordered one dose at a time or with a scheduled number

eX changes for sodium ions in the GI tract via enema

M onitor for decreased potassium, sodium retention, constipation, fecal impaction, gastric irritation and EKG for dysrhythmias

A ssess for Digoxin toxicity if client is taking Digoxin

N ormal Potassium level is 3.5-5.0 mEq/L - expected outcome

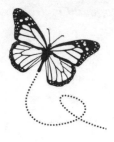

Don't waste your life in doubts and fears: spend yourself on the work before you, well assured that the right performance of this hour's duties will be the best preparation for the hours or ages that follow it.

RALPH WALDO EMERSON

Immunization Agents

PRECAUTIONS/CONTRAINDICATIONS WITH IMMUNIZATIONS

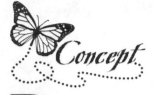

R isks that come with the immunizations (Weigh risks/data that come with vaccinating or not!).

I llnesses (with or without fever); Immunocompromised individuals.

S ubstance in any immunization that caused reactions in the past should not be used in any vaccine.

K now of a previous anaphylactic reaction to a vaccine is contraindicated for further doses of vaccine.

5 R'S FOR SAFE ADMINISTRATION

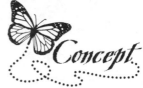

Ready for an allergic RESPONSE such as anaphylaxis by having emergency meds and equipment on standby.

Reconstitution of immunizations—Follow directions! Use within 30 minutes of being reconstituted.

Review and provide written vaccine information sheets for parents, children, and adults.

Review undesirable effects with clients/family members and when to notify provider regarding these.

Route, date, and site; type, manufacturer, lot number and expiration of vaccine; and name, address, and signature must be DOCUMENTED!

HEPATITIS A AND B VACCINES

Action: Produce antibodies that provide active immunity.

Indications: Prevent Hepatitis A and / or Hepatitis B.

Warnings: Hepatitis A–Pregnancy, acute febrile illness; Hepatitis B – Allergy to Baker's yeast

Undesirable Effects: Hepatitis A–local reactions, headache; Hepatitis B – Local soreness

Other Specific Information: Hepatitis A–Recommended for children in areas with high rates of hepatitis A and other high-risk groups. Give two doses for high-risk group. (Give two doses 6 months apart after age 12 months). Hepatitis B–Give within 12 hr after birth with additional doses at age 1 to 2 months and 6 to 18 months. Children who have not been vaccinated as infants should complete the series by 12 years of age. Give three doses for high-risk group.

Interventions: Refer to the "5 R's for Safe Administration".

Education: Review who should receive these vaccines and the undesirable effects.

Evaluation: Client will experience no problems with Hepatitis A or B.

Drugs: Hepatitis A vaccine (Havrix, Vaqta); Hepatitis B vaccine (Engerix-B, Recombivax HB)

HEPATITIS A & HEPATITIS B

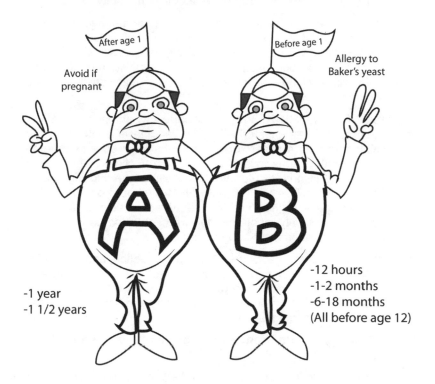

"Tweedle A and Tweedle B,

A takes 2 and B takes 3

A's after 1 and B's before 1"

INFLUENZA IMMUNIZATION

Action: Produce antibodies that provide active immunity.

Indications: Seasonal influenza vaccine is recommended one dose annually for all adults over age 50; healthcare providers including those who provide care for young children; individuals with chronic medical conditions such as asthma, cerebral palsy, and diabetes; individuals living in long-term care facilities, and individuals who are immunocompromised.

Warnings: Refer to **"RISK"** on concept page. Hypersensitivy to eggs/egg products. Live, attenuated influenza vaccine is contraindicated for administration as a nasal spray for adults over 50 and children < 2 years; immunocompromised clients, and/or clients who have a chronic disease. History of Guillain–Barre syndrome. Fluvirin should be used in children > 4 yrs old only. FluMist should be avoided in clients receiving salicylates. The live, attenuated vaccine (LAIV), given as a nasal spray, is only recommended for client who under age 50 and are not immunocompromised or pregnant.

Undesirable Effects: Inactivated: Mild local reaction, and fever; Live attenuated: Cough, fever, and headache. Rare: Risk for Guillain Barre syndrome resulting in ascending paralysis, starting with weakness of lower extremities, and progressing to difficulty breathing. Intranasal: upper respiratory congestion, malaise.

Other Specific Information: FluMist should be avoided in clients receiving salicylates.

Interventions: Do not administer FluMist concurrently with other vaccines, or in clients who have received a live virus vaccine within 1 month or an inactivated vaccine within 2 weeks of vaccine. (Refer to the **"5 R's for Safe Administration."**)

Education: Instruct client regarding undesirable effects and when to notify provider of care. Review the importance of being aware of the hypersensitivity to eggs/egg products. Review the importance of not taking FluMist with salicylates. Annually, starts age 6 months, administer trivalent inactiviated influenza vaccine (TIV). Starting at age 2 the live, attenuated influenza vaccine (LAIV) (nasal spray) may be used. October through November is the ideal time, and December is acceptable.

Evaluation: Client will not experience the flu.

Drugs: Influenza vaccine injection: (**Flu**arix, **Flu**virin, **Flu**zone); Intranasal: (**Flu**Mist)

INFLUENZA VACCINE

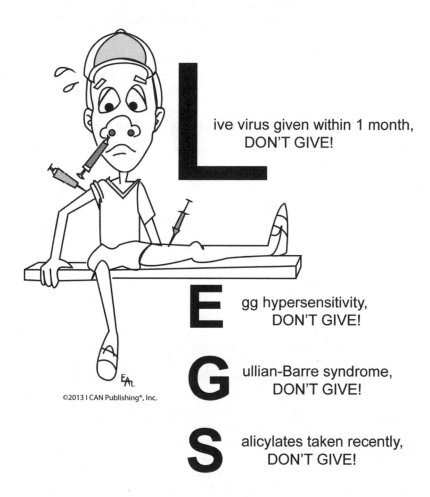

L ive virus given within 1 month, DON'T GIVE!

E gg hypersensitivity, DON'T GIVE!

G ullian-Barre syndrome, DON'T GIVE!

S alicylates taken recently, DON'T GIVE!

©2013 I CAN Publishing®, Inc.

In**FLU**enza vaccine: DO give in the nose (mist), arms and **LEGS!** DON'T give for any of the reasons above. Note that all of these immunizations have "**FLU**" in the name.

TAMIFLU

Action: Inhibits the enzyme neuramidase, which may alter virus particle aggregation and release.

Indications: Uncomplicated acute illness due to influenza infection in adults and children > 1 year of age who have had symptoms for < 2 days. Prevention of influenza in clients > 1 yr.

Warnings: Contraindicated in: Hypersensitivity; Children < 1 yr. Use cautiously in OB or lactation since safety is not established.

Undesirable Effects: Insomnia, vertigo, confusion, self-injurious behavior. Bronchitis, nausea and vomiting.

Other Specific Information: Drug-drug interactions—none significant

Interventions: Assess symptoms of influenza (sudden onset of fever, cough, headache, fatigue, muscular weakness, sore throat). Symptoms may need to be treated with additional support. Treatment should be started as soon as possible from the time of the initial sign of flu symptoms. May be administered with food or milk to decrease GI irritation. Tap closed bottle to loosen powder when preparing oral solution. Add total amount of water for constitution and shake closed bottle for 15 seconds. Remove childproof cap and push bottle adaptor into neck of bottle. Close bottle with childproof top tightly. Prior to using, shake well. Use within 10 days of constitution. If oral suspension is unavailable, capsules may be opened and mixed with sweetened liquids.

Education: Review with client and or family the importance of taking as soon as influenza symptoms appear and continue to take as prescribed. If miss a dose, take as soon as remember unless it is within 2 hours of the next dose. Do not take two doses at once. Remind client that oseltamivir should not be shared with anyone. Discuss with client that this is not a substitute for the flu shot. Clients should receive an annual flu shot based on the guidelines for immunization.

Evaluation: Client will experience a reduction of the duration of the flu symptoms.

Drugs: oseltamivir (Tami**flu**)

TAMIFLU

T ake as soon as symptoms are detected

A ssess for symptoms; (fever, cough, fatigue, headache, weakness)

M ilk and food before medication to decrease GI irritability

I mmunization should still be taken - this medication only decreases FLU symptoms; it doesn't prevent FLU!

F

L

U

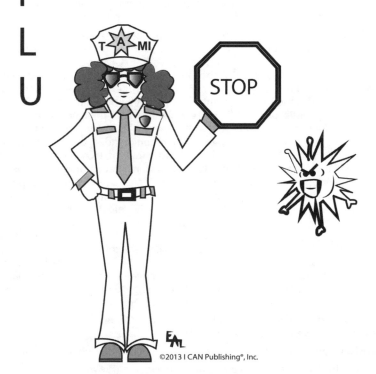

©2013 I CAN Publishing®, Inc.

PNEUMOCOCCAL VACCINE (PCV)

Action: Produce antibodies that provide active immunity.

Indications: Pneumococcal polysaccharide vaccine (PPSV)– Vaccinate adults who are immunocompromised, who have a chronic disease, who smoke cigarettes, have no spleen function (such as in sickle cell disease), who live in a long-term facility, or are at high risk of fatal infection, a second dose should be given at least five years following the first dose. CDC guidelines should be followed for revaccination. If there is no evidence of a vaccination, then one dose should be administered at age 65 years old. Pneumococcal conjugate vaccine (PCV)–Give doses at 2, 4, 6, and 12 to 15 months. Older infants and children start at 7-11 mo of age per protocol.

Warnings: Pregnancy. Hypersenstivity to all components including diphtheria toxoid; moderate to severe febrile illness; thrombocytopenia or coagulation disorder. Use cautiously in clients receiving anticoagulants; safe use in children $<$ 6 wks has not been established.

Undesirable Effects: Erythema induration, tenderness, nodule formation at injection site, fever. No serious adverse effects.

Other Specific Information: Antineoplastics, corticosteroids, radiation therapy, and immunosuppressants decrease antibody response. There are no requirements to wait between the doses of these or other inactivated vaccines.

Interventions: Shake before use, since product is a suspension. Refer to the **"5 R's for Safe Administration"** with the exception of the anaphylaxis, since no serious effects typically occur. The new AAP/CDC guidelines stipulated the use of the newest form of the pneumococcal vaccine, the heptavalent pneumococcal conjugate vaccine (PCV7) and recommended it "for use in all children 23 months of age and younger. Although other pneumococcal vaccines are available, PCV7 represents the first pneumococcal vaccine approved for use in children younger than age 2. The policy recommends that PCV7 be given concurrently with other recommended childhood vaccines at 2, 4, 6, and 12 to 15 months. The number of PCV7 doses required depends upon the age at which vaccination is initiated. The vaccine was also recommended for all children 24 to 59 months of age who are at especially high risk of invasive pneumococcal infection. This includes children with sickle cell disease, human immunodeficiency virus (HIV) infection, and other children who are immunocompromised. The pneumococcal vaccine is given as one dose for most people. The vaccine is injected as a liquid solution of 0.5 mL into the muscle (intramuscular or IM), typically deltoid muscle, or under the skin (subcutaneous or SC). The area injected is typically sterilized by rubbing alcohol onto the skin prior to the injection. If five or more years have passed since the first dose was received prior to turning 65 years old, then the client needs a dose of this vaccine at age 65.

Education: Discuss with client the protocol for taking this vaccine, and review schedule with parents for an infant.

Evaluation: Client will not experience the disease through active immunity.

Drugs: Pneumococcal 7-valent conjugate vaccine (Prevnar)

PNEUMOCOCCAL VACCINE
(PREVNAR)

"Prevnar prevents pneumococcal
So give when risk is forseen

In months 2, 4, 6, and year 65
Please get this vaccine

Prevent Pneumonia
And keep lungs clean!"

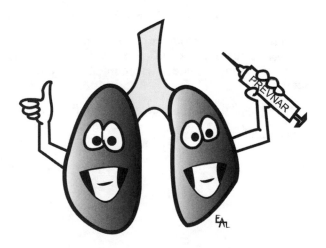

VARICELLA VACCINE

Action: Produce antibodies that provide active immunity.

Indications: Children who have not been vaccinated or have not had chickenpox. Adults who do not have evidence of previous infection.

Warnings: Pregnancy. Pregnant women should avoid being with children who were just recently vaccinated. Allergy to gelatin or neomycin; active infection; immunosuppression, including HIV or medication administered; cancer of the lymphatic system and cancer of blood.

Undesirable Effects: Local soreness, fever. Varicella-like rash, local or generalized such as vesicle on the body.

Other Specific Information: Salicylates should be avoided for 6 weeks following vaccination.

Interventions: Refer to the **"5 R's for Safe Administration"**. Assess for any allergies to gelatin or neomycin. Give one dose at 12 to 15 months and 4 to 6 years or 2 doses administered 4 weeks apart if administered after age 13. Two doses should be administered to adults who do not have evidence of previous infection. A second dose should be administered for adults who had only one previous dose.

Education: Instruct client regarding the undesirable effects and to avoid salicylates for 6 weeks following vaccination. Review the importance of not being around any pregnant woman following a **recent vaccination.**

Evaluation: Client will not experience any illness from varicella.

Drug: Varicella vaccine (Varivax)

VARICELLA
(CHICKEN POX VACCINE)

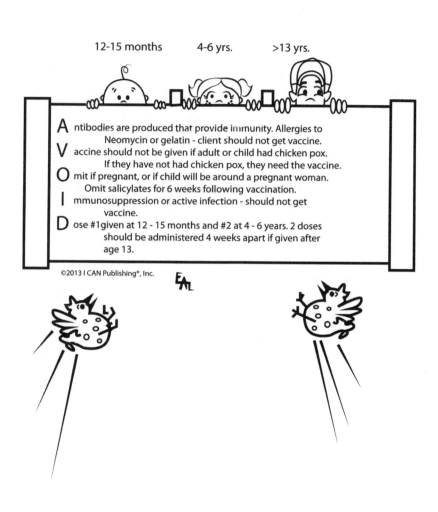

12-15 months   4-6 yrs.   >13 yrs.

A ntibodies are produced that provide immunity. Allergies to Neomycin or gelatin - client should not get vaccine.

V accine should not be given if adult or child had chicken pox. If they have not had chicken pox, they need the vaccine.

O mit if pregnant, or if child will be around a pregnant woman. Omit salicylates for 6 weeks following vaccination.

I mmunosuppression or active infection - should not get vaccine.

D ose #1 given at 12 - 15 months and #2 at 4 - 6 years. 2 doses should be administered 4 weeks apart if given after age 13.

©2013 I CAN Publishing®, Inc.

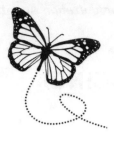

Do not go where the path may lead, go instead where there is no path and leave a trail.

RALPH WALDO EMERSON

I haven't failed. I've just found 10,000 ways that won't work.

THOMAS EDISON

Complementary Agents

NOTE: As a pharmacist, I would caution against the use of these agents. The manufacturers of these agents are not required to follow the Good Manufacturing Practice Act as pharmaceutical manufacturers are required. The integrity of these agents cannot be guaranteed. Users are at an increased risk for drug interactions if taking these agents with prescription medications. Buyer beware!

—NICOLE BLACKWELDER, PHARMD.

Editors' Note: We have included these agents because of the increasing use of complementary agents by clients. Also, complementary agents are included on the NCLEX-RN® exam.

—LORETTA AND SYLVIA

BLACK COHOSH

Action: Therapeutic effects are produced by glycosides isolated from the fresh or dried rhizome with attached roots. Exact action remains unclear.

Indications: Management of menopausal symptoms. Premenstrual discomfort. Dysmenorrhea. Mild sedative.

Warnings: Pregnancy and lactation. Use cautiously in: not studied in combination with hormonal therapies. Not studied in clients with hormone-dependent cancers (i.e., breast, endometrial, ovarian cancer); should not be used longer than 6 months use. Alcohol containing preparations should be used cautiously in clients with known intolerance or liver disease.

Undesirable Effects: Seizures when used in combination with evening primrose and chasteberry. Headache, dizziness: GI upset; Rash; weight gain, cramping.

Other Specific Information: Unknown effects when combined with hormone replacement therapy and antiestrogens (e.g., tamoxifen). If used with hepatotoxic drugs, liver damage may occur. Preparations containing alcohol may interact with disulfiram and metronidazole. May decrease the cytotoxic effects of cisplatin. May precipitate hypotension when taken with antihypertensive medications.

Interventions: Assess severity of menopausal symptoms. Evaluate BP if client is taking an antihypertensive drug due to the risk for hypotension. Assess for nausea and vomiting. Review for history of seizures, alcohol intake, and liver disease. Assess if female has irregular periods because black cohosh may induce a miscarriage. Administer with food to assist with decreasing nausea. **Do not confuse black cohosh with blue or white cohosh.**

Education: Review importance of not taking if pregnant. Discuss importance of not taking if currently on or going to start antihypertensive medication due to risk for hypotension. Recommend consulting with provider prior to taking if client has a history of seizures, liver dysfunction, excessive alcohol intake, cancer, or other medical problems. If nausea becomes a problem, take with food. Discuss the importance of not taking with other estrogen replacements without seeking support from provider of care. Review importance of continued medical management with Pap smears, mammograms, pelvic examinations, and blood pressure monitoring per protocol.

Evaluation: Client will not experience any menopausal vasomotor symptoms

Drugs: black cohosh (baneberry, black snakeroot, bugbane, phytoestrogen, rattle root, rattleweed, rattle top, squawroot)

BLACK COHOSH

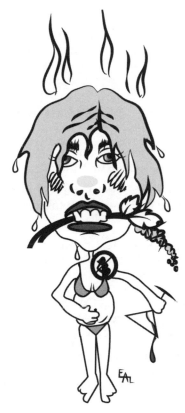

Black Cohosh Rhyme

Feeling menopausal
Stripping off my clothes
Don't take with Chasteberry
Or Evening Primrose

Black Cohosh is what I'm eating
Beware liver disease or seizing

My head hurts
And so does my tummy
I'm dizzy, cramping
And getting kinda chubby

If you're pregnant
Stay far away
No martinis or bikinis
Check my B/P today!

COENZYME Q10

Action: Co-Q10 has antioxidant and membrane-stabilizing properties. Co-Q10 is a free radical scavenger; protects cell membranes and DNA from oxidative damage. It is found in all human cells. Tissue is protected from ischemic cellular damage.

Indications: Allergies, asthma, respiratory disease; Alzheimer's, and schizophrenia. Gives energy to the heart especially in congestive heart failure.

Warnings: Hypersensitivity to Co-Q10.

Undesirable Effects: Anorexia, nausea, diarrhea, epigastric discomfort.

Other Specific Information: Oral antidiabetic agents may ↓ effectiveness of Co-Q10. Co-Q10 may ↓ response to warfarin.

Interventions: Cardiovascular assessment should be ongoing. Coenzyme Q 10 is oil soluble and is best absorbed when taken with oily or fatty foods, such as fish.

Education: Co-Q10 is perishable and deteriorates in temperatures above 115°F; a liquid form or oil form is preferable. Vitamin E helps preserve this coenzyme. Foods highest in vitamin E include mackerel, salmon and sardines; other foods include peanuts, spinach, and beef. Caution client not to perform intense exercise during Co-Q10 therapy due to potential damage of ischemic tissue. Instruct client with heart failure to inform health care provider of any clinical changes.

Evaluation: Client will have no signs of heart failure such as peripheral edema, hepatosplenomegaly, jugular vein distention, S3, and basilar crackles. The client will have a normal sinus rhythm on the ECG and will have an increased sense of well being. Client will have a decrease in the symptoms for which the herb was administered.

Drugs: Adelir, Co-Q10, Heartcin, Inokiton, Neuquinone, Taidecanone, Ubiquinone, Udekinon

Coenzyme Q10

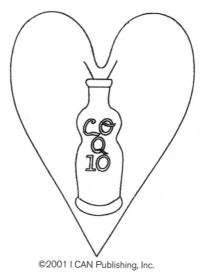

©2001 I CAN Publishing, Inc.

E —Vitamin helps preserve Co-Q10

N ausea, vomiting, anorexia—U E

al**Z** heimer's, schizophrenia; CHF—indications

Y ES, it has ANTI-AGING effects

M ackeral, Salmon, and Sardines—↑ in vitamin E

E ffectiveness of Co-Q10 is ↓ with oral antidiabetics

The energy for the heart is coming from the "Coke™ Co-Q10 bottle". "ENZYME" will help recall some key facts.

ECHINACEA

Action: Stimulates phagocytosis; increases mobility of leukocytes; increases respiratory cellular activity. This results in an increased immune, antiseptic, antiviral, immunostimulant, anti-inflammatory, and antibacterial effect. Has peripheral vasodilator properties.

Indications: Sore throat, colds, flu; low immune status; cancer. External ointments used for burns, ulcerations, eczema, herpes simplex, psoriasis, and wounds that heal poorly. Reduces recurrence of Candida albicans and decreases the growth of Trichomonas vaginalis.

Warnings: Externally, none known. Internally, progressive systemic diseases such as tuberculosis, multiple sclerosis, HIV (including AIDS), collagen diseases, or other autoimmune diseases. Alcoholics and clients with liver disease. Pregnancy, breastfeeding, children.

Undesirable Effects: Allergies may occur if client is allergic to plants in the daisy family.

Other Specific Information: Do not administer with immunosuppressants or hepatotoxic drugs. Many tinctures contain significant amount of alcohol, so avoid disulfiram or metronidazole.

Interventions: Monitor WBCs, vital signs, and breath sounds (respiratory diseases).

Education: Instruct client that herb should not be used longer than 8 weeks; 10–14 days of therapy is probably sufficient. If illness does not resolve after taking the herb, advise to notify provider.

Evaluation: WBCs will return to normal range. Temperature will return to normal range, and client will have a decrease in the symptoms for which the herb was administered.

Drugs: Coneflower Extract, Echinacea, Echinacea Angustifolia Herb, Echinacea Fresh Freeze-Dried, Echinacea Glycerite, Echinacea Herb, Echinacea Herbal Comfort Lozenges, Echinacea Purpurea

ECHINACEA

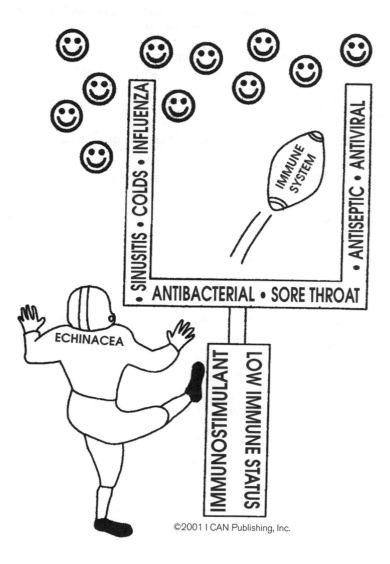

Echinacea is giving a powerful boost to the immune system so colds, flu, sore throats will heal quickly and smiles will return.

EVENING PRIMROSE

Action: The evening primrose oil stems from essential fatty acids that are crucial as structural elements for cells and as precursors of synthesis of prostaglandins. Linoleic acid is not manufactured by the body and must be provided through diet. The body relies on the metabolic conversion of linoleic acid (LA) to gamma linoleic acid (GLA). A deficiency in this process results in diabetes, cancer, CV disease, hypercholesterolemia, etc. This herb contains the highest amount of GLA of any food substance.

Indications: Rheumatoid arthritis, PMS, menopause, and diabetic neuropathy.

Warnings: Pregnancy, breast cancer, schizophrenia, or clients taking epileptogenic medications such as phenothiazines.

Undesirable Effects: Abdominal discomfort, nausea, headache, rash, immunosuppression may occur after use of GLA for > 1 yr.

Other Specific Information: Phenothiazines may ↑ risk of seizures.

Interventions: Use Oil of Evening Primrose for the best source of gamma linoleic acid.

Education: Instruct women with breast cancer or clients with a seizure disorder not to use this herb.

Evaluation: The client's symptoms will improve based on the therapeutic reason for taking the herb.

Drugs: Efamol, Epogram, Evening Primrose Oil, Mega Primrose Oil, My Favorite Evening Primrose Oil, Primrose Power

EVENING PRIMROSE

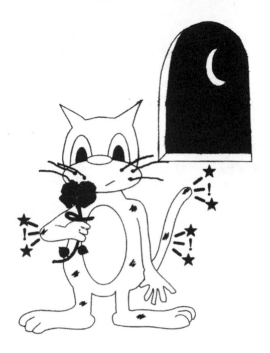

R heumatoid athritis, PMS, menopause: indications

O il of Evening Primrose—best source of GLA

S eizures ↑ risk if herb is taken with phenothiazines

E ducation—don't use if client has a history of breast cancer or seizures

Kat smells the primrose oil to enhance her amorous activities for the night. Of course if she were having hot flashes, the evening primrose would reduce those right along with the pain she may be having from rheumatoid arthritis.

FEVERFEW

Actions: Inhibits synthesis of prostaglandins and leukotrienes. Inhibits secretion of serotonin from platelet granules. These substances are known to increase in the brain during the early phase of migraine attack.

Indications: Migraine headaches, arthritis, fever, and menstrual disorders.

Warnings: Pregnancy or breast-feeding.

Undesirable Effects: Occasional mouth ulceration or gastric disturbance, dry and sore tongue, swollen lips, abdominal pain, vomiting, diarrhea, and flatulence. Post-feverfew syndrome (withdrawal syndrome characterized by moderate to severe pain and joint and muscle stiffness).

Other Specific Information: Use caution with anticoagulants; may ↑ bleeding.

Interventions: Recommend avoiding chewing the leaves since they can cause mouth ulcers.

Education: Discuss proper oral hygiene due to the risk of mouth ulcerations. Discuss the importance of reporting undesirable effects to provider. Even though feverfew is given for pain, the user can still operate heavy machinery. Treatment for at least a few months is recommended. Instruct client not to withdraw the herb abruptly.

Evaluation: Client's temperature will return to normal range and pain will subside.

Drugs: Feverfew, Feverfew Glyc, Feverfew Power

MYRA MIGRAINE

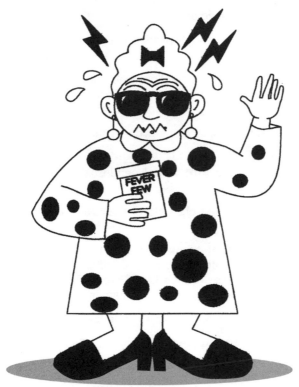

©2001 I CAN Publishing, Inc.

M ay cause mouth ulcers

Y ou can't use during pregnancy

R educes pain

A nticoagulants may cause bleeding

Myra Migraine is holding her jar of Feverfew leaves that reduce the pain of her headaches and photophobia. It has also stimulated Myra's appetite and her dress size is about to outgrow her "big hair".

FISH OIL

Action: Hypotriglyceridemic action.

Indications: To lower the body's production of triglycerides, may help depression.

Warnings: Do not use if one is allergic to fish or soybeans. Client needs to inform provider of care if they have diabetes or hypothyroidism. May increase risk of bleeding when taken in large doses.

Undesirable Effects: Stomach upset, chest pain, irregular heartbeats, flu-like symptoms, fever, chills.

Other Specific Information: ↓ triglycerides, may increase triglycerides if diet is not followed.

Interventions: Check total cholesterol (HDL and LDL, and VLDL) levels. Assess vital signs.

Education: Instruct client to avoid eating foods that are high in cholesterol or fat. Take with meals to avoid after taste. Client should avoid drinking alcohol. May reduce blood pressure slightly especially when used with other antihypertensive medications.

Evaluation: Serum triglyceride levels will be lowered.

Drugs: omega-3 polyunsaturated fatty acids (Fish Oil, Lovaza)

FISH OIL

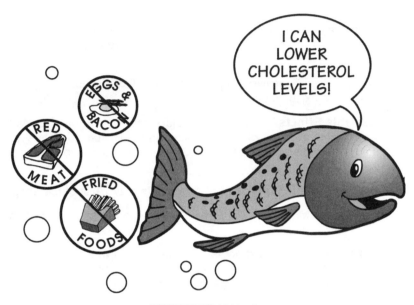

Fish oil lowers the body's production of triglycerides.

GARLIC

Action: Inhibits platelet aggregation (blood thinner). Decreases lipids and has antitumor effects. Lowers total serum cholesterol, triglycerides, and low-density lipoprotein (LDL), while increasing high-density lipoprotein (HDL). Garlic also has antitumor and antimicrobial effects.

Indications: Lowers high blood pressure and serum lipid levels; aids in the treatment of arteriosclerosis; yeast or wound infections; colds and flu.

Warnings: Hypersensitivity, peptic ulcer or reflux disease. Pregnant women due to oxytocic effects.

Undesirable Effects: The entire body can smell of garlic; diaphoresis; hypothyroidism; irritation of mouth, esophagus, or stomach; nausea/vomiting. Chronic use may lead to decreased hemoglobin production and lysis of RBCs.

Other Specific Information: Anticoagulants may ↑ risk of bleeding.

Interventions: Monitor CBC if client taking high-dose or long-term garlic.

Education: Aged garlic extract is desirable. May give the entire body a garlic odor. Odorless garlic supplements are available. Instruct client to watch for signs of bleeding (bleeding gums, bruising, petechiae) if taking with hemostatic agents.

Evaluation: The client will have a decrease in BP, lipid levels, or clinical symptoms for which the garlic was administered.

Drugs: Garlic, Garlic-Power, Garlique, Kwai, Kyolic, Odorless Garlic Tablets, One a Day Garlic, Sapec

GARLIC

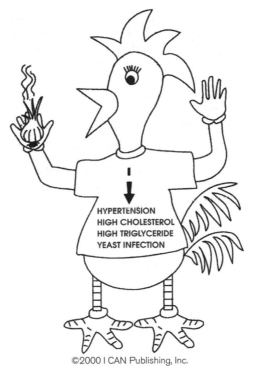

HYPERTENSION
HIGH CHOLESTEROL
HIGH TRIGLYCERIDE
YEAST INFECTION

©2000 I CAN Publishing, Inc.

O bserve for bleeding if taking anticoagulants

D oes also have antitumor and antimicrobial effects

O dorless garlic supplements are available

R eevaluate BP and lab reports

Garlic Chicken is much improved from her high cholesterol, triglycerides and high blood pressure. Garlic also helps her yeast infection.

GINGER

Action: Reduces spasms and cramps in the colon. A strong antioxidant and effective antimicrobial agent for sores and wounds. Inhibits platelet aggregation induced by ADP and epinephrine. Other studies have suggested that components in ginger may be gastroprotective against various chemical insults and stressors. It is postulated to be from increased mucosal resistance and potentiation of the defensive mechanism against chemicals or alterations in prostaglandins, providing more protective effects.

Indications: Nausea, motion sickness, indigestion, inflammation.

Warnings: Pregnant clients: Use only under medical supervision in clients receiving anticoagulants because it may affect bleeding time by inhibiting platelet function.

Undesirable Effects: Possible CNS depression or arrhythmias with overdose.

Other Specific Information: Anticoagulants may enhance risk of bleeding.

Interventions: Monitor for undesirable effects. Evaluate for signs of bleeding.

Education: Advise the female client to avoid use of ginger during pregnancy. Instruct client to watch for signs of bleeding when taking ginger. Explain that no consensus exists with respect to the exact dose.

Evaluation: Client will experience therapeutic results from the ginger (i.e., nausea will subside, indigestion will subside, etc.)

Drugs: Cayenne Ginger, Gingerall, Ginger Peppermint Combo, Ginger Power, Ginger Trips

GINGER

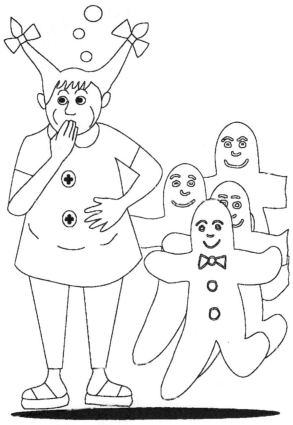

G ive to reduce spasms in colon

I ncreased risk of bleeding with anticoagulants

N ausea—use

Gingerbread men rush to the rescue of nausea and vomiting.

GINKGO BILOBA

Action: The herb produces arterial and venous vasoactive changes that increase the tissue perfusion and cerebral blood flow. Stimulates prostaglandin biosynthesis. Acts as an anti-oxidant.

Indications: Memory loss; early stages of Alzheimer's disease; poor circulation to extremities, intermittent claudication; antioxidant.

Warnings: Hypersensitivity; pregnancy, children; hemophilia or bleeding disorders; clients taking anticoagulants or antiplatelet agents.

Undesirable Effects: These are rare. Mild gastrointestinal upset in less than 1% of clients. Long-term use has been linked with rare occurrences of spontaneous subdural hematoma, intracerebral or intraocular hemorrhage.

Other Specific Information: Cigarette smoking and/or use of platelet-aggregation inhibitors may ↑ risk of subarachnoid hemorrhage. May interact with carbemazepine, phenobarbital, phenytoin, and TCAs.

Interventions: Administration for at least 2 weeks recommended. Children and adults taking medicinal doses should be seen by a qualified health care provider.

Education: Stay within recommended dosage and duration. Advise to take no aspirin or NSAIDs or alcohol; report unusual bleeding or bruising. Keep out of reach from children due to the potential risk of seizures with ingestion. Avoid contact with the fruit pulp or seed coats due to risk of dermatitis.

Evaluation: Substantial regression of major symptoms of chronic cerebral insufficiency including vertigo, senility, fatigue, lack of vigilance, and poor circulation to the limbs.

Drugs: Bioginkgo 24/6, Bioginkgo 27/7, Gincosan, Ginexin Remind, Ginkai, Ginkgoba, Ginkgo Go!, Ginkgold, Ginkgo Phytosome, Ginkgo Power, Ginkoba

GINKO

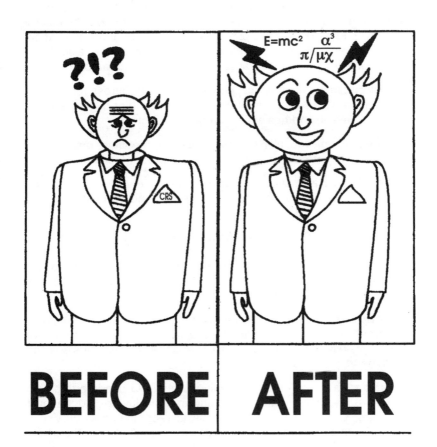

As indicated by the initials on his handkerchief, Gink **"can't remember shit**!" A few weeks on Ginko Biloba and he receives the benefits of increased memory and decreased depression. He can just feel the better blood flow through his brain and can now think like Einstein!

GINSENG

Action: Supports and enhances adrenal function, allowing for more consistent energy and better reaction to stress. Reduces cholesterol and triglycerides, decreases platelet adhesiveness and coagulation, and increases fibrinolysis. Antiarrhythmic effects have also been determined with ginseng similar to verapamil and amiodarone.

Indications: Improves stamina, concentration, and stress-resistance; adjunct in radiation and chemotherapy. Lowers blood glucose and cholesterol levels; and has antihypertensive effects.

Warnings: Cardiovascular disease, hyper/hypotension, diabetes, or clients receiving steroid therapy. Pregnancy, breast-feeding.

Undesirable Effects: High doses can cause jitters, headaches, and hypertension. Vaginal bleeding, skin eruptions, and pruritus have also been noted.

Other Specific Information: Antidiabetic agents should be used cautiously due to ginseng's hypoglycemic effect. MAO inhibitors given with ginseng may result in tremors, headache, and mania. Anticoagulants, aspirin, NSAIDs may inhibit blood clotting. Herb may interfere with digoxin's effects.

Interventions: Monitor for "Ginseng Abuse Syndrome" (i.e., nervousness, irritability, insomnia, morning diarrhea). This can occur if tea or coffee are taken with the herb. Monitor the diabetic client for signs and symptoms of hypoglycemia.

Education: Take 1 hour before eating. Vitamin C can interfere with absorption. Avoid caffeine. Take early in the day to reduce over stimulation. Generally up to 3 months is recommended. Advise a client with pre-existing medical problems to be evaluated by the health care provider prior to taking ginseng. Review undesirable effects and report to provider of health care.

Evaluation: Client will experience an increase in energy and an improvement of symptoms for which ginseng was administered.

Drugs: Bio Star, Cimexon, Gincosan, Ginsana, Ginsatonic, Neo Ginsana

GINSENG

FINISH

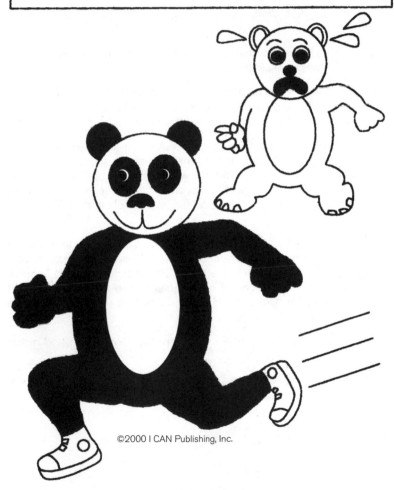

©2000 I CAN Publishing, Inc.

GINSENG BEAR GETS TO THE FINISH LINE FIRST! He has taken his tonic that improves stamina and fights fatigue. Needless to say, the second bear in the race did not take his ginseng.

GLUCOSAMINE

Action: May stop or slow osteoarthritis progression by stimulating cartilage and synovial tissue metabolism.

Indication: Osteoarthrisis. Temporomandibular joint (TMJ), arthritis, glaucoma.

Warnings: Shellfish allergy; Use cautiously with clients with diabetes or asthma.

Undesirable Effects: Nausea, heartburn, diarrhea, constipation. Headache, drowsiness, skin reactions.

Other Specific Information: May antagonize the effects of antidiabetics. May induce resistance to some chemotherapy drugs such as etoposide, teniposide, and doxorubicin.

Interventions: Evaluate for shellfish allergy prior to administering. Monitor pain (type, location, and intensity). Assess glucose levels via home monitoring device for clients with diabetes until response is determined. Evaluate for gastric discomfort. Assess bowel function and treat constipation with improved fluids and bulk in diet. Take prior to meals.

Education: Instruct client as to why the herbal supplement should not be used if they have a shellfish allergy. Review the reason why this herbal supplement should be taken on a regular basis to achieve effects. Notify provider of care if gastric discomfort develops. Caution diabetics to monitor glucose values to ascertain the impact on the glycemic control.

Evaluation: Client will experience an improvement in pain and range of motion.

Drugs: glucosamine (2-amino-2-deoxyglucose sulfate, chitosamine)

GLUCOSAMINE

Glucosamine is successful in decreasing pain from osteoarthritis and/or TMJ. Remember to educate the client not to take the drug if they have a shellfish allergy!

GOLDENSEAL

Action: Astringent, anti-inflammatory, oxytocic, antihemorrhagic, and laxative properties. Decreases the anticoagulant effects of heparin and acts as a cardiac stimulant. It increases coronary perfusion and inhibits cardiac activity. Antipyretic activity(greater than aspirin), antimuscarinic, antihistaminic, antitumor, antimicrobial, antihelmintic and hypotensive effects have also been documented.

Indications: GI disorders, gastritis, peptic ulceration, anorexia, postpartum hemorrhage, dysmenorrhea, eczema, pruritus, mouth ulcerations, otorrhoea, tinnitus, and conjunctivitis and as a wound antiseptic, diuretic, laxative, and anti-inflammatory agent.

Warnings: Clients with CV disease, particularly heart failure, arrhythmias, and during pregnancy.

Undesirable Effects: Asystole, bradycardia, CNS depression, contact dermatitis, diarrhea, GI cramping, heart block, leukocytosis, nausea, paresthesia, respiratory depression (with high doses), seizures, vomiting. Death may be caused by large alkaloid doses. Symptoms of overdose include GI upset, nervousness, depression, exaggerated reflexes, and convulsions that progress to respiratory paralysis and CV collapse.

Other Specific Information: Anticoagulants may reduce the beneficial effects of therapeutic anticoagulants. Antihypertensive agents may interfere or enhance hypotensive effects when taken with goldenseal or its extracts. Beta blockers, calcium channel blockers, digoxin may enhance or interfere with the cardiac effects of these drugs. Don't use together. CNS depressants (alcohol, benzodiazepines) may enhance sedative effects. Do not use with goldenseal.

Interventions: Monitor for signs of vitamin B deficiencies (megaloblastic anemia, peripheral neuropathy, seizures, cheilosis, glossitis, angular stomatitis, and infertility). Monitor for other undesirable effects.

Education: Recommend the client to avoid hazardous activities until CNS effects of the agent are known.

Evaluation: Client will experience therapeutic effects from the medication.

Drugs: Golden Seal Extract, Golden Seal Extract 4:1, Golden Seal Power, Golden Seal Root, Nu Veg Golden Seal Root, Nu Veg Golden Seal Herb

GOLDENSEAL

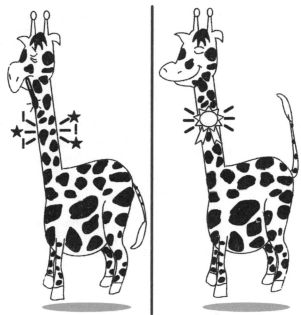

©2005 I CAN Publishing, Inc.

G I disorders and gastritis can benefit from this herb

O verdose—symptoms are GI upset, nervousness and seizures

L eukocytosis—undesirable effect

D o not administer anticoagulants, antihypertensive agents

E valuate for signs of vitamin B deficiency

N ot given to clients with CV disease

Gerry Giraffe has placed a golden seal on his infected throat and respiratory tract to help with his infection. His travel back to Africa will be improved since Goldenseal also treats traveler's diarrhea.

KAVA-KAVA

Action: The limbic system is inhibited by kavapyrones, an effect associated with suppression of emotional excitability and mood enhancement. Noted for promoting relaxation without loss of mental sharpness.

Indications: Anxiety disorders, stress, insomnia, muscle spasms, backache, neck ache, and pain from TMJ.

Warnings: Pregnant, breast-feeding, or children < 12. Use cautiously in clients with renal disease, neutropenia, or thrombocytopenia. Do not take if diagnosed with Parkinson's disease.

Undesirable Effects: Mild gastrointestinal disturbances; alterations in motor reflexes and judgment; visual disturbances. Dry, discolored flaking skin; reddened eyes (may be from cholesterol metabolism). Dopamine antagonism. ↓ patellar reflexes, pulmonary hypertension, and shortness of breath. ↓ bilirubin levels, plasma proteins, and urea. Weight loss. Long-term use−↓ platelet and lymphocyte count.

Other Specific Information: When taken with kava these interactions can occur. Alprazolam may cause coma. Benzodiazepines, alcohol, and other CNS depressants ↑ sedative effects. Levodopa ↑ Parkinsonian symptoms. Pentobarbitol may have ↑ effects.

Interventions: Monitor for undesirable effects.

Education: Warn against using with medicines referred to in "Other Specific Information." Do not take for more than 3 months without provider advice due to significant undesirable effects. Instruct client to take with food.

Evaluation: Client will experience a decrease in anxiety and an improvement in peaceful sleep.

Drugs: Aigin, Antares, Ardeydystin, Cefkava, Kavasedon, Kavasporal, Kavatino, Laitan, Mosaro, Nervonocton N, Potter's Antigian Tablets, Viocava

KAVA-KAVA

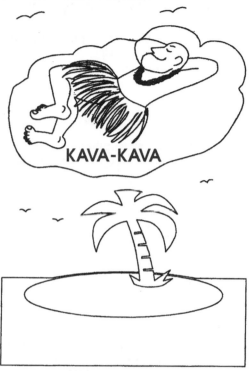

KAVA-KAVA

K ava interacts with CNS depressants

A dvise to take with food

V isual and mild GI disturbances: U E

A lprazolam given with Kava may cause

Kava-Kava has been restless, nervous, anxious, and unable to sleep, but she is now floating on her cloud of calm. She will not be able to stay on her cloud for too long, because this herb also acts as a diuretic.

MA HUANG (EPHEDRA SINICA)

Action: May activate the alpha and beta adrenergic receptors to constrict arterioles which will increase the heart rate and may cause bronchodilation, and decrease the appetite. The CNS will be stimulated.

Indications: Weight loss; increase athletic abilities; and used to decrease symptoms of influenza, colds, and allergies.

Warnings: Since it contains ephedrine, Ma Huang can stimulate the cardiovascular system and high doses can cause death from hypertension and dysrhythmias.

Undesirable Effects: Hypertension, dysrhythmias; euphoria, psychosis.

Other Specific Information: Interacts with any CNS stimulant to potentiate their effect. MAO inhibitors taken with Ma Huang may result in severe hypertension. Antihypertensive medications may have a decrease effect when taking with Ma Huang.

Interventions: Review with client any medications that are being currently taken. Monitor vital signs and emotional state.

Education: Review the importance of monitoring HR, BP, a feeling of euphoria, and/or being out of touch with reality and notifying provider of care.

Evaluation: Client will experience therapeutic effects from the medication with no undesirable effects.

Drugs: ma huang (Ephedra sinica)

MA HUANG
(EPHEDRA SINICA)

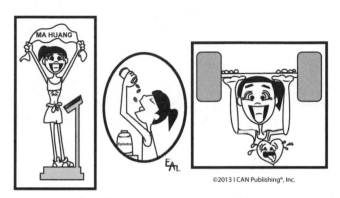

©2013 I CAN Publishing®, Inc.

W eight loss; increased athletic abilities, and used to decrease symptoms of influenza - Indications

E phedrine is in Ma Huang which can lead to cardiovascular stimulation and high doses can lead to death

I nteracts with CNS stimulants to potentiate their effect. MAOI's with Ma Huang may cause hypertension.

G ets a feeling of well being/ euphoria, and/or being out of touch with reality - Undesirable Effects

H eart Rate, BP - Monitor

T he alpha and beta adrenergic receptors may be activated to constrict arterioles which will Increase HR and decrease appetite. The CNS will be stimulated.

MILK THISTLE

Action: Hepatoprotective and antihepatotoxic actions over liver toxins. Silymarin, seeds from milk thistle, alters the outer liver membrane cell structure so that toxins cannot enter the cell. It also stimulates RNA polymerase A, which enhances ribosome protein synthesis and leads to activation of the regenerative capacity of the liver through cell development.

Indications: Alcoholic cirrhosis and hepatitis, antiinflammatory.

Warnings: Pregnant or breast-feeding clients. Caution with clients who have a hypersensitivity to plants belonging to the Asteraceae family.

Undesirable Effects: Mild laxative effect. Uterine and menstrual stimulation.

Other Specific Information: No interactions reported.

Interventions: Monitor liver function test results.

Education: Advise the client to consult with a medical professional in liver disease prior to starting this therapy. Report planned or suspected pregnancy. Instruct the client to report unusual symptoms immediately.

Evaluation: Client will experience therapeutic effects from the milk thistle.

Drugs: Beyond Milk Thistle, Milk Thistle Extract, Milk Thistle Phytosol, Milk Thistle Power, NU VEG Milk Thistle Power, Silymarin

MILK THISTLE

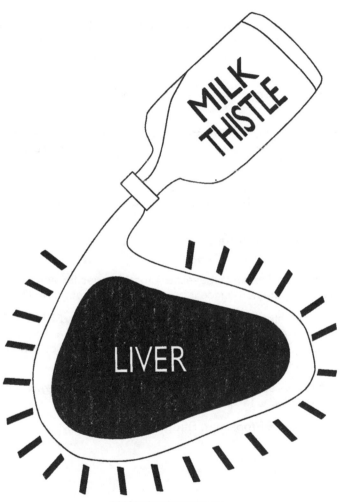

Milk Thistle alters the outer liver so that toxins cannot enter the liver cells.

SAW PALMETTO BERRY: SERENOA REPENS

Action: Lipidosterolic extract of S. repens (LSESR) appears to have an inhibitory effect on the binding of dihydrotestosterone (DHT) to androgen receptors in the prostate. LSESR also has an anti-inflammatory effect.

Indications: Benign prostate enlargement (BPH); may function as a mild diuretic.

Warnings: Pregnancy, breast-feeding, and women of childbearing age. Use cautiously in clients with medical problems other than BPH due to lack of data.

Undesirable Effects: Large amounts may cause diarrhea. In rare cases, stomach problems and headaches may occur. May create false-negative prostate-specific antigen (PSA) results.

Other Specific Information: ↑ side effects of estrogen or birth control pills. May ↓ iron absorption.

Interventions: Obtain a baseline prostate-specific antigen (PSA) before starting the herb since it can cause a false-negative PSA.

Education: Instruct client to take herb with AM and PM meal to ↓ GI effects. Client should use herb for BPH only after a diagnosis has been made and with the management of the provider of health care. Advise client to report any undesirable effects.

Evaluation: Client will experience a decrease in the symptoms for which the herb was taken.

Drugs: Permixon, Propalmex, Strogen

SAW PALMETTO

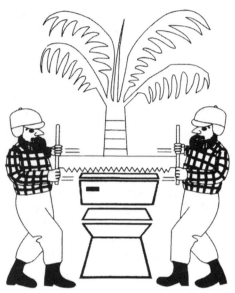

©2000 I CAN Publishing, Inc.

S tomach problems and headaches may occur

A lters PSA (prostate-specific antigen) test. May cause false negative

W atch for bloody urine

These two non-spring chicken men are sawing the toilet in half. They want to keep from spending their nights standing at the commode due to frequency of urination from enlarged prostate glands.

St. John's Wort

Action: The exact mechanism has not been determined. Inhibits the stress-induced increase in corticotropin-releasing hormone, adrenocorticotropic hormone, and cortisol; increases the nocturnal melatonin levels. St. John's Wort has an antiviral activity.

Indications: Mild to moderate depression, insomnia, anxiety, and PMS symptoms; wound healing, insect bites.

Warnings: Clients taking prescription antidepressants. Pregnant or breast-feeding clients; children.

Undesirable Effects: Photosensitivity in people with fair skin. Dizziness, constipation, dry mouth, GI distress, restlessness.

Other Specific Information: Alcohol, MAO inhibitors, narcotics, OTC cold and flu medications, sympathomimetics, tyramine-containing foods may ↑ MAO inhibition activity. Paroxetine may ↑ sedative-hypnotic effects with the herb. Serotonin syndrome may occur when used with SSRIs or tricyclic antidepressants. Do not use with drugs that cause photosensitivity (i.e., sulfonamides, tetracyclines, antipsychotics, etc.).

Interventions: The client's depression should be evaluated by a health care provider.

Education: Use over a period of several weeks or months to obtain the desired effect. Best under supervision of health provider. Should not be used at the same time as prescription antidepressants. Avoid foods high in tyramine such as red wines, beer, aged cheese, glandular meats (liver), colas and chocolate. Teach to say out of the sun.

Evaluation: Client's communication and behavior will indicate an improvement of depression.

Drugs: Hypercalm, Hypericum, Kira, Mood Support, St. John's Wort, Nutri Zac, Tension Tamer

ST. JOHN'S WORT

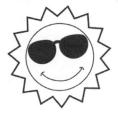

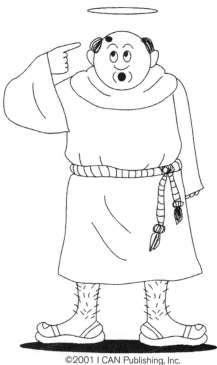

©2001 I CAN Publishing, Inc.

W atch the sun

O K for stings and bites

R educes viral infections

T aking MAOIs and SSRIs may cause serious U E

St. John's Wort on his head is making him anxious and unable to sleep.
St. John's Wort calms the emotions and is used for depression.

VALERIAN

Action: May act as a mild sedative. Historically used for over 1000 years for insomnia. Contains GABA in quantities sufficient to cause sedation.

Indication: Insomnia, anxiety, stress, muscle cramps, muscle spasms, menstrual cramps

Warnings: Women who are pregnant or nursing or children under 3 years old should not take this herb without medical advice.

Undesirable Effects: Drowsiness, headache. Benzodiazepine-like withdrawal symptoms if discontinuation occurs after long-term use.

Other Specific Information: Increased CNS depression with alcohol, antihistamines, sedative hypnotics and other CNS depressants. Alcohol-containing preparations may interact with disulfuram and metronidazole. Additive sedative effects can occur when used with herbal supplements with sedative properties such as kava, melatonin, SAMe, and St. John's wort.

Intervention: Assess for sleep habits and the reduction of stress and cramps. Assess the response in the elderly client where loss of balance and drowsiness my present a significant risk for injury from falls.

Education: May cause individual to test positive for benzodiazepines in a standard drug screen. Warn client to avoid use of other herbals or medications that have a sedative effect due to the combination resulting in drowsiness. Review the importance of not driving or operating heavy machinery immediately after taking valerian and not drinking alcohol while taking this herbal supplement. Discuss the importance of eliminating stimulants such as caffeine and to provide an environment at bedtime that promotes sleep.

Evaluation: Client will experience a restful night's sleep without stress, muscle cramps, or drowsiness upon awakening.

Drugs: Valerian, Valerian liquid, Valeriana officinalis, Valerian tea

NATURE'S VALIUM: VALERIAN

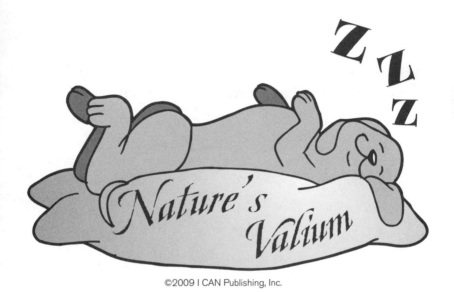

©2009 I CAN Publishing, Inc.

Ah … sleep! No cramps!

The pessimist sees difficulty in every opportunity. The optimist sees the opportunity in every difficulty.

WINSTON CHURCHILL

INDEX–ALPHABETICAL

INDEX–PHARMACEUTICAL

B

bacampicillin (Spectrobid) 144

beclomethasone 116, 118, 266
(Beclovent, Beconase, QVAR, Vancenase, Vanceril, Beconase, Vancenase)

benazepril (Lotension) 44

benztropine (Cogentin) 236, 368

bepridil (Vascor) 54

betamethasone 266
(Celestone, Diprosone, Uticort, Valisone)

betaxolol (Kerlone) 50

bethanechol 172
(Duvoid, Urabeth, Urecholine)

bisacodyl 246
(Carter's Little Pills, Dulcolax, Dacodyl, Feen-a-mint, Fleet Laxative, Therelax)

bisoprolol (Zebeta) 50

bitolterol (Tornalate) 114

black cohosh 500

bleomycin (Blenoxane) 190

botulinum toxin type A (Botox) 344

brompheniramine (Dimetapp) 112

bromocriptine (Parlodel) 366

Bronitin Mist 24

Bronkaid Mist 24

buclizine (Bucladin-S) 112

budesonide 116, 118, 266
(Rhinocort, Pulmicort)

bumetanide (Bumex) 66

buprenorphine 416
(Buprenex, Subutex)

bupropion 398, 420
(Wellbutrin, Wellbutrin SR, Zyban)

busulfan (Busulfex, Myleran) 184

buspirone (Buspar) 388

butenafine (Mentax) 164

butoconazole (Femstat 3) 164

C

calcitonin (Fortical, Miacalcin) 454

calcium carbonate 478

(Caltrate, Chooz, Equilet, OsCAL, Oystercal, Tums)

candesartan (Atacand) 46

capecitabine (Xeloda) 188

captopril (Capoten) 44

carbachol (Carboptic) 342

carbamazepine 380
(Apo-Carbamazepine, Atretol, Carbatrol, Epitol, Novo-Carbamaz, Tegretol, Tegretol CR, Tegretol-XR)

carbenicillin (Geocillin) 144

Carbidopa/Levodopa 364
(Sinemet)

carboplatin (Paraplatin) 184

carisoprodol (Soma) 322

carmustine (BiCNU, Gliadel) 184

carteolol (Cartrol) 50

carvedilol (Coreg) 50

cefaclor (Ceclor) 136

cefadroxil (Duricef) 136

cefamandole (Mandol) 136

cefazolin (Ancef, Kefzol) 136

cefdinir (Omnicef) 136

cefditoren pivoxil (Spectracef) 136

cefepime (Maxipime) 136

cefixime (Suprax) 136

cefmetazole (Zefazone) 136

cefonicid (Monocid) 136

cefoperazone (Cefobid) 136

cefotaxime (Claforan) 136

cefotetan (Cefotan) 136

cefoxitin (Mefoxin) 136

cefpodoxime (Vantin) 136

cefprozil (Cefzil) 136

ceftazidime (Fortaz) 136

ceftibuten (Cedax) 136

ceftizoxime (Cefizox) 136

ceftriaxone (Rocephin) 136

cefuroxime (Ceftin, Zinacef) 136

celecoxib (Celebrex) 216

cephalexin (Keflex) 136

cephapirin (Cefadyl) 136

U

urea (Ureaphil) 72
urokinase (Abbokinase) 94

V

Vaginal contraceptive ring 450
(NuvaRing)
valacyclovir (Valtrex) 168
valdecoxib (Bextra) 216
Valerian 534
valproic acid 378
(Depakote, Depakote ER,
Depakene, Epival)
valsartan (Diovan) 46
vancomycin 150
(Vancocin, Vancold)
Vaponefrin 24
vardenafil (Levitra) 460
varenicline (Chantix) 418
Varicella vaccine (Varivax) 496
vasopressin 278
(Pitressin Synthetic)
vecuronium (Norcuron) 330
venlafaxine 398
(Effexor/Effexor XR)
verapamil (Isoptin, Calan) 54, 358
Vinblastine (Velban) 192
Vincristine (Oncovin) 192
vinorelbine (Navelbine) 192

W

warfarin (Coumadin) 76

Z

zafirlukast (Accolate) 122
zalcitabine (HIVID) 178
zidovudine (Retrovir) 178
zileuton (Zyflo) 122
ziprasidone (Geodon) 408
zoledronic acid (Reclast, Zometa) 440

People learn in many different ways. We want to tell you about our FUN products and services because our business is to help you PASS!

www.icanpublishing.com

NURSING Made Insanely Easy! is a pocket-sized book, including images and many memory tools, streamlining nursing and allied health education with an EASY, totally different bottom-line approach to concepts.

E ssential concepts to assist learners to prepare for exams, exit exams, and NCLEX®.

A ssist nursing graduates to remember health and nursing concepts and apply to clinical decision making.

S pecial images per page with essential concepts on the opposite page.

Y our learning is memorable and fun, and helps focus on linking nursing concepts to clinical thinking.

For example, one look at "Cushy Carl" and you will remember the priority clinical assessments and nursing plan of care regarding the concepts for a client with Cushing's Syndrome forever.

NCLEX-RN® 101: How to Pass! A question book that has been developed with an emphasis on the NCLEX-RN® exam. The questions test your ability to apply clinical decision making strategies to answer application and analysis questions. Answers and rationales are provided for each question. These questions require multi-logical thinking strategies and closely reflect the NCLEX® standards. The book has been designed with analysis grids to assist you in tracking your growth and identify specific areas necessary for studying. Separate chapters have been developed for each of the Client Need categories that will be evaluated on the NCLEX-RN®. The alternate item format questions will help prepare for the interactive question types you will experience on the NCLEX® exam. There is also a free simulated NCLEX-RN® online with detailed rationales for all options with the book purchase.

Pharmacology NCLEX® Review is a one-day, live interactive review brought to your site for 50 participants or more. Call I CAN Publishing®, Inc. at 1-866-428-5589 for information and dates on our sites in many states or go to www.icanpublishing.com for additional information. If there is not a site in your state, we will be happy to establish one for you!

This course provides the SECRETS to NCLEX® and clinical practice success regarding pharmacology and clinical decision-making in a FUN and EASY one-day format. The book *Pharmacology Made Insanely Easy*, a packet of pharmacology material, and test questions evaluating pharmacology are included in the cost of this dynamic pharmacology review. Participants leave saying, "Wow, I finally get it!"

E-Question Bank is available at www.icanpublishing.com. The one test that is a must, "The Last One Before the BIG ONE"! This exam has 265 exam items accompanied with rationales for each of the options. These exam items have been developed within the framework of the NCLEX-RN® and represent the same percentage of each of the Client Needs as the NCLEX-RN®. Questions will be accompanied with I CAN Hints that will provide innovative clinical decision making strategies and memory strategies to assist with reviewing and applying the specific NCLEX® standards.

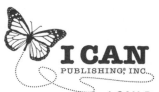

I CAN
PUBLISHING® INC.

I CAN Publishing®, Inc.
2650 Chattahoochee Drive • Suite 100
Duluth, GA 30097
866.428.5589

www.icanpublishing.com

Like us on Facebook